KEY TOPICS IN
NEONATOLOGY

The KEY TOPICS Series

Advisors:

T.M. Craft *Department of Anaesthesia and Intensive Care, Royal United Hospital, Bath, UK*
C.S. Garrard *Intensive Therapy Unit, John Radcliffe Hospital, Oxford, UK*
P.M. Upton *Department of Anaesthetics, Treliske Hospital, Truro, UK*

Anaesthesia, Second Edition

Obstetrics and Gynaecology, Second Edition

Accident and Emergency Medicine

Paediatrics, Second Edition

Orthopaedic Surgery

Otolaryngology

Ophthalmology

Psychiatry

General Surgery

Renal Medicine

Trauma

Chronic Pain

Oral and Maxillofacial Surgery

Oncology

Cardiovascular Medicine

Neurology

Neonatology

Forthcoming titles include:
Gastroenterology

Respiratory Medicine

Thoracic Surgery

Critical Care

Orthopaedic Trauma Surgery

KEY TOPICS IN
NEONATOLOGY

RICHARD H. MUPANEMUNDA
BSc BM MRCP(UK) FRCPCH
Honorary Senior Clinical Lecturer, Birmingham University
Consultant Neonatologist, Birmingham Heartlands Hospital NHS Trust
Birmingham, UK

MICHAEL WATKINSON
MA MB BChir MRCP(UK) FRCPCH
Honorary Senior Clinical Lecturer, Birmingham University
Consultant Neonatologist, Birmingham Heartlands Hospital NHS Trust
Birmingham, UK

Consultant Editor

DAVID R. HARVEY
MB FRCP FRCPCH
Professor of Paediatrics and Neonatal Medicine
Honorary Consultant Paediatrician
Imperial College School of Medicine, Hammersmith Campus
London, UK

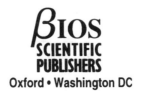

Oxford • Washington DC

© BIOS Scientific Publishers Limited, 1999

First published 1999, Reprinted 2000

A CIP catalogue record for this book is available from the British Library.

ISBN 1 85996 256 4

BIOS Scientific Publishers Ltd
9 Newtec Place, Magdalen Road, Oxford OX4 1RE, UK
Tel. +44 (0)1865 726286. Fax. +44 (0)1865 246823
World Wide Web home page: http://www.bios.co.uk/

Important Note from the Publisher
The information contained within this book was obtained by BIOS Scientific Publishers Ltd from sources believed by us to be reliable. However, while every effort has been made to ensure its accuracy, no responsibility for loss or injury whatsoever occasioned to any person acting or refraining from action as a result of information contained herein can be accepted by the authors or publishers.

The reader should remember that medicine is a constantly evolving science and while the authors and publishers have ensured that all dosages, applications and practices are based on current indications, there may be specific practices which differ between communities. You should always follow the guidelines laid down by the manufacturers of specific products and the relevant authorities in the country in which you are practising.

Production Editor: Jonathan Gunning.
Typeset by J&L Composition Ltd, Filey, UK.
Printed by T.J. International Ltd, Padstow, UK.

Front cover: Ashleigh Baldock being cared for in the Neonatal Intensive Care Unit, Birmingham Heartlands Hospital.

CONTENTS

[a] Contributed by R. Danha, Senior House Officer in Anaesthetics, Solihull Hospital, Solihull, UK.

[b] Contributed by M. Chaudhari, Specialist Registrar in Paediatric Cardiology, The Birmingham Children's Hospital, Birmingham, UK.

[c] Contributed by H.M. Goodyear, Consultant Paediatrician, Birmingham Heartlands Hospital NHS Trust, Birmingham, UK.

ABBREVIATIONS

17-OHP	17-hydroxyprogesterone
25-OHD	25-hydroxyvitamin D
1,25-$(OH)_2$D	1,25-dihydroxyvitamin D
3β-HSD	3β-hydroxysteroid dehydrogenase
A_1AT	α_1-anti-trypsin
AC	abdominal circumference
ACE	angiotensin converting enzyme
ADH	antidiuretic hormone
ADPCKD	autosomal dominant polycystic kidney disease
AFP	alpha-fetoprotein
AGA	appropriate for gestational age
AIDS	acquired immunodeficiency syndrome
APH	antepartum haemorrhage
ARDS	acute respiratory distress syndrome
ARPCKD	autosomal recessive polycystic kidney disease
ASD	atrial septal defect
AST	aspartate aminotransferase
AVSD	atrioventricular septal defect
BP	blood pressure
BPD	bronchopulmonary dysplasia
BSE	bovine spongiform encephalitis
BT	bleeding time
CAH	congenital adrenal hyperplasia
CBF	cerebral blood flow
CDC	US Centers for Disease Control and Prevention
CDG	carbohydrate-deficient glycoprotein
CDH	congenital diaphragmatic hernia
CF	cystic fibrosis
cGMP	cyclic guanylate monophosphate
CHB	complete heart block
CHD	congenital heart disease
CHF	congestive heart failure
CI	confidence interval
CM	conventional management
CMD	congenital muscular dystrophy
CMV	cytomegalovirus
CNS	central nervous system
CP	cerebral palsy
CPAP	continuous positive airway pressure
CPD	citrate, phosphate, dextrose
CPDA	citrate, phosphate, dextrose and adenine
CPK	creatine phosphokinase
CRP	C-reactive protein
CRS	congenital rubella syndrome

CSF	cerebrospinal fluid
CT	computerized tomography
CVH	combined ventricular hypertrophy
CVS	chorion villus sampling
DA	ductus arteriosus
DCA	dichloroacetate
ddI	didanosine
DHT	dihydrotestosterone
DIC	disseminated intravascular coagulation
DISIDA	di-isopropyl iminodiacetic acid
DMSA	dimercaptosuccinic acid
DNPH	dinitrophenylhydrazine
DORV	double outlet right ventricle
DPPC	dipalmitoyl phosphatidylcholine
ECG	electrocardiogram
ECHO	echocardiography
ECM	external cardiac massage
ECMO	extracorporeal membrane oxygenation
EDD	expected date of delivery
EDF	end-diastolic flow
EEG	electroencephalogram
ELBW	extremely low birthweight
ELISA	enzyme-linked immunosorbent assay
EMG	electromyogram
ENT	ear, nose and throat
ET	endotracheal
FBC	full blood count
FBS	fetal blood sampling
FDP	fibrin degradation products
FFP	fresh frozen plasma
FiO$_2$	fractional inspired oxygen concentration
FL	femoral length
FRC	functional residual capacity
G6PD	glucose-6-phosphate dehydrogenase
GABA	gamma-aminobutyric acid
GBS	group B streptococcus
GFR	glomerular filtration rate
GH	growth hormone
GOR	gastro-oesophageal reflux
HBeAg	hepatitis B 'e' antigen
HBIG	hepatis B immunoglobulin
HBsAg	hepatitis B surface antigen
HBV	hepatitis B virus
HCV	hepatitis C virus
HDN	haemorrhagic disease of the newborn
HFJV	high-frequency jet ventilation
HFOV	high-frequency oscillatory ventilation

HIE	hypoxic–ischaemic encephalopathy
HIV	human immunodeficiency virus
HLHS	hypoplastic left heart syndrome
HNIG	human normal immunoglobulin
HSV	herpes simplex virus
ICD	immune complex dissociation
ICROP	International Classification of Retinopathy of Prematurity
IDM	infant of diabetic mother
Ig	immunoglobulin
IGF	insulin-like growth factor
IGFBP	insulin-like growth factor binding protein
i.m.	intramuscular
IMD	inherited metabolic disease
IPPV	intermittent positive pressure ventilation
IPV	inactivated poliomyelitis vaccine
IQ	intelligence quotient
IRT	immunoreactive trypsin
ITP	idiopathic thrombocytopenic purpura
IU	international units
IUGR	intrauterine growth restriction
i.v.	intravenous
IVH	intraventricular haemorrhage
IVIG	intravenous immunoglobulin
IVS	intact ventricular septum
IVU	intravenous urography
LA/AO	left atrial to aortic root ratio
LBW	low birthweight
LCP	long-chain polyunsaturated fatty acids
LGA	large for gestational age
LIP	lymphoid interstitial pneumonia
LP	lumbar puncture
LV	left ventricle
LVH	left ventricular hypertrophy
MAG-3	mercapto-acetyl-triglycerine-3
MAP	mean airway pressure
MAS	meconium aspiration syndrome
MCUG	micturating cystourethrogram
mIU	milli international units
MIS	Müllerian inhibitor substance
MRI	magnetic resonance imaging
MRSA	methicillin-resistant *Staphylococcus aureus*
MSUD	maple syrup urine disease
mU	milli units
NEC	necrotizing enterocolitis
NICU	neonatal intensive care unit
NIPS	Neonatal Infant Pain Score
NKH	non-ketotic hyperglycinaemia
NNU	neonatal unit

NO	nitric oxide
NO_2	nitrogen dioxide
NOS	nitric oxide synthase
NTD	neural tube defect
nvCJD	new variant Creutzfeldt–Jakob disease
OA	oesophageal atresia
OI	oxygenation index
OPV	oral poliomyelitis vaccine
OR	odds ratio
$PaCO_2$	arterial carbon dioxide tension
PaO_2	arterial oxygen tension
PAS	periodic acid–Schiff reaction
PBF	pulmonary blood flow
PCKD	polycystic kidney disease
PCP	*Pneumocystis carinii* pneumonia
PCR	polymerase chain reaction
PCV	packed cell volume
PDA	patent ductus arteriosus
PE	pre-eclampsia
PEEP	positive end-expiratory pressure
PFO	patent foramen ovale
PG	prostaglandin
PHH	post-haemorrhagic hydrocephalus
PI	protease inhibitor
PIE	pulmonary interstitial emphysema
PIP	peak inspiratory pressure
PKU	phenylketonuria
Pl^{A1}	platelet A1 antigen
PLH	pulmonary lymphoid hyperplasia
PM	post-mortem
PNDM	permanent neonatal diabetes mellitus
p.o.	by mouth
PPHN	persistent pulmonary hypertension of the newborn
PROM	preterm rupture of membranes
PS	pulmonary stenosis
PT	prothrombin time
PTT	partial thromboplastin time
PUJ	pelvi-ureteric junction
PVH	periventricular haemorrhage
PVL	periventricular leucomalacia
PVR	pulmonary vascular resistance
RDA	recommended dietary allowance
RDS	respiratory distress syndrome
rHuEPO	recombinant human erythropoietin
ROP	retinopathy of prematurity
RSV	respiratory syncytial virus
RSVIG	respiratory syncytial virus immunoglobulin
RT	reptilase time

RTA	renal tubular acidosis
RVH	right ventricular hypertrophy
SaO$_2$	oxygen saturation
s.c.	subcutaneous
SCD	sickle cell disease
SCID	severe combined immunodeficiency
SGA	small for gestational age
sGC	soluble guanylate cyclase
SLE	systemic lupus erythematosus
SMA	spinal muscular atrophy
sPDA	symptomatic patent ductus arteriosus
SRY	sex determining region Y
SVT	supraventricular tachycardia
TA-GVHD	transfusion-associated graft-versus-host-disease
TAPVD	total anomalous pulmonary venous drainage
TAR	thrombocytopenia with absent radius
TB	tuberculosis
TDF	testis-determining factor
Te	expiratory time
TGA	transposition of great arteries
THAM	tris-hydroxymethyl-aminomethane
Ti	inspiratory time
TMI	transient myocardial ischaemia
TNDM	transient neonatal diabetes mellitus
TOF	tracheo-oesophageal fistula
TORCH	toxoplasmosis, other (particularly syphilis), rubella, cytomegalovirus, herpes
TPN	total parenteral nutrition
TPHA	*Treponima pallidum* haemagglutination assay
TRH	thyrotrophin-releasing hormone
TSH	thyroid-stimulating hormone
TT	thrombin time
U&E	urea and electrolytes
UAC	umbilical artery catheter
UDPGT	uridine diphosphate glucuronyl transferase
UTI	urinary tract infection
UVC	umbilical venous catheter
VCV	volume controlled ventilation
VDRL	venereal disease research laboratory
VKDB	vitamin K deficiency bleeding
VLBW	very low birthweight
VSD	ventricular septal defect
VT	ventricular tachycardia
VUR	vesico-ureteric reflux
VZV	varicella-zoster virus
VZIG	varicella-zoster immunoglobulin
WBC	white blood cell
WPW	Wolf–Parkinson–White syndrome
ZDV	zidovudine

PREFACE

Neonatology is a relatively new subspecialty in medicine, having largely come into being in the last three decades. This short period has, however, witnessed a dramatic reduction in neonatal mortality, particularly of very small preterm infants, due to the rapid advances in perinatal and neonatal medicine. Many areas of neonatology are still changing as new information becomes available, often leading to new diagnostic and therapeutic techniques. Although large formal neonatology textbooks serve as a very useful resource, they soon become dated as new information becomes available.

This book aims to provide the reader with a very up-to-date summary of the current concepts and practices in neonatal medicine. The field is covered in a series of self-contained, easily read topics set in a unique format which encourages the adoption of a problem-based approach ideal for day-to-day clinical practice. Although some topics reflect our personal clinical practice, the systematic approach to each topic is retained. Reference is made to related topics which allows the reader ready access to the subject matter of their choice unencumbered by extraneous detail.

As such, the text is an ideal revision aid for the neonatology components of the postgraduate paediatric examinations (including MRCP or DCH). It will also serve as a useful reference text for other professionals, both trainees and qualified, who are involved in the care of both well and sick newborns.

We are thankful to our colleagues for reading through various topics, in particular Dr R. Danha who read through most of the topics and was a source of great encouragement. Also our sincere appreciation to Tracey Fantham whose secretarial assistance made this book possible. Finally, we are especially thankful to the staff at BIOS for their helpful guidance from the outset, and their enduring patience despite the many broken deadlines.

We dedicate the book to our own 'ex-prems' Francesca, Grace and Henry.

Richard H. Mupanemunda
Michael Watkinson

ABDOMINAL DISTENSION

Abdominal distension is one of the commonest physical signs for which a medical opinion may be sought. The causes are legion, varying from physiological abdominal distension through a variety of benign causes to serious acute medical emergencies.

Aetiology

1. *Physiological*
   - Gaseous distension in infants receiving mechanical ventilation or continuous positive airway pressure (CPAP).
   - Delayed bowel action.
   - Lax abdominal muscles (e.g. prune belly syndrome).
   - Urinary retention.

2. *Pathological*
   - Ascites.
   - Hirschsprung's disease.
   - Intestinal obstruction (e.g. atresia or volvulus).
   - Intra-abdominal masses (organomegaly or tumours).
   - Iatrogenic (e.g. intraperitoneal extravasation of parenteral infusates).
   - Intra-abdominal haemorrhage.
   - Imperforate anus.
   - Meconium ileus or plug (associated with cystic fibrosis (CF)).
   - Necrotizing enterocolitis (NEC).
   - Pneumoperitoneum.

Presentation

This may be the sole abnormal physical sign in an otherwise well infant when physiological causes are responsible. On the other hand, pathological abdominal distension with bilious vomiting may present at birth or later in a sick infant with a shiny, silent, tense and tender abdomen with perforated NEC. In non-ventilated infants, this may be heralded by apnoeas and bradycardias or acute collapse. A ventilated infant with a rapidly increasing abdominal girth may have developed a pneumoperitoneum.

Investigations

- Abdominal radiograph.
- Abdominal ultrasound scan.
- Water-soluble contrast or barium enema study.
- Infection screen.
- Electrolytes.

Management

Infants presenting with meconium ileus or those passing a meconium plug should be screened for CF (immunoreactive trypsin (IRT) or DNA analysis for common CF mutations). Acute and subacute intestinal obstruction is managed by gastric decompression (nasogastric suction) and elective surgery in an appropriate centre. The infant should be in a stable condition prior to surgery. Infants with severe or perforated NEC may require more urgent surgical intervention and should receive adequate analgesia, broad-spectrum antibiotics including anaerobic cover (e.g. ceftazidime, vancomycin and metronidazole) and, if necessary, mechanical ventilation. Intra-abdominal collections (e.g. ascites) may be drained with a fine canula to decompress the abdomen, and the peritoneal fluid cultured. Adequate analgesia should always be administered where the infant may be in pain (e.g. i.v. morphine infusion at 20–40 µg/kg/hour for an infant with perforated bowel).

Further reading

Beasley SW, Hutson JM, Auldist AW. *Essential Paediatric Surgery*. London: Arnold, 1996.
Black JA, Whitfield MF. *Neonatal Emergencies: Early Detection and Management*, 2nd edn. Oxford: Butterworth-Heinemann, 1991.
O'Doherty N. *Atlas of the Newborn*, 2nd edn. Lancaster: MTP Press, 1985.
Philip AGS. *Neonatology: A Practical Guide*, 4th edn. Philadelphia: W.B. Saunders, 1996.
Reyes HM, Vidyasagar D (eds). Neonatal surgery. *Clinics in Perinatology*, 1989; **16**: 1.

Related topics of interest

ACID–BASE BALANCE

The acid–base balance is a vital dynamic index of an infant's wellbeing. The pH of plasma is 7.36–7.45 (33–44 nmol/l of H^+). An infant is acidotic if the pH is <7.26 and alkalotic if the pH is >7.46. If the pH is <7.26 and the carbon dioxide level is high, a respiratory acidosis is present, but if carbon dioxide is normal or low, a metabolic acidosis is present. If the pH is >7.46 with a low carbon dioxide level, a respiratory alkalosis is present (e.g. hyperventilation) and if the carbon dioxide level is normal, a metabolic alkalosis is present. Metabolic and respiratory alkalosis is uncommon and invariably iatrogenic (excess base administration or hyperventilation). Acidosis, on the other hand, is quite common and may be respiratory (high carbon dioxide), metabolic (low or normal carbon dioxide) or mixed (combination of both) with a negative base excess. The causes and management of these conditions are detailed in *Table 1* below.

There are several buffering systems in place to prevent the build up of excess acid (especially bicarbonate, haemoglobin, protein and phosphate). These systems are not fully developed in newborns and particularly preterm infants. There is a tendency, therefore, for newborns to develop acidosis (most commonly mixed acidosis). Excess acid may be generated from ongoing metabolic processes (including congenital metabolic errors of metabolism), enteral or parenteral intake, respiratory failure, decreased renal excretion of acid or the inappropriate renal loss of bicarbonate. The acid–base balance is best assessed by arterial blood gas analysis. When metabolic acidosis is present, it is important to identify the cause in order to give the specific therapy for it. A raised anion gap suggests the presence of an unmeasured organic acid (e.g. lactate). The anion gap is calculated as the sum of sodium and potassium, less the sum of chloride and bicarbonate (normal value: 6–14 mmol/l).

Table 1. Causes and management of alkalosis and acidosis

Condition	Causes	Management
Respiratory alkalosis	Hyperventilation	Reduce ventilatory support if ventilated
Respiratory acidosis		
Unventilated	Respiratory failure	Intubation and ventilation
Ventilated	Endotracheal tube blockage (raised $PaCO_2$, normal or low PaO_2)	Change endotracheal tube
	Endotracheal tube dislodged (raised $PaCO_2$, low PaO_2)	Re-intubate
	Pneumothorax (raised $PaCO_2$, and low PaO_2)	Aspirate pneumothorax and insert chest drain
Metabolic alkalosis	Excessive gastric losses, e.g. high atresia, pyloric stenosis	Replacement of gastric losses
	Excess base administration	Stop base administration
Metabolic acidosis	Hypoxia, anaerobic metabolism	Administer oxygen ± intermittent positive-pressure ventilation (IPPV)

Table 1. (continued)

Condition	Causes	Management
Metabolic acidosis	Anaemia	Blood transfusion
	Excessive respiratory effort	IPPV
	Hypotension and hypovolaemia	Colloid administration ± inotropes
	Renal bicarbonate loss	Bicarbonate replacement
	Excess acid administration parenterally	Reduce intake appropriately
	Infection	Broad-spectrum antibiotics after all appropriate cultures
	Inborn error of metabolism (persistent acidosis)	Assay serum amino acids, lactate and ammonia, with urinalysis for pH, acetone, ketoacids and urine amino and organic acids

Problems associated with marked acidosis

- Increased pulmonary vascular resistance.
- Inhibition of surfactant synthesis.
- Impaired myocardial contractility.
- Impaired diaphragmatic contractility.
- Impaired renal excretion of acid load.

Base administration

First check that the blood gases make sense and repeat if necessary, as excess heparin in a blood gas syringe may give erroneous readings. Administer base when the pH is <7.25 and the base deficit is greater than −10 mmol/l. The amount of base (in mmol) is calculated from the formula:

base deficit (mmol/l) × bodyweight (kg) × 0.4 (extracellular volume).

Give bicarbonate as a 4.2% solution (0.5 mmol/ml of solution) as a slow infusion (0.5 mmol/min). In the presence of a high $PaCO_2$ or hypernatraemia, THAM (tris-hydroxymethyl-aminomethane) may be preferable. A 7% THAM solution contains 0.5 mmol/ml. THAM, however, may cause apnoeas and should preferably be administered to ventilated infants. It is preferable to initially administer an amount of base sufficient to only *half correct* the calculated base deficit, with repeat gases to reassess the acid–base balance. For persistent acidosis a constant infusion of base may be required.

Problems associated with base administration

Provided appropriate doses of base are administered slowly, concerns regarding intracerebral haemorrhage associated with base administration may be allayed. However, over-correction of a metabolic acidosis may carry more risks than a persistent mild acidosis. Thus some patients with urea cycle defects may present with mild acidaemia, which should not be corrected as acidosis protects against NH_4 dissociation and toxicity.

Common patterns of blood gas abnormalities

- Respiratory alkalosis (acute): pH raised, $PaCO_2$ reduced, HCO_3 normal or slightly reduced.
- Respiratory alkalosis (chronic): pH normal or raised, $PaCO_2$ reduced, HCO_3 reduced.
- Respiratory acidosis (acute): pH decreased, $PaCO_2$ raised, HCO_3 normal or slightly raised.
- Respiratory acidosis (chronic): pH slightly decreased, $PaCO_2$ raised, HCO_3 raised.
- Metabolic acidosis: pH reduced, $PaCO_2$ reduced, HCO_3 reduced.
- Metabolic alkalosis: pH raised, $PaCO_2$ raised or normal, HCO_3 raised.

pH and corresponding hydrogen ion concentration

pH	$[H^+]$ (nanomolar)
6.9	126
7.0	100
7.1	79
7.2	63
7.3	50
7.4	40
7.5	32
7.6	25

Further reading

Driscoll P, Brown T, Gwinnut C, Wardle T. *A Simple Guide to Blood Gas Analysis*. London: BMJ Publishing, 1997.

Howell JH. Sodium bicarbonate in the perinatal setting revisited. *Clinics in Perinatology*, 1987; **14**: 807–16.

Seri I. Regulation of acid–base balance in the fetus and neonate. In: Polin RA, Fox WW (eds). *Fetal and Neonatal Physiology*, 2nd edn. Philadephia: W.B. Saunders, 1998; 1726–30.

von Planta I, Weil MH, von Planta M *et al*. Hypercarbic acidosis reduces cardiac resuscibility. *Critical Care Medicine*, 1991; **19**: 1177–82.

Related topics of interest

ACUTE COLLAPSE

This is one acute medical emergency where swift and appropriate response can make a major difference to outcome. Irrespective of the cause, the major objectives should be to re-establish adequate gas exchange and maintain the cardiovascular circulation.

Aetiology
- Overwhelming sepsis.
- Pneumothorax.
- Aspiration of vomitus.
- Major haemorrhage (e.g. intra-abdominal, intrapulmonary or intracranial).
- Severe NEC (± perforation).
- Metabolic and endocrine disorders.
- Congenital heart disease (e.g. hypoplastic left heart syndrome, interrupted aortic arch).
- Compromised airway in the ventilated infant (blocked or displaced endotracheal tube).

Presentation
Sudden onset of bradycardia, hypotension, pallor or cyanosis in either a previously well or already unwell infant. There may, in addition, be vomitus in the mouth, blood coming from the oropharynx or trachea, abdominal distension and hypothermia. The infant may look extremely ill with laboured or absent respiratory effort, mottled skin, marked hypotonia and cold peripheries. Bloody stools may be passed at the same time, suggesting intra-abdominal pathology (NEC). Occasionally seizures may also be noted.

Investigations
- Fibreoptic cold light chest transillumination for pneumothoraces.
- Chest and abdominal radiographs.
- Arterial blood gases.
- Blood glucose.
- Urea and electrolytes (U&E).
- Full blood count (FBC).
- Clotting screen.
- Head ultrasound scan.
- Infection screen (blood, urine ± cerebrospinal fluid (CSF)).
- Metabolic screen (obtain acute blood and urine samples and store accordingly).

Management
Near normal gas exchange, adequate tissue perfusion and normal pressure should be re-established and maintained as rapidly as possible. If the respiratory effort is inadequate and the infant is not already ventilated, clear the oropharynx and commence bag and mask (or T-piece) ventilation with 100% oxygen. Check pulse and peripheral pulses. If absent, commence external cardiac massage (ECM). If the infant is unresponsive

after 1 min, intubate and continue ECM with bagging. Ensure that the bag and mask or T-piece set-up is connected to oxygen *and* that it is turned on! Transilluminate the chest wall to exclude a large tension pneumothorax and drain (needle aspiration) if present. If still unresponsive, check the endotracheal tube position and administer 0.3 ml of 1:1000 adrenaline via the endotracheal tube. If this produces a satisfactory response in the pulse and oxygenation (saturations >95%), discontinue ECM and continue with respiratory support and connect to a mechanical ventilator. Check arterial blood gases and blood glucose and adjust ventilation accordingly. Give dextrose and/or base as required. Obtain chest and abdominal X-rays.

Administer colloid if the peripheral circulation is inadequate, followed, if necessary, by inotropes (dopamine or dobutamine at 5–20 μcg/kg/min). Once the infant is stable, work out the most likely cause, if it is not already evident. Consider performing a head ultrasound scan in a newborn where intraventricular haemorrhage (IVH) might be a possibility. If a haemorrhage has occurred, check clotting and administer fresh frozen plasma (FFP) or cryoprecipitate (if fibrinogen <1 g/l). If sepsis is likely, complete a septic screen (with LP if stable) and cover with broad-spectrum antibiotics. If the cause is obscure, consider rarer metabolic disorders, especially if there is persistent acidosis, hypoglycaemia or inordinate neurological depression. Suspect adrenal insufficiency if dehydration, low sodium (<130 mmol/l), high potassium (>5 mmol/l) and ± hypoglycaemia are present. Maintain respiratory support with full monitoring over several hours and gradually wean according to the status of the infant and results of the investigations.

If an infant remains unresponsive to full cardiopulmonary resuscitation for 4–5 min, give 1:1000 adrenaline (0.4–1 ml i.v.) and consider giving base if the resuscitation efforts are still unsuccessful after 10 min (3–5 mmol of 4.2% $NaHCO_3$ i.v.). Needle both sides of the chest in case bilateral pneumothoraces are present. Continue with resuscitation efforts for at least 20 min.

Unsuccessful resuscitations

Always try and obtain consent for a post-mortem (PM). A coroner may need to be informed. Where inherited metabolic disease is a possibility, obtain urine (amino and organic acids), blood (amino acids, DNA studies), skin (fibroblast cultures), muscle and/or liver biopsies. Freeze urine, spin blood, and separate red cells and plasma and freeze separately. Snap freeze liver and muscle samples in liquid nitrogen or store at 4°C in tissue culture medium or plain saline, but transfer to the most appropriate storage medium at the earliest opportunity.

Further reading

American Academy of Pediatrics/American Heart Association. *Textbook of Neonatal Resuscitation*. Dallas: American Heart Association, 1994.

Black JA, Whitfield MF. *Neonatal Emergencies: Early Detection and Management*, 2nd edn. Oxford: Butterworth-Heinemann, 1991.

Burchfield DJ, Berkowitz ID, Berg RA *et al*. Medications in neonatal resuscitation. *Annals of Emergency Medicine*, 1993; **22**: 435.

Emery JL, Variend S, Howat AJ *et al*. Investigation of inborn errors of metabolism in unexpected infant deaths. *Lancet*, 1988; **ii**: 29.

Meerstadt PWD, Gyll C. *Manual of Emergency X-ray Interpretation*. Philadelphia: W.B. Saunders, 1995.

Reece RM (ed). *Manual of Emergency Pediatrics*, 4th edn. Philadelphia: W.B. Saunders, 1992.

Surtees R, Leonard JV. Acute metabolic encephalopathy: a review of causes, mechanisms and treatment. *Journal of Inherited Metabolic Disease*, 1989; **12**: 42.

Willett LD, Nelson RM Jr. Outcome of cardiopulmonary resuscitation in the neonatal intensive care unit. *Critical Care Medicine*, 1986; **14**: 773.

Related topics of interest

Acid–base balance (p. 3)
Inherited metabolic disease – investigation and management (p. 156)
Pulmonary haemorrhage (p. 259)
Resuscitation (p. 282)
Shock (p. 302)

ANAEMIA

The cord haemogloblin concentration in term infants averages 17 g/dl (range 14–20 g/dl) and 14 g/dl (range 13–18 g/dl) in preterm infants. Delayed clamping of the cord and holding the infant below the level of the placenta at birth will significantly raise the haemoglobin concentration. After birth, erythropoietin production is switched off by the greater availability of oxygen, reticulocytosis falls from 5% (at birth) to less than 1% and the haemoglobin level falls to a nadir of 7–10 g/dl by 8–10 weeks, remaining stable for several weeks, before gradually increasing. The fall in haemoglobin is more rapid and more marked in preterm infants, with the nadir of haemoglobin concentration varying inversely with gestational age. In term infants this decline and rise in haemoglobin concentration has been labelled physiological as the infants are asymptomatic. In preterm infants the fall in haemoglobin concentration is often so marked that some infants require erythrocyte transfusions and thus this 'anaemia of prematurity' is labelled non-physiological. It is characterized by reticulocytopenia, bone marrow hypoplasia and erythropoietin levels that are low relative to the degree of anaemia.

Anaemia may present at birth or during the first week of life (early anaemia), or later (later onset anaemia), depending on the aetiology. Anaemia presenting after the first day of life commonly follows haemorrhage or haemolysis (non-immune), while the anaemia due to impaired red cell production often presents after the first month of life.

Early onset anaemia

This is a haemoglobin level of <13 g/dl (PCV <40%) during the first week of life. This is primarily a haemorrhagic anaemia resulting from repeated blood sampling during intensive care of very low birthweight infants with small total blood volumes.

Aetiology

- Twin-to-twin transfusion.
- Fetomaternal transfusion.
- Fetal haemorrhage: placenta praevia, abruption, vasa praevia or placental incision at Caesarian section.
- Fetoplacental transfusion at birth.
- Chronic or acute fetal haemolysis: rhesus disease, α-thalassaemia.
- Perinatal neonatal haemorrhage: intracranial, subaponeurotic fractures, ruptured spleen or liver, umbilical cord rupture or accidents.
- Iatrogenic losses: repeated blood sampling.

Clinical features

1. *Acute blood loss*
- Pallor.
- Hypotension.
- Poor capillary refill.
- Tachycardia.
- Tachypnoea.

2. *Chronic blood loss*
- Pallor.

- Tachycardia.
- Congestive cardiac failure.
- Hepatosplenomegaly.
- Jaundice.
- Hydrops fetalis.

Investigations

- Full blood count and film.
- Blood group and Coombs' test.
- Maternal Kleihauer test.
- Coagulation screen.
- Cranial ultrasonography (intracranial haemorrhage) and/or abdominal ultrasonography (concealed internal haemorrhage).
- Exclude red cell abnormalities: haemoglobin electrophoresis (haemoglobinopathies) and red cell enzymopathies.
- Serum bilirubin.

Management

Always look for the underlying cause and rectify this if possible. For acute blood loss and shock, rapid resuscitation is paramount. Give blood (10–30 ml/kg of group O rhesus negative or blood harvested from placenta) at once. Alternatively, give 4.5% human albumin or plasma as volume expanders until blood is available. Repeat colloid administration (albumin or blood) until blood pressure normalizes and correct acidosis. For severe hydrops fetalis due to rhesus isoimmunization (cord haemoglobin <11 g/dl, cord bilirubin >80 μmol/l, or rate of rise of bilirubin >10 μmol/l/hour, with positive Coombs' test) carry out an exchange transfusion. The primary aim is to correct the anaemia and raise serum albumin and not remove bilirubin. Remember to maintain the airway and if necessary give oxygen.

Later onset anaemia

This is a haemoglobin level of <10 g/dl after the first week of life. This is primarily a hypo-regenerative anaemia resulting from the inability of the immature haematopoietic tissue to react adequately to hypoxia.

Aetiology

- Anaemia of prematurity: impaired erythropoiesis and reduced red cell survival.
- Iatrogenic: repeated blood sampling.
- Chronic haemolysis which may be subdivided into immune haemolysis (isoimmunization), congenital red cell defects (morphological, enzymatic and haemoglobin abnormalities) and acquired red cell defects (secondary to toxins, drugs or infection).
- The haemoglobin abnormalities may be synthetic defects (thalassaemias) or structural defects (haemoglobin variants).

- Bleeding: intracranial or intra-abdominal haemorrhage, NEC, disseminated intravascular coagulation (DIC).
- Severe infection.
- Iron deficiency (after 6–8 weeks).
- Vitamin E deficiency (haemolytic anaemia).
- Other essential vitamin or mineral deficiencies (folic acid, vitamin B12, copper and zinc deficiencies).
- Maternal autoimmune disease (systemic lupus erythematosus (SLE), autoimmune haemolytic anaemia).
- Failure of red cell production, for example Diamond–Blackfan syndrome (autosomal recessive inheritance) characterized by reticulocytopenia (<0.2%) and anaemia, but normal leucocyte and platelet production.

Clinical features

- Apnoeic attacks.
- Tachycardia.
- Poor feeding.
- Poor weight gain.
- Increased oxygen requirements in oxygen-dependent infants.

Investigations

- Full blood count, film and reticulocyte count.
- Serum bilirubin (total and conjugated).
- Coagulation screen (if actively bleeding).
- Serum biotin, copper and zinc (perioral dermatitis).
- Check stools for occult blood.

Management

Transfuse with packed cells if symptomatic. For oxygen-dependent infants with chronic lung disease, transfuse to raise the haemoglobin to 12–14 g/dl (PCV >45%). For anaemia of prematurity, transfuse if haemoglobin is <8 g/dl. Give iron (2 mg/kg/day from 4 weeks until weaned), folic acid (0.1 mg daily orally from day 10 until 3 months post-term) and vitamin E (5–25 IU/day orally).

There are several formulae for estimating the blood transfusion requirements of anaemic infants:

(a) Transfusion of 3 ml of packed red cells per kg bodyweight will raise the baby's haemoglobin by 1 g/dl.
(b) Transfusion of 10 ml of packed cells per kg will raise PCV by 10%.
(c) Volume of packed red cells (PCV = 80%) to be transfused = desired rise in haemoglobin × weight in kg × 3.

Prevention

Recombinant human erythropoietin (rHuEPO) has recently been licensed for the treatment of anaemia of prematurity in several European countries (e.g. Recormon®, Boehringer Mannheim, UK). rHuEPO at doses of 750 units/kg/week (given as three doses of 250 units/kg by s.c. injection (i.v.

shorter half-life) on 3 days per week) with oral iron supplementation at 6 mg/kg/day (initiated at 2 mg/kg/day and gradually increased) from the first week of life for 6 weeks, reduces the need for transfusion for later onset anaemia in infants of <34 weeks gestation (birthweight 750–1500 g). Some restrict rHuEPO administration to all infants of <28 weeks gestation, but only those <3rd percentile at 28–32 weeks gestation. Sick ventilated infants or those having daily venesection of >1.2 ml/day may receive a high-dose rHuEPO regimen consisting of 1400 units/kg/week given as 200 units/kg/day by i.v. infusion beginning within 72 hours of birth and continued for 2 weeks; thereafter the standard regimen may be continued for the remaining 4 weeks. rHuEPO has been demonstrated to be both safe and cost-effective.

Further reading

Brown MS. Physiologic anaemia of infancy: normal red cell values and physiology of neonatal erythropoiesis. In: Stockman JA, Pochedly C (eds). *Developmental and Neonatal Hematology*. New York: Raven Press, 1988; 244–74.

Doyle JJ, Zipursky A. Neonatal blood disorders. In: Sinclair JL, Bracken MB (eds). *Effective Care of the Newborn Infant*. Oxford: Oxford University Press, 1992; 426–53.

Lilleyman JS, Hann IM (eds). *Paediatric Haematology*. Edinburgh: Churchill Livingstone, 1992.

Nathan DG, Orkin SH. *Nathan and Oski's Hematology of Infancy and Childhood*, 5th edn. Philadelphia: W.B. Saunders, 1997.

Obladen M, Maier RF. Erythropoietin therapy in preterm infants. In: Hansen TN, McIntosh N (eds). *Current Topics in Neonatology, Number 2*. London: W.B. Saunders, 1997; 108–24.

Oski FA, Naiman JL. *Hematologic Problems in the Newborn*, 3rd edn. Philadelphia: W.B. Saunders, 1982.

Related topics of interest

ANAESTHESIA AND POST-OPERATIVE ANALGESIA

Neonates presenting for surgery are usually in urgent need of such treatment. They are also at a period when significant physiological and maturational changes of transition from fetal to extrauterine life are occurring. The special problems relating to this age group which may influence anaesthetic management are:

- Thermoregulation.
- Cardiovascular function.
- Neonatal airway and respiratory function.
- Renal function.
- Glucose homeostasis.

Thermoregulation

Heat loss occurs by conduction, convection, radiation and evaporation, the major mechanism being radiation. Anaesthesia interferes with heat production by inhibiting shivering and non-shivering thermogenesis. Hypothermia delays recovery from anaesthesia, prolongs the effects of muscle relaxants and increases oxygen consumption. If heat loss is not minimized aggressively, the anaesthetized neonate readily becomes hypothermic.

Cardiovascular function

The neonatal heart has much less contractile power since the myocardial cell has half as much contractile mass as an adult cell. Augmenting preload does not increase cardiac output but increasing heart rate does. Sympathetic innervation is incomplete but parasympathetic innervation is complete, resulting in increased susceptiblity to bradycardia. The commonest cause of bradycardia in the newborn is hypoxia.

Neonatal airway and respiratory function

The neonate has a narrow subglottic area which limits the size of the endotracheal tube. A large abdomen, weak intercostal muscles and the horizontal configuration of the ribs pose additional mechanical disadvantage. The ability of the neonate to breathe spontaneously is limited and ventilation should always be controlled. Premature infants less than 45–55 post-conceptual weeks are at risk of life-threatening apnoeas following anaesthesia, and they are more prone to ventilatory dysfunction from the effect of residual anaesthetic agents.

Renal function

Renal function is immature at birth and this may prolong the effects of drugs administered during anaesthesia. Renal excretion of drugs is influenced by glomerular filtration, tubular excretion and reabsorption. In newborns, the glomerular filtration rate (GFR) is only 20% of that of adults, but this rapidly increases to 50% by day 10 of life and approaches adult values towards the end of the first year of life. Both full-term and preterm infants have a limited ability to handle sodium loads, the preterm infant being an obligate sodium loser. A careful selection of both the composition and volume of fluids given intra-operatively is required since neonatal renal function is limited.

Glucose homeostasis

This is not well developed in the early postnatal period and predisposes the neonate, especially the preterm infant, to the risk of both hyper- and hypoglycaemia. The stress of surgery and uncontrolled exogenous glucose therapy are the two most important causes of hyperglycaemia in the perioperative period. Normoglycaemia can be maintained by restricting the amount of exogenously administered glucose to 4–6 mg/kg/min and frequently monitoring blood glucose levels.

Preoperative preparation

This is aimed at stabilizing the sick neonate so that he/she can be transported to theatre and anaesthetized without undue haemodynamic compromise. Adequate i.v. access should be established and in the critically ill neonate, an arterial line should be inserted. If the neonate has indwelling umbilical arterial and venous lines, their location should be confirmed radiologically prior to transport.

Preoperative starvation orders

For elective procedures, the last milk feed is allowed up to 4 hours preoperatively and clear liquid up to 2 hours preoperatively. In case surgery is delayed, an i.v. infusion with a dextrose-containing solution must be commenced to maintain normoglycaemia.

Transport to theatre

This may pose significant risks, especially to the small, sick, ventilated preterm infant. Monitoring must be continued throughout the period of transfer. The trip to and from theatre involves lifting the infant (and all attached equipment) into and out of the transport incubator four times within a short space of time. The most commonly encountered problems include:

- Accidental extubation.
- Cold stress (hypothermia).
- Dislodging of arterial and venous lines.
- Dislodging chest drains and surgical drains.
- Changing ventilator modalities (five ventilator changes in all for a round trip).
- Adverse effects of ambulance transportation if surgery is performed off site.

Intra-operative care

- Full remote continuous monitoring of all vital parameters should be continued during surgery.
- Take meticulous care to avoid hypothermia.
- Monitor fluid balance carefully to avoid hypo- and hypervolaemia.
- Replace significant blood losses intra-operatively (small total blood volume).

- Check blood gases and blood glucose during prolonged procedures.
- High-risk infants (e.g. with BPD) undergoing minor procedures such as hernia repair have fewer respiratory complications if the surgery is done under regional anaesthesia (i.e. epidural anaesthesia) rather than a general anaesthetic.

Post-operative analgesia and pain control

Neonates are often denied post-operative analgesia because they are susceptible to the respiratory depressant effects of narcotics and they cannot vocalize pain. It is also especially difficult to assess pain in neonates and, in particular, ventilated infants. Regional blocks performed intra-operatively provide analgesia during the immediate post-operative period. Systemic narcotics are the most commonly used agents for management of pain and morphine may be considered the prototype. Neonates requiring post-operative ventilation are ideal candidates for narcotic analgesia. The suppression of respiration due to narcotics promotes synchronous mechanical ventilation. However, greater skill and judgement is required in the use of narcotics for pain management in newborns who are not ventilated. The newborn must be observed closely with apnoea monitoring. Equipment and personnel for emergency airway management and treatment with naloxone should be readily available. However, for minor degrees of discomfort or pain, opiates may be avoided and mild analgesics, e.g. paracetamol (10 mg/kg/dose given 4-hourly) may suffice.

Further reading

Alexander SM, Todres ID. The use of sedation and muscle relaxation in the ventilated infant. *Clinics in Perinatology*, 1998; **25**: 63–78.

Cote CJ, Ryan JF, Todres ID, Goudsouzian NG (eds). *A Practice of Anaesthesia for Infants and Children*, 2nd edn. Philadelphia: W.B. Saunders, 1993.

Gavilanes AWD, Heineman E, Herpes MJHM, Blanco CE. Use of neonatal intensive care unit as a safe place for neonatal surgery. *Archives of Disease in Childhood, Fetal and Neonatal Edition*, 1997; **76**: F51–3.

Krishna G, Ernhardt JD. Anaesthesia for the newborn ex-preterm infant. *Seminars in Paediatric Surgery*, 1992; **1**: 32–4.

Zeigler JW, Todres ID. Intubation of newborns. *American Journal of Diseases of Childhood*, 1992; **146**: 147–9.

Related topics of interest

APNOEAS AND BRADYCARDIAS

Apnoea in the newborn infant is defined as a pause in breathing of more than 20 seconds or a shorter pause associated with bradycardia or hypoxaemia. This condition increases in incidence at lower gestations. Thus below 30 weeks gestation three out of four infants will have recurrent apnoeas and bradycardias, the incidence falling to less than 1 in 10 by 35 weeks gestation and 0.08% in term infants. Apnoeas may represent a central disturbance in the regulation of breathing with airflow and respiratory effort ceasing at the end of expiration (central apnoea). Alternatively, the upper airway may intermittently become totally occluded while the infant continues to make ever-increasing, regular respiratory effort in an attempt to overcome the obstruction (obstructive apnoea). Some infants, however, may have 'mixed apnoeas' which resemble central apnoea initially with cessation of respiration followed by intermittent but ineffective respiratory effort indicative of airway obstruction.

Most apnoeas are of the mixed type, with initial central episodes being followed by pharyngeal soft tissue collapse. Furthermore, upper airway protective reflexes may result in apnoea. Thus gastro-oesophageal reflux or pharyngeal incoordination may also induce apnoeas.

Aetiology

1. Abnormal airway
- Choanal atresia.
- Micrognathia.
- Tracheomalacia.
- Upper airway incoordination (neurological abnormality).

2. CNS disorders
- Brainstem immaturity.
- Intracranial haemorrhage.
- Seizures.
- Hypoxic–ischaemic encephalopathy.
- Congenital malformations.
- Maternal medication during pregnancy and labour.
- Central hypoventilation syndromes.

3. Metabolic disorders
- Hypoglycaemia.
- Hypocalcaemia.
- Hyponatraemia.
- Inherited metabolic disease.

4. Systemic disorders
- Anaemia.
- Sepsis.
- Hypoxia.
- Cardiac failure.

5. Miscellaneous
- Overheating.
- Recent general anaesthesia.

Bradycardias often accompany apnoeas but may be unassociated with apnoea and may not be due to central hypoxaemia. Marked bradycardia (pulse <80/min) may be deleterious and requires therapy.

Investigations

1. *Well infants*
- Blood glucose (exclude hypoglycaemia).
- FBC (exclude anaemia).
- Oesophageal pH monitoring (exclude reflux).
- Electroencephalogram (EEG) (exclude seizures).

2. *Unwell infants*
- Full infection screen (blood culture, lumbar puncture, urine culture, chest X-ray).
- Blood gases.
- Serum calcium, magnesium and electrolytes.
- Cranial ultrasound scan.
- Abdominal X-ray (exclude NEC).

Management

The primary aim is to correct any underlying disorders, intermittently stimulate the infant during the events and maintain monitoring. There is no evidence that well infants with mild apnoea (<10 per day) and quick responses to tactile stimulation need any more specific therapy. Therapy is summarized thus:

- Gentle stimulation if not self-resolving.
- Monitor for hypoxaemia and administer supplemental oxygen if necessary.
- Use bag and mask if response to supplemental facial oxygen is poor.
- Transfuse if anaemic (keep haemoglobin $\geq 12\,g/dl$).
- Administer methylxanthines – i.v. aminophylline (loading dose 5 mg/kg, maintenance 4.4 mg/kg/day) or oral theophylline (loading dose 5 mg/kg/day in three divided doses, then up to 8 mg/kg daily – therapeutic range 28–84 mmol/l (5–15 mg/l)). Alternatively, caffeine (which is less toxic) may be given orally (loading dose 10 mg/kg and a once daily maintenance of 2.5 mg/kg, equivalent to 20 mg caffeine citrate/kg and 5 mg caffeine citrate/kg, loading dose and maintenance, respectively). Caffeine and theophylline are equally effective.
- If methylxanthines fail, add doxapram starting at 0.5 mg/kg/hour, increasing to 2.5 mg/kg/hour, intravenously or orally. Load with 2.5–3.0 mg/kg i.v. over 15–30 min followed by maintenance therapy.
- If drug therapy fails, try nasal CPAP (4–6 cmH$_2$O).
- If CPAP fails, intubate and ventilate at low pressures and rates.

Prognosis   In otherwise uncomplicated preterm infants, there is no evidence that apnoeas cause long-term neurological impairment when other complicating factors are controlled.

Further reading

Henderson-Smart DJ. Apnea of prematurity. In: Beckerman RC, Brouillette RT, Hunt CE (eds). *Respiratory Control Disorders in Infants and Children.* Baltimore: Williams & Wilkins, 1992; 161–77.

Henderson-Smart DJ. Recurrent apnoea. In: Yu VYH (ed). *Bailliere's Clinical Paediatrics, Pulmonary Problems in the Perinatal Period and their Sequelae.* London: Bailliere Tindall, 1995; 203–22.

Polin RA, Fox WW (eds). *Fetal and Neonatal Physiology,* 2nd edn. Philadelphia: W.B. Saunders, 1998.

Spitzer AR (ed). *Intensive Care of the Fetus and Neonate.* St. Louis: C.V. Mosby, 1996.

Related topics of interest

ASSESSMENT OF GESTATIONAL AGE

Antenatal

The measurement most frequently used to assess fetal gestation is the bi-parietal diameter at around 16 weeks gestation. The 95% confidence interval of such a measurement is 0.8 weeks. If a scan is done between 6 and 10 weeks, measurement of the crown-rump length is at least as accurate, but thereafter curling of the fetus may make this a difficult measurement. A combination of these measurements, combined if necessary with fetal femur length, is used for assessment at different gestations.

The accuracy of gestational assessment by scanning drops off dramatically as pregnancy progresses because of biological variation in growth. Later scans are useful for following an individual's growth, but a late first scan contributes little to gestational assessment. Ultrasonographic biometry in early pregnancy is a more accurate assessment of gestation and the expected date of delivery than maternal dates, even when the mother is certain!

Postnatal

In 1970, Dubowitz developed a scoring system for the assessment of gestational age in infants less than 5 days old based upon morphological and neurological characteristics. It is limited by the fact that only six babies of <30 weeks gestation were included, and that, at its best, the confidence interval of the score was ±14 days. Thus, even in the best hands, an assessment of a baby's gestation as (say) 32 weeks means that the assessor is 95% sure that the true gestation is between 30 and 34 weeks. The confidence limits are even wider (>2.5 weeks) at lower gestations (or birthweight <1500 g), the very ones that concern us most nowadays. Furthermore, the handling of sick preterm babies for this assessment is a problem. Parkin recognized this and developed a simplified score based only on morphological criteria that could be assessed with very minimal handling, but the confidence intervals of his score were ±18 days. Further doubt was cast when experienced Norwegian paediatricians reported confidence intervals of ±5 and ±6 weeks for the two scores, respectively. The Ballard score is an abbreviated version of the Dubowitz scoring system and is therefore subject to the same limitations. Notwithstanding the above limitations, a new expanded Ballard scoring system has been developed for very low birthweight and extremely low birthweight infants. The updated Ballard included 61 infants less than 26 weeks and 89 between 26 and 31 weeks gestation. This sytem provides a means of gestational assessment for all infants of gestational ages greater than 20 weeks. For the most immature infants, the assessment is more accurate when performed during the first 12 hours of life. Other additional ways of estimating gestational age include nerve conduction studies and examination of the anterior vascular capsule of the lens.

Nowadays with accurate dating by antenatal ultrasound, there is neither need nor justification for a detailed postnatal assessment of gestation. However, the above methods of assessing gestational age may be extremely useful in the minority of pregnancies where the mother deliberately conceals her pregnancy, is unable (due to language or communication difficulties) or unwilling to divulge the requisite information, or is particularly unreliable (e.g. a drug abusing mother with unfavourable social circumstances). Thus familiarity with at least one of the above assessment systems is advantageous.

Further reading

Ballard JL, Khoury JC, Wedig K *et al*. New Ballard score expanded to include extremely premature infants. *Journal of Pediatrics*, 1991; **119**: 417–23.

Dubowitz LMS. *The Neurological Assessment of the Preterm and Full-term Infant, 2nd edn. Clinics in Developmental Medicine No. 148*. Cambridge: Cambridge University Press, 1998.

Dubowitz LMS, Dubowitz V, Goldberg C. Clinical assessment of gestational age in the newborn infant. *Journal of Pediatrics*, 1970; **77**: 1–10.

Hitter H, Gorman W, Rudolph A. Examination of the anterior vascular capsule of the lens. II. Assessment of gestational age in infants small for gestational age. *Journal of Pediatric Ophthalmology and Strabismus*, 1981; **18**: 52.

Mongelli M, Wilcox M, Gardosi J. Estimating the date of confinement: ultrasonographic biometry versus certain menstrual dates. *American Journal of Obstetrics and Gynecology*, 1996; **174**: 278–81.

Parkin JM, Hey EN, Clowes JS. Rapid assessment of gestational age at birth. *Archives of Disease in Childhood*, 1976; **51**: 259–63.

Pearce MJ, de Chazal R. Establishing gestational age. In: Dewbury K, Meire H, Cosgrove D (eds). *Ultrasound in Obstetrics and Gynaecology*. Edinburgh: Churchill Livingstone, 1993; 211–21.

Vogt H, Haneberg B, Finne PH, Stensberg A. Clinical assessment of gestational age in the newborn infant – an evaluation of two methods. *Acta Paediatrica Scandinavica*, 1981; **70**: 669–72.

Related topics of interest

Extreme prematurity (p. 80)
Intrauterine growth restriction (p. 165)
Maternal drug abuse (p. 182)

Neurological evaluation (p. 206)
Postnatal examination (p. 244)

BIRTH INJURIES

The continuing advances in antenatal and perinatal care have led to a progressive fall in fetal deaths due to trauma during delivery. However, birth injuries still cause a significant neonatal morbidity of which neonatal staff should be aware. Difficult delivery by any method is a prime risk factor but so is a very rapid delivery. An increased risk is also attached to preterm delivery, Caesarean delivery and multiple pregnancy.

Head and neck

Facial and superficial injuries

Facial bruising, cyanosis, subconjunctival and petechial haemorrhages, which all resolve soon after birth, are common with face and brow presentations, as well as when the cord is wound tightly around the neck. Similarly, the use of forceps commonly leaves superficial bruising on the face which rapidly resolves. Scalp or facial cuts from scalpel injuries may follow Caesarian births and significant facial injuries may require an expert opinion.

The presenting part of the scalp often gives the skull an elongated and pointed appearance (caput succedaneum) which gradually settles. Prolonged traction during vacuum extraction may cause considerable injury to the fetal scalp with haemorrhage, skin necrosis and infection leading to permanent scars.

Scalp electrodes may also produce lacerations which may also become infected. Subperiosteal haemorrhages produce haematomas (cephalhaematomas) which are limited by the suture lines (parietal and occipital bones, mainly). The fluctulant swelling eventually calcifies and resolves. Significant cephalhaematomas may be associated with anaemia, underlying skull fracture and the attendant hyperbilirubinaemia. Apart from some local toilet and perhaps analgesia when the integrity of the skin has been breached, no treatment is usually required for the above injuries.

Vacuum extraction may result in a more serious, often unrecognized subaponeurotic haemorrhage (bleeding beneath the epicranial aponeurosis) leading to significant anaemia and even shock. The immediate management involves volume replacement with blood (or colloid if blood unavailable).

Intracranial injuries

Significant intracranial haemorrhage and injury may also result from perinatal trauma, most commonly as subarachnoid or subdural haemorrhages and less commonly periventricular/intraventricular (PVH/IVH), intracerebral and intracerebellar haemorrhages. PVH/IVH primarily occurs in preterm infants. Haemorrhage within the subarachnoid space arises from small blood vessels (mainly venous) within the subarachnoid space. Subarachnoid haemorrhages are commonly silent but may be accompanied by seizures and, rarely, rapid neurological deterioration. Diagnosis is by lumbar puncture (uniformly blood-stained CSF) and computerized tomography (CT) scan (better able to exclude other types of haemorrhages especially in the posterior fossa). Prognosis is usually good.

Subdural haemorrhages may occur following excessive moulding forces on the head, producing dural tears and rupture of the closely applied vessels (mostly with difficult delivery of the head, breech deliveries and in association with severe birth asphyxia). Symptoms vary from irritability, seizures, apnoea, altered consciousness, bulging fontanelle, brain stem compression and cranial nerve dysfunction (e.g. third nerve palsy with unilateral fixed dilated pupils) associated with a rapid fall in haemoglobin. Diagnosis is by ultrasound scan (large subdurals produce midline shift) or CT scan (investigation of choice). Perform coagulation studies and correct any defects and administer vitamin K. Large subdurals over the surface of the brain with midline shifts or posterior fossa collections with major neurological signs should be decompressed (craniotomy and aspiration of clot or subdural tap). In the absence of concomitant birth asphyxia, small subdural haemorrhages are associated with a good outcome but large, especially infratentorial, haemorrhages may be fatal.

Neurological complication

Facial nerve palsy. The use of forceps may result in excessive pressure being applied on the facial nerve as it lies against the mandible, resulting in a temporal usually unilateral weakness of the facial nerve. The eye cannot be shut on the affected side. The mouth is pulled forward to the opposite side when the infant cries. Complete resolution is common during the first weeks of life. There may be transient feeding difficulties and artificial tears required till recovery occurs. Distinguish from prenatal nerve injury from which there may be little or no recovery.

Cervical spine and cord injuries

Injuries to the cervical spine and spinal cord

The spinal cord is especially prone to injury as it can only stretch 0.5–1 cm, compared to the spine which can stretch up to 5 cm. Therefore cervical bony disruption is always associated with severe spinal cord transectional injury. Injuries commonly occur at the C1–2 level (cephalic delivery) or C6–7/C8–T1 levels (breech delivery). The hyperextended fetus ('flying-fetus') has a high risk of cord injury due to its unusual posture if delivered vaginally. The infant is initially hypotonic, hypoventilates and may have absent reflexes. Breathing may be diaphragmatic (unless the phrenic nerve is also paralysed) and a paraparesis or quadriparesis is common in survivors. Magnetic resonance imaging (MRI) scans are the investigation of choice.

Injuries to the brachial plexus

If the spinal cord escapes injury, its nerve roots may still sustain injury especially in the brachial plexus with a prevalence of approximately 1 in 2500 births. Excessive pulling on the upper limbs or the head, shoulder dystocia, and excessive flexion of the neck during both vertex and breech deliveries may all result in injury to the brachial plexus. Injury to the cervical sympathetic nerves produces myosis, ptosis and enophthalmos (Horner's syndrome) and unilateral diaphragmatic paralysis follows damage to the ipsilateral phrenic nerve.

Erb's palsy

This is the commonest manifestation of brachial plexus injury and results from traumatic stretching of C5 and C6 nerve roots during delivery (e.g. traction on head during a shoulder dystocia). The affected arm is adducted and internally rotated with the elbow extended. The forearm is pronated and the wrist flexed (waiters tip position). The biceps jerk is absent and the Moro reflex is asymmetrical. Exclude diaphragmatic paralysis, fractured clavicle and cervical spine injury. Spontaneous recovery is usual. Physiotherapy prevents joint contractures. In selected cases, surgery to the plexus may aid recovery.

Klumpke's paralysis

This follows lower brachial plexus (C8 and T1) injury and affects small muscles of the hand, wrist and finger flexors (claw hand deformity) and sympathetics (Horner's syndrome). The Moro reflex is reduced on the affected side. Exclude fractures of spine, clavicle, proximal humerus and arm (X-ray the whole limb, shoulder and spine). Preserve full range of passive motion with physiotherapy till spontaneous recovery occurs (6–18 months). However, less than one in five have *full* neurological recovery though functional outcome is good.

Visceral, cutaneous and limb injuries

Abdominal injury

This may occur in the presence of abdominal distension, particularly in association with massive hepatosplenomegaly, malpresentation (especially breech) and rough handling during manipulation. Intra-abdominal haemorrhage may result with attendant shock. Subcapsular haemorrhage may remain 'latent' for a few days until rupture of the capsule which is heralded by shock. Manage as for haemorrhagic shock and treat any underlying coagulopathy. Request a surgical review.

Perineal injury

Breech delivery is associated with vulval or scrotal bruising and haematomata. In males, testicular viability may be threatened by marked scrotal oedema and consequent impaired testicular perfusion. Treatment is symptomatic and pain relief. Exclude congenital torsion of the testes which requires immediate surgery.

Injury to the limbs

Long bones may sustain mid-shaft fractures (most commonly clavicular) and epiphyseal avulsions (mainly humerus and femur) during difficult deliveries. While long-bone mid-shaft fractures are generally recognized immediately when they occur (by obstetrician), epiphyseal separations often go undetected until the inflammatory phase (healing phase) commences. Risk factors include large infants (e.g. infants of diabetic mothers), difficult instrumental deliveries, congenital disorder (e.g. osteogenesis imperfecta) and being the first born.

The affected limb is swollen, tender and shows minimal movement because of pain (pseudoparalysis). Epiphyseal separation may mimic septic arthritis/osteomyelitis. Note, radial nerve may be injured if humerus is fractured producing wrist drop. Confirm fractures with appropriate radiographs. Mid-shaft fractures only require simple splinting (seek orthopaedic review) and no treatment (save analgesia) is required for fractured clavicles (often only recognized after callus has formed). If septic arthritis can not be ruled out easily, treat as such with intravenous antibiotics until the picture becomes clearer.

Cutaneous bruising and soft tissue injury

Malpresentations (commonly breech) may result in extensive bruising of the presenting part due to the additional manipulations during the delivery. Preterm infants bruise easily and may develop significant haemorrhage into their muscles if handled roughly during manipulation. This also applies to term infants with coagulation defects. Hypovolaemia, anaemia and hyperbilirubinaemia may result. Management is symptomatic (e.g. blood transfusion or phototherapy).

Further reading

Geirsson RT. Birth trauma and brain damage. *Bailliere's Clinical Obstetrics and Gynaecology*, 1988; **2**: 195.

MacKinnon JA, Perlman M, Kirpalani H *et al*. Spinal cord injury at birth: diagnostic and prognostic data in 22 patients. *Journal of Pediatrics*, 1993; **122**: 431.

Medlock MD, Hanigan WC. Neurologic birth trauma: intracranial, spinal cord, and brachial plexus injury. *Clinics in Perinatology*, 1997; **24**: 845–57.

Related topics of interest

BLEEDING DISORDERS

Bleeding disorders during the neonatal period are quite common, particularly in preterm infants. Normal haemostasis requires vascular integrity, normal platelet function and a functional coagulation system (clotting factors or procoagulants, procoagulant inhibitors and fibrinolysis). In otherwise healthy infants, the commonest causes of bleeding are thrombocytopenia secondary to transplacental passage of maternal platelet antibodies, vitamin K deficiency and, less commonly, congenital coagulation factor deficiencies.

Clinical features
- Infants with isolated platelet disorders normally appear well except for progressive petechiae, bruising or mucosal bleeding.
- Vitamin K deficiency haemorrhagic disease or inherited coagulation defects occur in seemingly healthy infants with large bruises or localized bleeding (e.g. umbilical cord or large cephalhaematoma).
- Bleeding secondary to disseminated intravascular coagulation (DIC) or liver disease generally occurs in sick infants with multiple bleeding sites.
- Severe congenital coagulation factor deficiencies present with bleeding from the mucous membranes, umbilicus, peripheral blood sampling sites, following circumcision, and into the scalp forming large cephalhaematomas. A minority present with IVH as the first manifestation.

Investigating the bleeding infant

One should start with a careful history of family bleeding problems, outcome of previous pregnancies, maternal illnesses (especially infections), maternal and neonatal drug administration and ascertainment of vitamin K administration. Laboratory investigations should include:

- FBC and film (screen platelet numbers, presence of fragmented red cells).
- Coagulation screen
    Prothrombin time (PT).
    Partial thromboplastin time (PTT) – very heparin-sensitive.
    Thrombin time (TT).
    Reptilase time (RT) – fibrin degradation products (FDPs) but not heparin affect RT. Normal RT with prolonged PTT and TT suggest heparin contamination, while prolonged RT, PTT and TT suggest DIC.
    Plasma fibrinogen concentration (normal 1.56–4 g/l).
    Bleeding time (BT) – rarely needed.

Abnormalities in the above tests usually guide the selection of additional tests such as specific factor or procoagulant assays. For a male child in whom haemophilia A or B is suspected, specific factor assays must be performed regardless of the coagulation screen (PTT) results.

General management Appropriate management depends on the correct identification of the haemostatic defect. Commonly FFP (10–20 ml/kg), platelet concentrates (10–20 ml/kg), and cryoprecipitate (1 bag, which contains ~250 mg fibrinogen and 80–120 units of factor VIII), are used, and, where a specific defect is apparent, the specific factor concentrates are administered.

Thrombocytopenia

Defined as a platelet count of <100 000 × 10^9/l, thrombocytopenia is very common in newborns and may be found in ~20% of infants admitted to the NICU. It is most commonly found in SGA infants. Thrombocytopenic bleeding is uncommon if the count is ≥40 × 10^9/l. Bleeding may occur due to severe thrombocytopenia or impaired platelet function.

Aetiology

1. *Increased peripheral consumption of platelets*
   - Disseminated intravascular coagulation (DIC) or consumption coagulopathy. DIC is confirmed by marked thrombocytopenia, prolonged PT, PTT, marked hypofibrinogenaemia (<1 g/l), elevated FDPs, and peripheral blood film schistocytes. Treatment starts with removing trigger factors, then providing supportive therapy (FFP, platelet concentrate or cryoprecipitate), exchange transfusion, and rarely, heparinization.
   - IUGR.
   - NEC.
   - Sepsis.
   - Giant haemangioma (Kasabach–Merritt syndrome).
     Local consumption of platelets and coagulation factors occurs, resulting in a bleeding tendency. Steroids are beneficial.
   - Exchange transfusion.
   - Polycythaemia.
   - Thrombosis.
   - Inherited metabolic disease.

2. *Decreased platelet survival*
   - Neonatal alloimmune thrombocytopenia. Maternal IgG alloantibodies are directed against paternally derived antigens on the baby's platelets, which are absent from the mother's platelets. In >75% of cases the Pl^{A1} (HPA-1a) alloantigen (present on the platelets of 98% of the general population), is implicated. The incidence is 1:3000–5000. It commonly presents as isolated thrombocytopenia (<10 × 10^9/l) in a well infant with petechiae, gastrointestinal

haemorrhage, or serious intracranial haemorrhage. Transfuse washed and irradiated maternal platelets or matched platelets from unrelated donor. Random donor platelets will give temporary respite in the bleeding infant. Steroids and i.v. IgG may also be beneficial.

- Autoimmune neonatal thrombocytopenia. This results from the transplacental passage of IgG platelet antibodies from mothers with idiopathic thrombocytopenic purpura (ITP), SLE, or hyperthyroidism. Antibody is directed against maternal and neonatal platelets. Cord platelet count is rarely $<50 \times 10^9/l$ but the lowest platelet count occurs several days after birth. Treatment is with i.v. IgG (1 g/kg) and if bleeding, irradiated platelets (10–20 ml/kg). Prednisolone (2 mg/kg/day) is also beneficial.
- Drug-induced (e.g. quinine, hydralazine, tolbutamide, thiazides).
- Hypersplenism. Usually mild with platelet counts of $50–100 \times 10^9/l$.

3. *Decreased production (<5%)*
- Amegakaryocytic thrombocytopenia (e.g. Wiskott– Aldrich syndrome).
- Aplastic anaemia (e.g. Fanconi anaemia, thrombocytopenia with absent radius (TAR) syndrome).
- Infiltrative disorders (e.g. congenital neuroblastoma).

4. *Platelet function disorders*
- Acquired. Mainly drugs (e.g. indomethacin).
- Congenital. e.g. Bernard–Soulier syndrome, Glanzmann's disease.

Congenital coagulation factor deficiencies

These are rare and only severe deficiencies present in the neonatal period. The majority are X-linked disorders. Examples include:

- Haemophilia A (factor VIII deficiency) with an incidence of 1:20 000.
- Christmas disease (factor IX deficiency).
- Factor VIII-related antigen, Von Willenbrand's disease.
- Fibrinogen deficiency (afibrinogenaemia or hypofibrinogenaemia).
- Factor XIII deficiency.

Vitamin K deficiency

Haemorrhagic disease of the newborn (HDN) classically occurs within the first week of life, but a late form can develop up to 26 weeks. Death and handicap can result from intracranial bleeding, often after minor herald bleeds of the umbilicus or mucous membranes. It is caused by a deficiency of vitamin K-dependent clotting factors (factors II, VII, IX, X), and hence is prevented by vitamin K administration at birth.

- In HDN the PT is prolonged.
- Vitamin K as phytomenadione (Konakion) 1 mg i.m. at birth prevents both early and late HDN.
- Konakion MM is licensed for oral administration. The recommended dose is 2 mg orally at birth, a further 2 mg 4–7 days later for all babies, and a further 2 mg dose at 1 month for exclusively breast-fed babies. A single oral dose at birth does not protect all breast-fed babies against late HDN. Repeated therapeutic doses of oral vitamin K are safe, but babies with malabsorption, diarrhoea, vomiting, or babies whose mothers forget later doses may not be protected.
- Studies in the UK in the early 1990s suggested that i.m. vitamin K (compared to oral vitamin K) was associated with a two-fold increase in childhood cancer. The UK National Cancer Registry challenged this. A similar Swedish study found no such association. American data has shown no rise in childhood leukaemia or cancer since i.m. vitamin K was introduced there. However, further UK studies have not been able to exclude completely a small risk of an increased incidence of leukaemia, and national guidelines have not been established.
- Emergency treatment in a bleeding baby is with fresh frozen plasma (FFP) and 1 mg of vitamin K i.v.
- It is estimated in the UK that if vitamin K were not given to other than high-risk infants (i.e. preterm infants, infants with a complicated delivery or who are ill or who have liver disease or difficulty absorbing feeds, especially if breast-fed), 60–80 infants would suffer a bleed (15–20 suffering intracranial haemorrhages, and 10–20 brain damage) and 4–6 would die annually.

Further reading

Hann IM, Gibson BES, Letsky EA (eds). *Fetal and Neonatal Haematology*. London: Baillière Tindall, 1991.

McNinch A, Draper G. Vitamin K for neonates: the controversy. *British Medical Journal*, 1994; **308:** 867–8.

Nathan DG, Orkin SH (eds). *Nathan and Oski's Hematology of Infancy and Childhood*, 5th edn. Philadelphia: W.B. Saunders, 1997.

Von Kries R. Neonatal vitamin K prophylaxis: the Gordian knot still awaits untying. *British Medical Journal*, 1998; **316:** 161–2.

Related topics of interest

BLOOD GLUCOSE HOMEOSTASIS

Perinatal metabolic adaptation

During fetal life, glucose is the principal energy substrate and provides 50% of the total energy needs. The fetal glucose consumption is 5 mg/kg/min. At birth, the newborn switches from a state of net glucose uptake and glycogen synthesis to one of independent glucose production. The ability of an infant to maintain normoglycaemia then depends on the adequacy of glycogen stores, glycogenolysis, gluconeogenesis and the production of alternative metabolic substrates (e.g. free fatty acids, lactate and ketone bodies). This process by which the body mobilizes glucose and other fluids is called counter-regulation. The main counter-regulatory hormones are glucagon and adrenaline. However, the brain does not solely depend on glucose for its energy supply, but on a number of other alternative metabolic fuels including lactate, fatty acids and ketone bodies. The blood glucose concentration is therefore only one component of the infant's metabolic milieu and cannot be interpreted in isolation. Blood glucose homeostasis is thus controlled by the opposing actions of insulin and counter-regulation (mainly glucagon) and its failure produces hypo- or hyperglycaemia.

Hypoglycaemia

Definition

A normal range for blood glucose in healthy term newborns has not been adequately described. Consequently, there is no universally acceptable definition of hypoglycaemia. Values are influenced by gestation, birthweight, postnatal age and feeding practice. Current evidence suggests that a blood glucose level persistently <2.6 mmol/l is associated with neurodevelopmental impairment. This limit, however, is derived from preterm infants.

Hypoglycaemia may be described as symptomatic (i.e. associated with clinical signs of apnoea, cyanosis, jitteriness, lethargy, abnormal cry or convulsions) or asymptomatic (without clinical signs). Symptomatic hypoglycaemia in term or preterm infants is associated with adverse neurodevelopmental sequelae. Preterm infants may be more (not less!) susceptible to the detrimental effects of hypoglycaemia. Symptomatic hypoglycaemia should be treated rapidly whatever the measured blood glucose level, as there is no definitive threshold for an 'unsafe' blood glucose level.

Incidence

This varies with the definition. A review of literature suggests incidences of 0–8% in term infants (when hypoglycaemia was defined as blood glucose <1.6 mmol/l in infants <48 hours old) and 3–15% in preterm infants (when hypoglycaemia was defined as blood glucose <1.1 mmol/l).

Conditions predisposing to hypoglycaemia

- Sepsis.
- Asphyxia.

- Cold stress.
- Congenital heart disease (CHD).
- Erythroblastosis fetalis.
- Infants of diabetic mothers (IDMs) (transient hyper-insulinism).
- Large for gestation term infants, birthweight >90th centile (hyperinsulinism).
- Prematurity (reduced glycogen and fat stores, elevated insulin:glucose ratio, impaired counter-regulation).
- Small for gestational age (SGA) infants (reduced fat and glycogen stores, impaired counter-regulation, hyperinsulinism).
- Intravenous administration of >10 g glucose/hour during labour.
- Prolonged oral and short-term i.v. administration of β-agonists to suppress preterm labour.

Screening for hypoglycaemia

- There is no need to screen healthy term infants.
- Reagent strip methods (e.g. Dextrostix (Ames) or BM stix (Boehringer)) are prone to errors at low glucose levels and are unsuitable for diagnosing neonatal hypoglycaemia. Therapy should not be instituted on the basis of these tests alone – always confirm with blood glucose measurement.
- Glucose electrode-based analysers are accurate even at low glucose levels.

Causes of refractory hypoglycaemia

1. *Hyperinsulinism*
- Nesidioblastosis (B-cell dysregulation syndrome).
- Beckwith–Wiedemann syndrome.
- Islet cell adenoma.

2. *Endocrine deficiency*
- Hypopituitarism.
- Cortisol deficiency.
- Glucagon deficiency.
- Growth hormone deficiency.

3. *Inherited metabolic diseases*
- Disorders of carbohydrate metabolism (e.g. galactosaemia, glycogen storage disease type I).
- Disorders of fatty acid metabolism (e.g. medium chain acyl-CoA dehydrogenase deficiency).
- Disorders of amino acid metabolism (e.g. proprionic acidaemia, methylmalonic acidaemia).

Investigations for refractory hypoglycaemia

During an episode of hypoglycaemia, perform:
- Blood glucose.
- Insulin (C-peptide, proinsulin).
- Cortisol.
- Growth hormone.

It may be necessary to also assay β-hydroxybutyrate, amino acids, glycerol, pyruvate, ketones, free fatty acids and lactate.

Prevention of hypoglycaemia

- Avoid preventable risk factors (e.g. cold stress).
- Early (<3–4 hours) enteral feeding in healthy term or preterm infants should be given priority.
- At-risk, well newborns unable to feed orally should be fed by gavage within 1–3 hours of birth.
- For at-risk newborns, breast milk is nutritionally most appropriate and the safest (unless mother has HIV infection).
- If enteral feeds are contraindicated (e.g. extreme prematurity, cardio-respiratory distress, birth asphyxia), give 10% dextrose i.v. at a rate approximating the endogenous rate of hepatic glucose production (i.e. 3–5 mg/kg/min for term appropriate for gestational age (AGA) infants; 4–6 mg/kg/min for preterm AGA infants; and 6–8 mg/kg/min for SGA infants). **Note:** 60 ml/kg/day of 10% glucose = 4.2 mg glucose/kg/min. Amount of glucose administered in mg/kg/min = concentration of glucose infusion (%) × rate of infusion (ml/hour) ÷ weight of baby ÷ 6.
- Check capillary glucose 3–4-hourly for the first 24 hours.

Treatment

1. Asymptomatic hypoglycaemia
- Send sample for true blood glucose, if possible.
- Feed the infant (breast, bottle or gavage).
- Correct any precipitating factors (e.g. hypothermia).
- Repeat reagent strip test (BM stix or Dextrostix) within 1 hour.
- If accurate ward-based glucose electrode measurement or laboratory glucose measurement is <1.5 mmol/l, treat as for symptomatic hypoglycaemia.
- Continue at least 3-hourly capillary glucose measurements until consistently ≥3 mmol/l (12–24 hours).

2. Symptomatic hypoglycaemia
- This is an emergency. Measure blood glucose immediately but do not wait for result!
- Commence 10% glucose i.v. infusion giving a 3 ml/kg 10% glucose priming bolus followed by an infusion of 8 mg/kg/min. Do not give intermittent glucose boluses alone!
- If venous access is difficult, give glucagon 0.1 mg/kg i.m. or Hypostop (a 40% glucose gel), 0.5 ml/kg massaged into buccal mucosa.
- Adjust the rate of infusion until plasma glucose is corrected and stabilized.
- If fluid overload is likely, change to 15% glucose or a greater concentration (via central line).

- Gradually reduce glucose infusion while increasing volume of enteral feeds.

3. Refractory hypoglycaemia. Glucose requirements of >12 mg/kg/min suggest transient or permanent hyperinsulinism. The following may help:

- Hydrocortisone 5 mg/kg i.v./i.m. 12-hourly.
- Glucagon 200 μg i.v. intermittently or as a continuous infusion (10 μg/kg/hour).
- Diazoxide 10 mg/kg/day at 8-hourly intervals (maximum 25 mg/kg/day) concurrently with chlorothiazide (to prevent fluid retention and potentiate the action of diazoxide). Diazoxide inhibits pancreatic insulin secretion, increases gluconeogenesis and reduces peripheral glucose utilization.
- Somatostatin or octreotide (the long-acting analogue) at 5 μg/kg 6-hourly.

If the above medical measures are unsuccessful, refer to a specialist centre for more detailed investigations (pancreatic ultrasonography, coeliac angiogram) and possible surgery (partial or total pancreatectomy).

Hyperglycaemia

Definition

Hyperglycaemia is defined as a blood glucose level >8 mmol/l.

Causes

- Stress (e.g. asphyxia).
- Drug therapy (dexamethasone, aminophylline).
- Excess glucose administration in total parental nutrition.
- Intolerance to a 'normal' glucose load especially in VLBW infants.
- Permanent (PNDM) or transient neonatal diabetes mellitus (TNDM).

Management

- Reduce the amount of glucose being infused by reducing the volume or concentration of glucose.
- Exclude sepsis as a cause.
- Take steps to avoid an osmotic diuresis and electrolyte disturbance from glycosuria.
- Occasionally, insulin therapy is required (0.05–0.1 units/kg/hour) – danger of unrecognized serious hypoglycaemia.

Neonatal diabetes

PNDM or TNDM are extremely rare, with an incidence of 1 in 400 000 in the UK. Commonly, the infants are VLBW at term and develop hyperglycaemia requiring insulin during the first 6 weeks of life, resolving in 3–6 months. There is a predisposition to impaired glucose tolerance and type 2 diabetes in later life. Paternal uniparental isodisomy of chromosome 6 (inheritance of both number 6 chromosomes from the father) is implicated.

Further reading

Bourchier D, Weston P, Heron P. Hypostop for neonatal hypoglycaemia. *New Zealand Medical Journal*, 1992; **105**: 22.

Cornblath M, Schwartz R. Hypoglycaemia in the neonate. *Journal of Pediatric Endocrinology*, 1993; **6**: 113–29.

Cornblath M, Schwartz R, Aynsley-Green A, Lloyd JK. Hypoglycaemia in infancy: the need for a rational definition. *Pediatrics*, 1990; **85**: 834–7.

Cowett RM. Neonatal glucose metabolism. In: Cowett RM (ed). *Principles of Perinatal Neonatal Metabolism*. New York: Springer-Verlag, 1991; 356–89.

DiGiacomo JE, Hay WW. Abnormal glucose homeostasis. In: Sinclair JC, Bracken MB (eds). *Effective Care of the Newborn Infant*. Oxford: Oxford University Press, 1992; 590–601.

Hawdon JM, Ward Platt M, Aynsley Green A. Prevention and management of neonatal hypoglycaemia. *Archives of Disease in Childhood*, 1994; **70**: F60–5.

Related topics of interest

Fluid and electrolyte therapy (p. 87)
Infants of diabetic mothers (p. 136)
Inherited metabolic disease – investigation and management (p. 156)
Inherited metabolic disease – recognizable patterns (p. 161)
Intrauterine growth restriction (p. 165)
Nutrition (p. 221)

BLOOD PRESSURE

The normal blood pressure profile in newborns, and in particular extremely low birthweight (ELBW) (<1000 g) infants, has not been completely described. While blood pressure can be measured directly and accurately, the appropriate level of mean blood pressure at which intervention is appropriate remains controversial. Even more controversial is how hypotension should be managed. Hypertension which is persistent is, by comparison, rare in neonates.

Blood pressure should be measured on a regular or continuous basis in all sick infants. Non-invasive Doppler or oscillometric devices may be used. Automatic oscillometric devices (e.g. Dinamap) tend to overestimate blood pressure in sick ELBW infants and are unreliable in the presence of limb oedema. Indwelling arterial catheters give more reliable measurements.

Hypotension

Hypotension is one of the commonest cardiovascular problems encountered in the management of very low birthweight (VLBW) infants soon after birth and it affects a significant proportion of all admissions to the neonatal intensive care unit (NICU). The definition of hypotension is disputed.

- The British Association of Perinatal Medicine and Royal College of Physicians defined hypotension as a mean systemic blood pressure less than an infant's gestational age in completed weeks.
- The major concern about hypotension is due to its association with IVH, periventricular leucomalacia (PVL) and poor neurodevelopmental outcome.

1. *Clinical features*
- Tachycardia.
- Metabolic acidosis.
- Impaired renal function (pre-renal failure).
- Decreased pulmonary blood flow (PBF) (impaired gas exchange).
- Capillary refill time >3 s (best sites are on the forehead and midpoint of sternum).
- Wide central–peripheral temperature gap (>2 °C), but less reliable during the first 3 days of life.

2. *Causes*
(a) Cardiovascular disorders
- Myocardial dysfunction.
- Marked tachycardia (e.g. supraventricular tachycardia (SVT)).
- Cardiac failure (e.g. patent ductus arteriosus (PDA)).
- Hypovolaemia (e.g. acute blood loss).
- Immaturity of cardiovascular regulatory mechanisms.
(b) Pulmonary disorders
- Pulmonary air leaks (e.g. tension pneumothorax).
- Excessive ventilation pressures (high thoracic pressure reduces venous return).

(c) Gastrointestinal disorders
- Perforation and peritonitis.
- NEC (hypovolaemia).
- Gross ascites or oedema (hypovolaemia).

(d) Sepsis (vasoparalysis from endotoxin or excessive production of endogenous vasodilators such as nitric oxide)

(e) Drug therapy (vasodilators)
- Tolazoline.
- Prostacyclin.
- Opiates.
- Magnesium sulphate.
- β-blockers.

(f) Artefact (air in intra-arterial catheter or transducer, erroneous measurements)

3. *Management*
- Replace blood volume with colloid or blood in the infant with an obvious recent acute blood loss (e.g. cord accident or feto-maternal haemorrhage) – the infant is very pale.
- The hypotensive, hypothermic, pale, sick newborn infant may benefit from volume expansion (fresh frozen plasma (FFP), human albumin, saline or blood) at 10–20 ml/kg over 30 min. If blood pressure remains suboptimal, commence dopamine (10 μg/kg/min) and gradually increase to 20 μg/kg/min in 5 μg/kg/min increments.
- Add dobutamine (10 μg/kg/min) and increase to 20 μg/kg/min if blood pressure remains suboptimal.
- Alternatively, or in addition, hydrocortisone may be added in VLBW infants (2.5 mg/kg i.v. 6-hourly for 48 hours, then 1.25 mg/kg 6-hourly for 48 hours, and finally 0.625 mg/kg 6-hourly for 48 hours).
- For refractory hypotension, add an infusion of noradrenaline (0.05–0.5 μg/kg/min).
- Asphyxiated infants may respond better to inotropes as opposed to volume expansion with colloids.
- Perform cardiac echocardiography in infants with severe hypotension to ascertain myocardial function and rule out associated congenital heart disease (CHD).

4. *Special notes*
- The routine administration of colloid to preterm infants of <32 weeks gestation is of no proven value.
- Dopamine is more effective than dobutamine in raising mean arterial blood pressure.
- At a high dose, the α-adrenergic effects of dopamine produce decreased renal blood flow, decreased PBF (from pulmonary vasoconstriction) and increased myocardial oxygen consumption.

- Dobutamine, with a predominantly β-adrenergic effect, increases left ventricular output and is less likely to increase pulmonary vascular resistance (PVR) when compared with dopamine.
- Normal saline (0.9% sodium chloride solution) is as effective as 5% albumin in treating hypotension in preterm infants (<34 weeks gestation).
- Early hypotension (within the first few hours of life, <24 hours) is *not* usually due to hypovolaemia.
- The use of human albumin in critically ill patients is currently debatable as it may increase mortality.

Hypertension

Hypertension is defined as a blood pressure of >100/75 in term infants and >80/45 in preterm infants. Infants must be at rest and the cuff width should be at least two-thirds of upper arm length.

1. Clinical features
- Tachypnoea.
- Lethargy.
- Abnormal muscle tone.
- Impaired renal function.
- Congestive cardiac failure.
- Haematuria and proteinuria.
- Oedema (salt and water retention).
- Seizures (hypertensive encephalopathy).

2. Causes
(a) Raised intracranial pressure
- IVH.
- Cerebral oedema (e.g. asphyxia).
(b) Stress (pain or cold)
(c) Sodium and fluid retention
- Renal failure.
- Excess sodium administration.
- Adrenal disorders (e.g. congenital adrenal hyperplasia (CAH)).
(d) Drug therapy
- Dexamethasone.
- Dopamine.
(e) Renin-angiotensin mediated
- Renal artery stenosis.
- Coarctation of the aorta.
- Obstructive uropathy.
- Cystic/dysplastic kidneys.

Renal artery occlusion accounts for >75% of neonatal hypertension with renal artery stenosis accounting for ~20% of cases.

3. Management

Treatment depends on the cause, but a renal cause will be found in over four out of five cases. Renal ultrasound scan, dimercaptosuccinic acid (DMSA), mercapto-acetyl-triglycer-ine-3 (MAG-3) renogram and renal angiogram may all be required (see 'Renal and urinary tract disorders').

- To control hypertension acutely, use diazoxide 3–5 mg/kg i.v. or hydralazine 0.5–1 mg/kg i.v. followed by maintenance therapy with oral agents.
- Captopril is useful in severe hypertension (100–300 μg/kg/dose 8-hourly) but watch renal function.
- Mild hypertension may respond to diuretics (especially with fluid overload) or β-blockers (e.g. propranolol 0.5–4 mg/kg/day given 6–8-hourly).
- Echocardiography will demonstrate coarctation of the aorta (upper limb BP > lower limb BP).
- Neonatal hypertension commonly has a treatable cause and a good prognosis.

Further reading

Bourchier D, Weston PF. Randomized trial of dopamine compared with hydrocortisone for the treatment of hypotensive very low birthweight infants. *Archives of Disease in Childhood, Fetal and Neonatal Edition*, 1997; **76:** F174–8.

Hope P. Pump up the volume? The routine early use of colloid in the very preterm infants. *Archives of Disease in Childhood, Fetal and Neonatal Edition*, 1998; **78:** F163–5.

Joint Working Party of the British Association of Perinatal Medicine and Research Unit of the Royal College of Physicians. Development of audit measures and guidelines for good practice in the management of neonatal respiratory distress syndrome. *Archives of Disease in Childhood*, 1992; **67:** 1221–7.

Klarr JM, Faix RG, Pryce CJE, Bhatt-Mehta V. Randomized, blind trial of dopamine versus dobutamine for treatment of hypotension in preterm infants with respiratory distress syndrome. *Journal of Paediatrics*, 1994; **125:** 117–22.

Miall-Allen VM, De Vries LS, Whitelaw AGL. Mean arterial blood pressure and neonatal cerebral lesions. *Archives of Disease in Childhood*, 1987; **62:** 1068–9.

Versmold H, Kitterman J, Phibbs R, Gregory GA, Tooley WH. Aortic blood pressure during the first 12 hours of life in infants with birthweight 610 to 4220 grammes. *Paediatrics*, 1981; **67:** 607–13.

Weindling AM. Blood pressure monitoring in the newborn. *Archives of Disease in Childhood*, 1989; **64:** 444–7.

Related topics of interest

BRONCHOPULMONARY DYSPLASIA

Bronchopulmonary dysplasia (BPD) was first described by Northway in 1966 as coarse reticular radiographic changes seen following ventilator therapy for respiratory distress syndrome (RDS). Later, Bancalari's definition (1979) required a history of assisted ventilation, radiographic abnormalities, oxygen dependence at 28 days, with continuing respiratory symptoms. A newer definition has been proposed as oxygen dependency at 36 weeks post-conceptional age in addition to radiographic findings and a history of assisted ventilation. This definition is increasingly being used.

Pathogenesis   The pathogenesis of BPD is complex and multifactorial.

- Pulmonary oxygen toxicity is a major contributor as high concentrations of oxygen induce lung inflammation and the release of chemotactic factors which attract pulmonary leucocytes to the lung, leading to the release of more inflammatory mediators and proteolytic enzymes. The preterm infant has lower levels of antiproteases, and of antioxidant enzymes, and is therefore more susceptible to oxygen toxicity and to BPD than the full term infant.
- There is a correlation between the development of BPD and the severity of the initial lung disease, partly because infants with the most severe lung disease require the highest ventilator pressures. *Barotrauma* is the term used for pressure-induced injury. Recent studies, however, suggest that excessive variations in lung volumes during mechanical ventilation are the principal mechanism of iatrogenic lung injury. This mechanism is known as *volutrauma*.
- Several other factors contribute to the pathogenesis of BPD. The presence of a symptomatic patent ductus arteriosus (PDA), excessive fluid administration early in the neonatal course, pulmonary air leak, vitamins A and E deficiency, early i.v. lipid infusions, family history of asthma, intrauterine infection, *Ureaplasma urealyticum,* male gender and white race have all been postulated.
- The currently favoured mechanism involves the interaction of all the above risk factors. Simply put, IPPV produces shearing and stretching forces which disrupt the pulmonary epithelium, exposing the subepithelial connective tissue and vascular bed to oxidative damage. The accompanying release of chemotactic mediators recruits inflammatory cells, which lead to further damage by releasing lysosomal proteases. This leads to extensive damage to the pulmonary epithelium, endothelium and extracellular lung matrix. The resulting proliferation of fibroblasts and collagen deposition produce alveolar and interstitial destruction with marked architectural remodelling of the lung.

- Histopathology shows alveolar type II cell hyperplasia, intra-alveolar and interstitial fibrosis, alveolar wall rupture, peribronchial and peribronchiolar fibrosis, obliterative fibroproliferative bronchiolitis and areas of hyperinflated sacs alternating with dispersed foci of atelectasis. The overall picture indicates a process of simultaneous acute and chronic lung destruction, progressing to an abnormal healing phase with fibroproliferative lung damage, diminished alveolization and increased pulmonary vascular resistance.

Clinical features

1. Respiratory system
- Tachypnoea with elevated minute ventilation.
- Increased work of breathing and oxygen consumption.
- Relative hypoxia with CO_2 retention.
- Lobar emphysema and atelectasis resulting from air trapping.
- Large airway collapse from tracheobronchomalacia.
- Increased pulmonary resistance and reduced compliance.
- Ventilation–perfusion mismatch.
- Bronchial hyperreactivity and wheezing attacks.

2. General and systemic
- Growth failure (lower energy intake and high energy expenditure).
- Modest elevation of systemic blood pressure.
- Pulmonary hypertension (and eventually cor pulmonale).
- Increased incidence of central and obstructive apnoeas.
- Increased incidence of late sudden death (up to sevenfold).

Prevention
- The most effective way of preventing BPD is avoiding preterm delivery and RDS.
- Antenatal steroids decrease the incidence of RDS and requirement for assisted ventilation by 40–60%, increase the concentration of antioxidant enzymes in the preterm lung and thus decrease the incidence of BPD.
- Surfactant therapy decreases mortality with little effect on the frequency of BPD.
- Early postnatal steroids commencing at 12 hours of age for 1–12 days, or between 7 and 14 days of age, have reduced the incidence of, and deaths from, BPD. However, the effect of steroids on long-term neurodevelopmental outcome remains uncertain, with some recent studies suggesting an excess of neuromotor abnormalities in the treated infants.
- Modes of ventilation may also influence the development of BPD. The use of early nasal CPAP and tolerance of high $PaCO_2$ significantly reduces the incidence of BPD. 'Gentler' ventilation with virtually no upper limit to allowable

levels of arterial CO_2 tension (permissive hypercapnia) has a tendency to decrease the incidence of BPD.

Management

1. General

- Once a diagnosis of BPD is established, use the lowest peak inflation pressures and rates to reduce ongoing lung injury in infants receiving assisted ventilation. As hypoxia increases pulmonary vascular resistance and right ventricular strain, maintain adequate oxygenation (PaO_2 >7 kPa or saturations >95%). Allow $PaCO_2$ to rise as long as the pH is satisfactory (>7.25).
- Transfuse packed red cells if haematocrit falls below 40% (haemoglobin <12 g/dl).
- Nursing in prone position improves oxygenation and decreases pulmonary resistance. Following extubation, those requiring ≤30% oxygen can receive their supplemental oxygen via a nasal cannula connected to a low-flow meter starting at 0.2–0.5 l/min and reducing progressively to less than 0.05 l/min before discontinuing oxygen therapy.
- If necessary, infants may be discharged home on oxygen therapy which reduces hospital stay and treatment costs.
- Gastro-oesophageal reflux (GOR) is common and this should be managed expectantly.
- Severe bronchiolitis and pneumonia caused by respiratory syncytial virus (RSV) can be life-threatening. Prophylaxis with RSV immunoglobulin (RSVIG), though expensive, reduces the incidence of RSV infection in infants with BPD.

2. Steroids

- Inflammation has an important early role in the pathogenesis of BPD.
- Steroids exert their effect by reducing the tracheobronchial alveolar inflammatory response and pulmonary oedema, thereby facilitating gas exchange, improving airway patency, lung compliance and facilitating weaning from assisted ventilation.
- The recommended starting dose of dexamethasone is in the region of 0.5–0.6 mg/kg/day, gradually tapered over 3–6 weeks. More than one course may be given.
- Steroids are associated with several complications, including glucose intolerance, elevated blood pressure, impaired growth, myocardial hypertrophy, gastroduodenal perforation, a leucocytosis (especially neutrophilia), suppression of the hypothalamo–pituitary–adrenal axis, risk of developing renal calcification and nephrocalcinosis (especially in conjunction with frusemide), and possibly causing new periventricular echodensities.

- After stopping steroids, catch-up growth is usual, the cardiac hypertrophy resolves and adrenal responsiveness is regained.

3. *Diuretics*
- There is significant interstitial pulmonary oedema in BPD.
- The reported benefits of diuretic therapy include improvements in minute and alveolar ventilation, oxygenation, lung compliance, pulmonary resistance, ventilator requirements, duration of oxygen and ventilator therapy and hospital mortality.
- Frusemide causes potent diuresis with associated electrolyte imbalance, hypercalciuria, nephrocalcinosis, nephrolithiasis and secondary hyperparathyroidism. The renal calcification resolves after cessation of frusemide therapy. Alternate-day therapy may be as effective but without the adverse metabolic consequences.
- Thiazides are less potent diuretics which also improve lung mechanics and are preferred for maintenance therapy. Chlorothiazide/hydrochlorothiazide with spironolactone/amiloride all given twice daily are generally used.

4. *Bronchodilators*
- The rationale for using bronchodilators is that infants with BPD have reactive airways disease and bronchiolar smooth muscle hypertrophy.
- Both β-agonists (e.g. salbutamol) and muscarinic antagonists (e.g. ipratropium bromide) improve lung mechanics (compliance and resistance) and oxygen in the short term.

5. *Nutrition*
- As growth failure is common in infants with BPD, nutritional intervention is of major importance.
- The input of dieticians is often necessary to provide energy intakes of ≥150 calories/kg/day.
- Lung repair is impaired by under-nutrition.

Long-term outlook
- Most post-neonatal hospital deaths in VLBW infants occur in infants with BPD.
- Up to 50% of those still ventilator-dependent at 6 months will die.
- The mortality following discharge from hospital is 11–20% and the risk of sudden infant death is seven-fold that of controls without BPD.
- There is a tendency for lung mechanics (compliance and resistance) to improve with age as the airways grow and new alveoli are formed. The risk for developing chronic obstructive or reactive airways disease remains in later life.

- There is clear evidence of adverse cardiovascular sequelae in infants with severe BPD. There may be transient systemic hypertension responsive to antihypertensive therapy or severe systemic hypertension associated with increased mortality. Some infants develop pulmonary hypertension and right ventricular hypertrophy and eventually cor pulmonale, which can be readily monitored by echocardiography and angiography. Pulmonary hypertension is a serious complication but may be ameliorated by oral hydralazine or nifedipine.
- Growth failure proportional to the duration and severity of BPD is also common (found in 30–40%), due mainly to the increased work of breathing, chronic hypoxia, diuretic and steroid therapy, and reduced calorie intakes.
- Neurodevelopmental problems may be identifed in up to 40% of infants but this is not related to the duration of oxygen or ventilator therapy.
- BPD remains a major cause of neonatal morbidity and mortality, being associated with chronic respiratory insufficiency, repeated hospitalizations, growth failure and neurodevelopmental problems.

Further reading

Barrington KJ, Finer NN. Treatment of bronchopulmonary dysplasia. *Clinics in Perinatology*, 1998; **25:** 177–202.

Bhutta T, Ohlsson A. Systematic review and meta-analysis of early postnatal dexamethasone for prevention of chronic lung disease. *Archives of Disease in Childhood, Fetal and Neonatal Edition*, 1998; **79:** F26–33.

Ehrenkranz RA, Mercurio MR. Bronchopulmonary dysplasia. In: Sinclair JC, Bracken MB (eds). *Effective Care of the Newborn Infant*. Oxford: Oxford University Press, 1992; 399–424.

Walsh WF, Hazinski TA. Bronchopulmonary dysplasia. In: Spitzer AR (ed.). *Intensive Care of the Fetus and Neonate*. St Louis: CV Mosby, 1996; p. 641.

Related topics of interest

CARDIAC ARRHYTHMIAS

Normal rhythm

The heart rate of a healthy neonate shows considerable variations depending on the state of sleep or activity. The normal resting heart rate of the newborn varies between 110 and 150 beats/min with a mean heart rate of 120. Sinus arrhythmia occurs in most normal neonates. Benign supraventricular and ventricular ectopic beats are also common and most subside spontaneously in the absence of structural heart defects. Persistently abnormal rhythms, for example bradycardia (<100 beats/min), tachycardia (>150 beats/min) or ectopic rhythms need cardiac evaluation even in the absence of other cardiac symptoms.

Abnormal rhythms

Tachyarrhythmias

1. Sinus tachycardia. This is a result of a faster rate of sinus node discharge, higher than normal for the age (>150 beats/min in neonates). Common causes are fever, pain, sepsis, blood loss, shock, hyperthyroidism and drugs (e.g. catecholamines and caffeine). Electrocardiogram (ECG) shows regular rhythm with normal P-wave axis, P-QRS-T wave sequence and normal QRS duration. Therapy is aimed at treating the underlying cause.

2. Supraventricular tachycardia (SVT). Paroxysmal SVT is characterized by rapid heart rates, usually between 200 and 300 beats/min. Episodes usually begin and end abruptly and the duration of tachycardia is variable. Short episodes of SVT are well tolerated in most neonates. Sustained SVT presents as pallor, irritability, poor feeding and respiratory distress and can progress to heart failure with cardiovascular collapse within 24–48 hours after onset. There is a 20% recurrence risk which drops significantly after 1 year of age.

Wolf–Parkinson–White (WPW) syndrome is responsible for up to 40% of SVT in neonates. The majority of neonates with SVT have no structural cardiac abnormality. However, up to 25% will have an associated heart defect. Ebstein's anomaly, corrected transposition of great arteries, tricuspid atresia and cardiac rhabdomyomas are the more common associations. The diagnosis is confirmed by ECG which shows a heart rate of >>200/min, and abnormal P-wave morphology and P-wave axis with normal QRS duration. In the case of WPW syndrome, ECG during sinus rhythm shows a short P–R interval, presence of a delta wave and wide QRS complex changing to inverted (retrograde) P-waves and narrow QRS complexes during tachycardia.

Management of SVTs

1. SVT with cardiovascular collapse. This is managed with synchronized cardioversion: 0.5 J/kg. If the tachycardia persists, repeat cardioversion with a double dose, that is, 1.0 J/kg. If conversion to sinus rhythm is still not accomplished, reconsider the diagnosis of SVT in consultation with the cardiologist.

2. SVT without cardiovascular compromise. Vagal manoeuvres, for example application of an ice bag to the face, can convert SVT to sinus rhythm. Adenosine is the drug of choice with an initial dose of 50 μg/kg as a rapid i.v. bolus with constant ECG monitoring. If there is no response, give a second dose of 100 μg/kg after 1–2 min. A third dose of 150 μg/kg can be given after a further 1–2 min. Adenosine is a potent blocker of A–V nodal conduction with an extremely short half-life (<10 s) and can successfully terminate acute attacks of SVT in up to 90% of cases. Intravenous infusion of amiodarone or flecanide forms the second line of therapy for refractory episodes of SVT.

3. Long-term therapy. Maintenance treatment is required to prevent recurrent episodes of SVT, especially when the attacks are frequent, long lasting and difficult to control and also after an episode of SVT associated with cardiovascular compromise. Digoxin (for non-WPW SVT) or β-blockers (propranolol or sotalol) are commonly used for this purpose. Most infants outgrow their SVT by the age of 1 year, when maintenance therapy can be discontinued.

4. Ventricular tachycardia (VT). VT is uncommon in neonates and is characterized by tachycardia with wide and abnormal QRS complexes (>0.08 s), A–V dissociation and secondary ST and T-wave changes. In neonates, VT is seen with cardiac tumours, myocardial diseases, prolonged QT syndrome, asphyxia, acidosis, hypokalaemia or hyperkalaemia. VT associated with cardiovascular compromise needs synchronized cardioversion, beginning with 2 J/kg followed by 4 J/kg if no response occurs. During cardioversion the patient ideally should be intubated and ventilated with 100% oxygen with adequate sedation and analgesia. Underlying acid–base and electrolyte abnormalities should be promptly corrected. Cardiac evaluation and maintenance therapy should be planned in close consultation with the paediatric cardiologist. β-blockers are commonly used in patients with prolonged QT syndrome for prevention of VT.

Bradyarrhythmias

1. Sinus bradycardia. This is defined as a heart rate of <100 beats/min with a normal P-wave preceding each QRS complex. Persistent sinus bradycardia in neonates is seen with hypoxia, hypothermia, acidosis, hypothyroidism, hyper-kalaemia, raised intracranial pressure and obstructive jaundice. Therapy should be aimed at the precipitating cause.

2. Complete heart block (CHB). CHB is characterized by independent beating of atria and ventricles. ECG reveals regular P-waves (constant P–P interval) and regular QRS complexes (constant R–R interval), but with complete A–V dissociation and slow ventricular rate. Congenital CHB occurs in 1 in 25 000 live births. Up to 30% of cases can be associated with structural heart disease, for example atrioventricular septal defects or corrected transposition of great arteries. There is a strong association of connective tissue disorders (SLE) in mothers of neonates with congenital CHB. Most mothers are asymptomatic at the time of delivery but about two-thirds will go on to develop evidence of connective tissue disorder later. The majority of patients with congenital CHB are asymptomatic at birth. Symptoms of heart failure develop with persistent bradycardia. Occasionally, in its most severe form, congenital CHB presents as hydrops fetalis necessitating early delivery. Symptomatic neonates require isoprenaline infusion followed by pacemaker implantation. The prognosis is good for isolated CHB. However, it is unfavourable in infants with persistent bradycardia (<50 beats/min), associated structural heart defects or a prolonged Q–T interval on ECG.

Further reading

Burton DA, Cabalka AK. Cardiac evaluation of infants. *Pediatric Clinics of North America*, 1994; **41**: 991–1011.

Gilette PC, Garson A. Clinical Pediatric Arrhythmias: Electrophysiology and Pacing, 2nd edn. Philadelphia: W.B. Saunders, 1998.

Park MK. *Pediatric Cardiology for Practitioners*, 3rd edn. Chicago: Year Book Medical Publishers, 1996.

Park MK, Guntheroth WG. *How to Read Pediatric ECGs*, 2nd edn. Chicago: Year Book Medical Publishers, 1987.

Silove ED. Assessment and management of congenital heart disease in the newborn by the district paediatrician. *Archives of Disease in Childhood*, 1994; **70**: F71–4.

Related topics of interest

CHILDBIRTH COMPLICATIONS AND FETAL OUTCOME

Labour is the whole process whereby the products of conception are expelled from the mother. Modern management of labour has greatly reduced the maternal and fetal morbidity and mortality previously associated with childbirth, by applying careful monitoring techniques aimed at anticipating the complications and potential risks from both predictable and unpredictable acute emergencies. These include malpresentation, malposition, cord accidents, dystocia and trauma.

Dystocia

Dystocia signifies difficult labour. A difficult labour is one where the hazards significantly exceed those of minimal-risk labours. There should be an assessment of the adequacy of the passages in relation to the size of the fetus. Pelvic anomalies or an unusually large baby will both cause potentially difficult deliveries.

1. Maternal risks
- Trauma (uterine, pelvic and perineal).
- Excessive blood loss.

2. Fetal risks
- Fractured clavicle(s) or limb(s).
- Erb's palsy.
- Injury to the cervical spine.
- Severe birth asphyxia (seizures, impaired neurodevelopmental outcome).
- Intracranial haemorrhage.
- Death.

Malpresentation

Malpresentation includes breech, transverse or oblique lie with shoulder presentation, face, brow, compound and cord presentation. Abnormal presentations occur in about 4% of singleton deliveries, the vast majority (3%) being breech. They account for significant mortality in both mother and fetus.

1. Maternal risks
- Prolonged labour.
- Ruptured uterus.
- Increased risk of infection.
- Trauma to vagina, cervix, perineum and uterus.
- Risks of emergency anaesthesia and Caesarean section.
- Obstructed labour (vesicovaginal and rectovaginal fistula in developing nations).
- Venous thrombosis and fatal pulmonary embolism in puerperium.

2. Fetal risks
- Fetal death.
- Meconium aspiration.

- Cord prolapse and severe asphyxia.
- Traumatic instrumental delivery.
- Injuries to spine or abdominal contents.
- Prolonged rupture of membranes and infection.

Breech presentation and labour

Between 30 and 40% of singletons present by breech between 20 and 25 weeks, and 15% at 32 weeks, but by 34 weeks most have undergone spontaneous version to a cephalic presentation. Subsequent reversion to breech is rare, occurring in 4%. Conditions predisposing to breech include multiple pregnancy, oligohydramnios or polyhydramnios, abnormal uterine shape, hydrocephaly, intrauterine fetal death or rarely pelvic tumours.

There are three types of breech presentation:

- extended or frank breech,
- flexed or complete breech,
- footling or incomplete breech.

Frank breech occurs in 60–70% of cases and has a low incidence of cord prolapse due to the snug fitting of the presenting part which engages early. Flexed breech has a four times higher incidence of cord prolapse than frank breech and it is higher still in footling breech presentation. Breech presentation is the commonest association with prolapse of the cord, occurring in 40–50% of cases.

1. Maternal risks
- Sepsis.
- Trauma to the vagina, cervix and perineum.
- Ruptured uterus from external cephalic version.
- Risks of emergency anaesthesia and Caesarean section.

2. Fetal risks
- Prematurity.
- Cord tears.
- Placental abruption and asphyxia.
- Fetal distress and death (following external cephalic version).
- Perinatal mortality may be four times higher than that of vertex presentation.
- Increased risk of congenital abnormality (6.3% incidence versus 2.4% in non-breech cases).
- Lower Apgar scores (three times as common as with cephalic presentation).
- Occipital injury and intracranial haemorrhage.
- Brachial plexus injury and cord transection.
- Fractures of long bones and the skull.

Malposition

Malposition of the fetal head is present when it engages the pelvis in the occipitoposterior position. This occurs in 10% of cephalic presentations and causes difficulties in approximately

10%. The diagnosis is suggested by severe backache in labour with early rupture of membranes. The head presents a larger diameter in the maternal pelvis and may become arrested in the occipitoposterior position deep in the pelvis.

1. Maternal risks
- Prolonged labour.
- Instrumental delivery or Caesarean section.
- Perineal trauma and bruising.
- Complications of instrumental or Caesarean deliveries.

2. Fetal risks
- Fetal distress.
- Birth asphyxia.
- Trauma and facial bruising.
- Feeding difficulties (following facial trauma).

Cord presentation and prolapse

This has an incidence of 1 in 200–300. While the membranes are intact, the condition is labelled cord presentation, but becomes cord prolapse when the sac ruptures.

1. Aetiology
- Malpresentation especially breech presentation.
- Prematurity (small fetus and relatively copious liquor).
- Multiparity (head not engaged till labour starts).
- Operative manoeuvres e.g. manual rotation.
- Cord abnormality (long cord or low placental insertion).

2. Management. Immediate delivery is the ideal if the fetus is alive and sufficiently mature. Cord presentation must be treated with the same urgency as cord prolapse. A corrected mortality of 10–17% has been reported but only 5.5% if delivery was effected within 10 min.

3. Fetal risks
- Severe asphyxia.
- Death.

Further reading

Foley MR, Strong TH. Obstetric Intensive Care: A Practical Manual. Philadelphia: W.B. Saunders, 1997.
Whitefield CR (ed). *Dewhurst's Textbook of Obstetrics and Gynaecology for Postgraduates*, 5th edn. Oxford: Blackwell Science, 1995.

Related topics of interest

CHROMOSOMAL ABNORMALITIES

Despite their relative infrequency, chromosomal abnormalities constitute a significant work-load in the care of newborns. Autosomal chromosomal abnormalities are present in up to 4 in every 1000 births, with sex chromosome abnormalities occurring in up to 3 births per 1000. Of the autosomal abnormalities, approximately 1.5 in every 1000 are trisomies (mainly trisomy 21) with balanced translocations largely accounting for the remainder. Up to 50% of miscarriages, however, may have associated chromosomal abnormalities.

Trisomies

Trisomy 21 (Down's syndrome)

This is the commonest autosomal anomaly with an overall incidence of 1 in 600–700 births. The incidence varies with maternal age from approximately 1 in 1200 births at age 20 years to 1 in 100 births at age 40 years, but with a rapid rise thereafter to 1 in 40 births at age 45 years. Up to 95% are due to an extra chromosome 21 because of non-disjunction during oogenesis in the mother. In 2.5%, there are chromosomal translocations (mostly 14/21), the remainder being mosaics.

Clinical features

1. Facial. Upward slanting eyes, prominent epicanthic folds, protruding tongue, flat nasal bridge, Brushfield's spots, short neck, flat occiput.

2. Limbs. Short broad hands, short incurved little fingers, single palmar creases, gap between first and second toes, increased risk of congenital hip dislocation.

3. Cardiovascular. Atrial and ventricular septal defects and atrioventricular canal defects are the commonest. Cardiac defects are present in 40% of cases.

4. Gastrointestinal. Gut stenoses and atresias (especially duodenal) are more common, including Hirschsprung's disease.

5. Neuromuscular. Hypotonia, feeding difficulties, motor delay.

Management

Inform parents of the diagnosis at the earliest opportunity. Confirm the diagnosis with chromosomal analysis. Give parents information on prognosis and general management. Parents may wish to establish links with the local Down's Syndrome Association. Genetic counselling about risks to future children and prenatal diagnosis is essential. The risk of having an affected child is significantly influenced by the maternal age, being 1 in 2300 at age 18 years, but 1 in 100 at 40 years. After one trisomic child (mother under 40 years) the recurrence risk is 1%, but the risk is 10% if the mother is a

14/21 translocation carrier (2% if the father is the translocation carrier) and 100% if either parent is a balanced Robertsonian 21/21 translocation carrier.

Trisomy 18 (Edwards' syndrome)

This is relatively rare with an incidence of 1 in 5000 and poor prognosis, only 1 in 10 surviving the first year of life. The incidence increases with maternal age. The recurrence risk is 1%.

Clinical features

1. *Prenatal.* Intrauterine growth restriction.

2. *Facial.* Small chin and mouth, long head, low-set and malformed ears, wide epicanthic folds and ptosis.

3. *Limbs.* Second finger overlaps third, and fifth may overlap fourth. Rocker bottom feet, hypoplastic nails and flexion deformities are common.

4. *Urogenital.* Cryptorchidism and renal defects.

5. *Cardiovascular.* Atrial septal defects or patent ductus arteriosus.

6. *Neurodevelopmental.* Severe mental retardation.

Trisomy 13 (Patau syndrome)

This is even rarer with an incidence of 1 in 7000 and poor prognosis, most infants dying during the first year of life. The recurrence risk for another chromosomal anomaly is 1%, but is lower for trisomy 13.

Clinical features

1. *Facial.* Small triangular head with sloping forehead, small eyes with frequent colobomata of the iris and cleft lip and palate.

2. *Limbs.* Polydactyly, overlapping fingers, rocker bottom feet.

3. *Cardiovascular.* Congenital heart defects in 80%.

4. *Urogenital.* Renal abnormalities.

5. *Gastrointestinal.* Gut malrotation.

Trisomy 22

Clinical features

1. *Facial.* Preauricular skin tags, beaked nose, anteverted nostrils, antimongoloid slant to the eyes, cleft palate, short neck.

2. *Limbs.* Broad thumbs.

3. *Cardiovascular.* Congenital defects in 50%.

| Cat eye syndrome | Cat eye syndrome (commonly associated with anal atresia and colobomata) is a partial trisomy of the long arm of chromosome 22. |

Trisomy 8

This is quite uncommon, most being mosaic for trisomy 8/normal karyotype.

| Clinical features | 1. *Facial.* Coarse features with broad nasal root, thick lips, prominent forehead and protuberant ears. |
| | 2. *Limbs.* Deep grooves on the soles and palms, mild camptodactyly, limited elbow extension. |

Trisomy 9

This is a relatively uncommon chromosome abnormality. Neonatal mortality is high and most survivors are severely mentally retarded. Cytogenetic analysis delineates two groups: mosaic and non-mosaic complete trisomy 9. The outcome is dismal for infants with complete trisomy 9. Mosaicism for trisomy 9 is predictive of longer survival but the degree of mosaicism does not predict survival or the degree of impairment. Other chromosome variations are found with increased frequency in cases or their parents.

Clinical features	1. *Facial.* Large bulbous nose (in >50%), widely spaced and deep-set eyes, epicanthic folds, antimongoloid slant of the eyes, microphthalmia, downturned mouth, micrognathia, protruding ears with abnormal antihelix, hypoplastic phalanges, extra neck skin folds, microcephaly and large fontanelles.
	2. *Prenatal.* Intrauterine growth restriction.
	3. *Other.* Mental retardation, skeletal anomalies, congenital heart defects, genital anomalies, intracranial and renal cysts.

Chromosomal deletion syndromes

Deletion of short arm of 5 (5p-) (Cri du chat syndrome)

In addition to the characteristic cry, other features are usually apparent.

| Clinical features | 1. *Facial.* Characteristic small head with small round face, widely spaced eyes, antimongoloid slant to the eyes, with marked epicanthic folds, low-set ears, cleft lip and palate. |
| | 2. *Other.* Renal and cardiac abnormalities. |

Deletion of short arm of 4 (4p-) (Wolf–Hirschhorn syndrome)

This syndrome has a dismal prognosis with half the affected infants dying before 6 months of age. Severe growth restriction is characteristic.

Clinical features

1. Facial. Fish mouth, cleft lip and palate, colobomata of the iris, low-set simple ears, pre-auricular pits and tags are common. Hypertelorism, a prominent glabella and absence of an angle between the broad nasal bridge and forehead commonly co-exist, giving the face a 'Greek warrior helmet' appearance.

2. Neurodevelopmental. Grand mal epilepsy and neurodevelopmental delay.

Deletion of the long arm of 18 (18q-)

This commonly gives a distinct syndrome which can be diagnosed on clinical grounds.

Clinical features

1. Facial. Characteristic mild facial flattening with prominent protruding jaw with downturned and 'carp-like' mouth. Hypertelorism, nystagmus, epicanthic folds with pale discs and prominent ears with narrow external canal associated with deafness.

2. Limbs. Fingers are tapered and thumbs are proximally implanted with dimples over extensor surfaces of joints.

Turner's syndrome (45, XO)

With an incidence of approximately 1 in 5000 births, this syndrome has by comparison a favourable prognosis.

Clinical features

1. Prenatal. Nuchal swelling or hydrops.

2. Facial. Webbed neck (pterygium colli), low trident posterior hairline.

3. Limbs. Lymphoedema of dorsum of hands and feet, increased carrying angle at the elbow, convex deep-set nails.

4. Cardiovascular. Cardiac defects especially coarctation of the aorta (20%).

5. Other. Widespread nipples and broad chest, renal anomalies, good neurodevelopmental outlook.

Further reading

Arnold GL, Kirby RS, Stern TP, Sawyer JR. Trisomy 9: review and report of two new cases. *American Journal of Medical Genetics*, 1995; **56**: 252–7.

Baraister M, Winter RM. *Colour Atlas of Congenital Malformation Syndromes*. London: Mosby-Wolfe, 1996.

Gilbert P. *The A–Z Reference Book of Syndromes and Inherited Disorders*, 2nd edn. London: Chapman & Hall, 1996.

Hall JG (ed). Medical genetics I & II. *Pediatric Clinics of North America*, 1992; **39 (1&2)**.

Harper PS. *Practical Genetic Counselling*, 3rd edn. Oxford: Butterworth-Heinemann, 1991.

Jones KL. *Smith's Recognizable Patterns of Human Malformation*, 5th edn. Philadelphia: W.B. Saunders, 1997.

Related topics of interest

Congenital malformations and birth defects (p. 70)
Intrauterine growth restriction (p. 165)
Prenatal diagnosis (p. 253)

COMPLICATIONS OF MECHANICAL VENTILATION

While artificial mechanical ventilation has been lifesaving for infants with respiratory failure and a variety of other conditions, it is associated with a significant morbidity and several potential complications. The incidence of complications varies between centres due partly to differences in patient demographics and the indications for assisted ventilation. Overall complication rates of 8–24% are reported. Complications may occur both in the short term or after prolonged periods of ventilation.

Short-term complications

- Oropharyngeal trauma.
- Pneumothorax.
- Pneumomediastinum.
- Pneumoperitoneum.
- Right upper lobe collapse.
- Subcutaneous emphysema.
- Pulmonary interstitial emphysema (PIE).
- Iatrogenic hypotension (excessive ventilatory pressures).

Clinical presentation
- Oropharyngeal bleeding or pulmonary haemorrhage.
- Sudden deterioration after a period of stability (tube blockage/pneumothorax).
- Acute collapse/shock (pneumothorax and/or pneumopericardium).
- Abdominal distension of rapid onset (pneumoperitoneum).
- Gradual worsening of gas exchange (PIE).

Investigations
- Chest transillumination.
- Chest X-ray.
- Arterial blood gases.

Management
Chest transillumination allows rapid detection of significant pulmonary air leaks especially if unilateral. If the situation is not clear, a chest radiograph should be performed. In emergencies, the chest should be needled and a chest drain inserted if a symptomatic air leak is detected. While very small pneumothoraces and pneumomediastinal air collections may be observed, all other symptomatic air leaks should be drained. PIE may be managed by adopting a low-pressure fast-rate strategy including high frequency oscillatory ventilation. A collapsed right upper lobe may be cleared by withdrawing the endotracheal tube from the right main bronchus. In rapid acute deteriorations associated with bradycardia and hypoxaemia, it is worth changing the endotracheal tube electively in case it has become blocked or dislodged.

Long-term complications

- Palatal deformities (oral intubation).
- Nasal deformities (nasal intubation).
- Accidental extubation.
- Pneumothorax.
- Tube blockage.
- Laryngotracheomalacia.
- Bronchocutaneous fistula.
- Tracheal traumatic granulomas.
- BPD.
- Endobronchial intubation and atelectasis.
- Side-effects of prolonged sedation and medication.
- Repeated pulmonary infections.
- Periventricular leucomalacia (PVL).
- Poor somatic growth.
- Post-extubation stridor.
- Vocal cord palsy.
- Dysphonia.

Clinical presentation   Acquired airway narrowing (e.g. subglottic stenosis) frequently presents as post-extubation stridor and/or failed extubation (with respiratory distress and apnoeas). Vocal cord palsies may present with post-extubation respiratory distress or dysphonia. BPD often presents as an insidious prolonged ventilator and oxygen dependency. Early persistent hypocapnia in preterm infants is now recognized to be a risk factor for developing BPD, severe intraventricular haemorrhage, cystic PVL and cerebral palsy.

Management   Significant orofacial deformities may require plastic surgery and should be referred for expert opinion. Steroids (dexamethasone) may be tried for post-extubation stridor as 1–2 mg/kg/day p.o. or i.v. given 6-hourly, beginning 24 hours prior to extubation and continuing for 24–48 hours afterwards. If this is unsuccessful, an ear, nose and throat (ENT) opinion should be obtained with a view to laryngoscopy and possible surgery. Apart from the orofacial deformities from prolonged intubation which may require plastic surgery, many of the acquired airway problems (e.g. vocal cord palsy and dysphonia) tend to resolve with time.

Further reading

Contencin P, Narcy P. Size of endotracheal tube and neonatal acquired subglottic stenosis. Study Group for Neonatology and Pediatric Emergencies in the Parisian Area. *Archives of Otolaryngology, Head and Neck Surgery*, 1993; **119**: 815–19.

Gannon CM, Wiswell TE, Spitzer AR. Volutrauma, $PaCO_2$ levels, and neurodevelopmental sequelae following assisted ventilation. *Clinics in Perinatology*, 1998; **25**: 159–75.

Jobe AH. Hypocarbia and bronchopulmonary dysplasia. *Archives of Pediatrics and Adolescent Medicine*, 1995; **149**: 615.

Richardson ME. *Otolaryngology, Pediatric Volume*, 3rd edn. St Louis: Mosby, 1998.

Rivera R, Tibballs J. Complications of endotracheal intubation and mechanical ventilation in infants and children. *Critical Care Medicine*, 1992; **20**: 193–9.

Scottile FD. Complications of mechanical ventilation. In: Lumb PD, Bryan-Brown CW (eds). *Complications in Critical Care Medicine*. Chicago: Year Book Medical Publishers, 1988; 27–33.

Related topics of interest

Bronchopulmonary dysplasia (p. 38)
Intubation (p. 170)
Mechanical ventilation (p. 185)
Respiratory distress (p. 275)
Respiratory distress syndrome (p. 278)
Resuscitation (p. 282)
Stridor (p. 307)

CONGENITAL DIAPHRAGMATIC HERNIA

Congenital diaphragmatic hernia (CDH) has been described, studied and treated for over four centuries. Despite the great advances made in the care of infants with CDH, the mortality remains high at 30–60% and survival averages 60%. Approximately 4–10% of all infant deaths from congenital anomalies are caused by CDH. The reported incidence ranges from 1 in 1000 to 1 in 12 000 (prevalence 3.3 per 10 000 births). Chromosomal anomalies are present in 5–30% of cases. Left-sided defects are six times more common than right-sided ones.

Associated malformations are found in 40–50% of cases, with structural cardiac anomalies being the commonest (seen in 30%). Renal and genital anomalies are predominant in males, while central nervous system (CNS), heart, gastrointestinal and liver defects are more common in females. The cause of CDH is, however, still largely unknown.

Pathophysiology	CDH results in a diaphragmatic defect and lung hypoplasia. Both lungs are structurally affected, the ipsilateral more severely than the contralateral lung. There are fewer bronchi, respiratory bronchi and alveoli, resulting in a global reduction in the gas exchange area. As vascular branching parallels development of the airways, the arterial branches in CDH are also reduced. Thus in CDH there is a reduction in the cross-sectional area of the pulmonary vascular bed and an increase in muscularization of these vessels, leading to the development of persistent pulmonary hypertension which adversely affects the outcome. Functionally, the surfactant system and ability of CDH lungs to deal with oxygen-free radicals are also impaired.
Prenatal diagnosis	A low maternal serum alpha-fetoprotein (AFP) may be associated with CDH (and also trisomy 18 and 21). The gold standard for antenatal diagnosis of CDH is now a level 3 ultrasound examination. Once CDH is diagnosed, look for associated anomalies as these alter the prognosis. Amniocentesis should also be performed, as up to 20% may have chromosomal defects (from microdeletions to trisomy 18, 13 and 12p tetrasomy).

Predictors of mortality

- Polyhydramnios.
- A gestational age of <25 weeks at diagnosis.
- Prenatally diagnosed CDH may have a higher incidence of associated anomalies and therefore a poorer prognosis.
- The presence of an intrathoracic stomach is associated with increased mortality of up to 10-fold.
- A contralateral lung-to-head circumference ratio of less than 0.62 (corrected for gestational age).
- A small lung-to-thoracic transverse area ratio.
- Left ventricular hypoplasia, a reduced left-to-right ventricular size (left ventricular mass index); a calculated left ventricular mass of <2 g/kg is predictive of death.

- The presence of a structural cardiac anomaly especially when detected prenatally.
- A chromosomal anomaly (prognosis depends on the chromosomal defect).
- A preoperative functional residual capacity (FRC) of <9 ml/kg.

Presentation

This depends on the severity of the defect and the side affected. Large left-sided defects present in the immediate postnatal period with respiratory distress (grunting, tachypnoea, recession and cyanosis) with a scaphoid abdomen. Right-sided defects tend to be less severe as the liver 'plugs' the defect preventing abdominal contents from entering the chest. Bowel sounds are present in the chest and the apex beat displaced in left-sided defects. Small right hernias may be chance findings on a chest X-ray.

Postnatal diagnosis

Chest X-ray is diagnostic with dilated loops of bowel in left hemithorax or an opaque hemithorax (before bowel is filled with air). Main differential diagnosis is cystic adenomatoid malformation of the lung, especially if radiographic findings are right-sided or position of the stomach is below the diaphragm.

Management

1. At birth. Avoid mask ventilation during resuscitation as this will result in visceral distension compromising ventilation and cardiac function. Intubate and ventilate if respiratory distress is present. Use the lowest possible airway pressure to maintain a preductal saturation of ≥90%. Pass a large bore tube to decompress the stomach.

Administration of prophylactic surfactant therapy is beneficial in patients who have had CDH diagnosed prenatally, as is prenatal steroid (dexamethasone) therapy. Secure umbilical arterial and central venous access for pressure monitoring and drug infusions.

2. Pre-operative stabilization. Confirm the diagnosis by a chest radiograph. Ensure circulatory adequacy and normoglycaemia. Correct hypovolaemic and/or metabolic acidosis with 4.5% albumin, THAM (tris-hydroxymethyl-aminomethane) or bicarbonate therapy. If ventilation is needed, intubate, paralyse, sedate and provide analgesia (i.v. infusion of morphine or fentanyl). Use the lowest airway pressure compatible with adequate oxygenation. Maintain preductal saturations of 85–90%, keeping peak airway pressure <30 cmH$_2$O. The strategy of hyperventilation-induced alkalosis (raising pH to >7.5 and reducing PaCO$_2$ to <30 mmHg (4 kPa) should be abandoned as it produces iatrogenic lung injury. It has also been associated with adverse neurological outcome. Less aggressive mechanical ventilation should be used to avoid overdistending the contralateral lung and the secondary effects of barotrauma. As long as the pH can be buffered with bicarbonate or THAM, ignore $PaCO_2$. This strategy of 'permissive hypercapnia' is currently favoured as it is associated with improved survival and decreased extracorporeal membrane oxygenation (ECMO) utilization.

High-frequency oscillatory ventilation (HFOV) and high-frequency jet ventilation (HFJV) may at times offer additional benefit, though this is inconsistent. It may be preferable to use HFOV for infants with hypoxaemia and hypercapnia unresponsive to conventional ventilation or only responsive to high pressure ventilation (peak airway pressure $>30\,cmH_2O$).

All infants should have an echocardiogram to exclude congenital heart defects, measure the left-ventricular mass index and determine the direction of ductal shunting. Right-to-left or bidirectional shunting suggests pulmonary hypertension, which may respond to systemic pressor therapy and inhaled nitric oxide (NO) therapy. To date, however, there is no convincing evidence that inhaled NO improves the outcome in CDH.

Infants with persistent pulmonary hypertension of the newborn (PPHN) and severe respiratory failure non-responsive to maximal medical treatment may be referred to ECMO support provided they do not have severe pulmonary hypoplasia. ECMO may be used before, during and after surgical repair of the defect. However, surgical repair on ECMO is associated with a greater mortality from haemorrhagic complications. Although there is a broad opinion that ECMO *improves* the outcome in CDH, this has not been proven, a recent UK trial showing no significant difference in survival between the ECMO-treated infants and those receiving conventional therapy.

As surgical repair of the diaphragmatic defect commonly produces a deterioration in lung compliance and gas exchange, most centres now adopt a strategy of non-urgent or deferred repair. Infants are no longer repaired on an emergency basis, with much greater emphasis being placed on pre-operative ventilation and stabilization up to and including ECMO support. Deferred surgery *does not* improve survival but helps to select survivors from non-survivors prior to undergoing the expense and stress of surgical repair. The timing of surgery depends on the degree of stability or liability of the pulmonary vascular bed. Repair may be deferred for several days and documenting resolution of pulmonary hypertension (by Doppler echocardiography) may suggest an optimal time for repair. Finally, prior to transfer for surgery, other associated anomalies (including chromosomal) should be excluded.

Operative repair   This is often through a subcostal oblique incision and a primary repair is often possible. If the defect is too large, a synthetic patch may be used. Closures that create undue tension compromise the surgical repair, complicate the post-operative ventilatory management, result in re-herniation of the diaphragm, and cause dehiscence or wound hernias. Fetal surgery including *in utero* tracheal ligation, endoscopic intrauterine surgery and open surgery are all still very experimental. Lung transplantation for severe pulmonary hypoplasia is a distant option.

Long-term outcome   Many survivors of CDH experience considerable morbidity as a consequence of their abnormal pulmonary development, severe respiratory failure and surgical repair of their defects. Foregut dismotility is common (20–89%), manifest as delayed gastric emptying and gastro-oesophageal reflux (GOR) (10–60%). There is a high incidence of chronic lung disease (up to 60%) secondary to the primary lung hypoplasia, barotrauma and oxygen toxicity, chronic aspiration from GOR and development of reactive airways disease, all resulting in frequent recurrent hospitalizations. Somatic growth failure is common (chronic lung disease, GOR, poor oral intake), 30–40% remaining below the 5th percentile for weight. Short-term neurodevelopmental delays have also been noted. Post-surgical complications include adhesive bowel obstruction and recurrence of the hernia defect.

Further reading

Davis CF, Sabharwal AJ. Management of congenital diaphragmatic hernia. *Archives of Disease in Childhood, Fetal and Neonatal Edition*, 1998; **79**: 1–3.
Glick PL, Irish MS, Holm BA (eds). New insights into the pathophysiology of congenital diaphragmatic hernia. *Clinics in Perinatology*, 1996; **23**: 4.
Jaffray B, MacKinlay GA. Real and apparent mortality from congenital diaphragmatic hernia. *British Journal of Surgery*, 1996; **83**: 79–82.
Katz AL, Wiswell TE, Baumgart S. Contemporary controversies in the management of congenital diaphragmatic hernia. *Clinics in Perinatology*, 1998; **25**: 219–48.

Related topics of interest

Congenital malformations and birth defects (p. 70)
Extracorporeal membrane oxygenation (p. 78)
Persistent pulmonary hypertension of the newborn (p. 237)

Prenatal diagnosis (p. 253)
Pulmonary hypoplasia (p. 261)
Respiratory distress (p. 275)

CONGENITAL HEART DISEASE – CONGESTIVE HEART FAILURE

Congestive heart failure (CHF) is a clinical syndrome characterized by the inability of the heart to pump enough blood to meet the metabolic requirements of the tissues. Severe CHF results in inadequate perfusion of vital organs, culminating in cardiovascular collapse or shock.

Clinical features of CHF in neonates

1. *History.* Feeding difficulty characterized by:
   - Slow to feed (>>30 min).
   - Pallor and sweating with feeding.
   - Breathlessness and irritability during feeding.
   - Failure to gain weight.

2. *Physical examination*
   (a) Signs of impaired myocardial function and compromised tissue perfusion
   - Tachycardia (heart rate >150/min), gallop rhythm, weak and thready pulse.
   - Cardiomegaly (clinical and radiographic).
   - Reduced urine output (<1 ml/kg/hour).
   - Metabolic acidosis.
   - Vascular collapse/shock: pale, mottled skin, cold extremities, prolonged capillary refill time (>3 s), increased toe–core temperature difference (>2°C), and impalpable pulses.
   (b) Signs of pulmonary congestion
   - Tachypnoea (respiratory rate >60/min).
   - Subcostal or intercostal recession.
   - Wheezing or basal rales.
   - Cyanosis.
   - Wet lung fields on chest X-ray.
   - Frank pulmonary oedema.
   (c) Signs of systemic venous congestion
   - Hepatomegaly (>3 cm or progressive).
   - Excess weight gain (>30 g/24 hours) despite feeding difficulties.

Differential diagnosis of CHF in neonates

1. *Non-cardiac causes*
   - Asphyxia.
   - Septicaemia.
   - Anaemia.
   - Polycythaemia.
   - Hypoglycaemia.
   - Fluid overload.
   - Arteriovenous fistulae.

2. *Cardiac causes*

(a) Left ventricular outflow tract obstruction
- Hypoplastic left heart syndrome (HLHS).
- Critical aortic stenosis.
- Coarctation of the aorta.
- Interrupted aortic arch.

Neonates with these conditions are usually normal at birth, as systemic perfusion and pulses are maintained by the patent ductus arteriosus (PDA). Cardiac failure and cardiogenic shock sets in with postnatal constriction of the ductus as systemic and coronary perfusion is impaired. Severe heart failure is usually seen in the first week of life.

(b) Left-to-right shunts
- Large PDA.
- Large VSD.
- Truncus arteriosus.
- Atrioventricular septal defects (AVSD).
- Total anomalous pulmonary venous connection (non-obstructed).

Presentation is beyond the first week of life as pulmonary vascular resistance falls. Features of increased pulmonary blood flow and sympathetic over-stimulation are predominant.

(c) Structurally normal heart with left ventricular dysfunction
- Cardiac arrhythmias.
- TMI of the newborn.
- Cardiomyopathies (infective, storage disorders, endocardial fibroelastosis, infant of diabetic mother).

Evaluation of a neonate with CHF

1. Perform the A-B-C of neonatal cardiopulmonary resuscitation.
2. Correct electrolyte and acid–base abnormalities.
3. Exclude non-cardiac causes.
4. Determine possible underlying cardiac aetiology and mechanism of CHF.

A schematic representation of the evaluation of an infant with CHF is given in *Figure 1*:

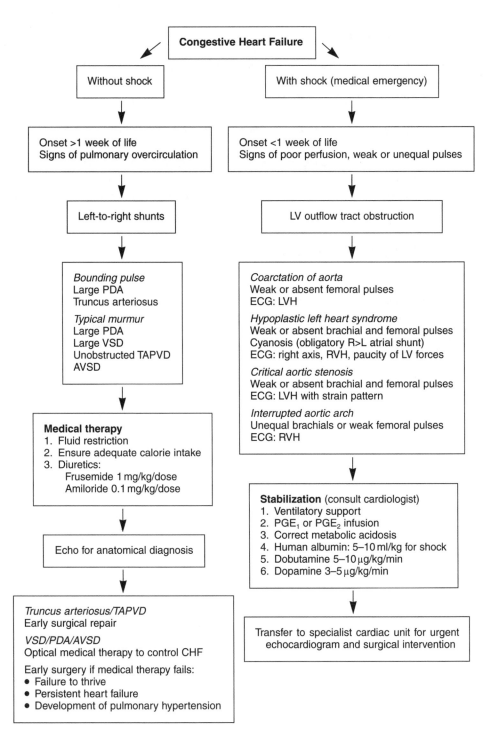

Figure 1. Schematic representation of the evaluation of an infant with CHF.

Further reading

Burton DA, Cabalka AK. Cardiac evaluation of infants. *Pediatric Clinics of North America*, 1994; **41**: 991–1011.

Castaneda AR, Jonas RA, Mayer JE, Hanley FL. Cardiac Surgery of the Neonate and Infant. Philadelphia: W.B. Saunders, 1994.

Park MK. *Pediatric Cardiology for Practitioners*, 3rd edn. Chicago: Year Book Medical Publishers, 1996.

Silove ED. Assessment and management of congenital heart disease in the newborn by the district paediatrician. *Archives of Disease in Childhood*, 1994; **70**: F71–4.

Snider AR, Serwer GA. *Echocardiography in Pediatric Heart Disease*. St. Louis: Mosby Year Book, 1990.

Related topics of interest

CONGENITAL HEART DISEASE – CYANOTIC DEFECTS

The incidence of congenital heart disease (CHD) is about 8 per 1000 live births and one-third of these cases present in the neonatal period. The common modes of presentation are:

- Cyanosis.
- Heart murmur.
- Congestive cardiac failure/vascular collapse.
- Cardiac arrhythmias.

Symptomatic heart disease in the neonate presents as cyanosis, cardiac failure or cardiovascular collapse. Asymptomatic heart disease is usually diagnosed when incidental finding of a heart murmur, abnormal pulses or abnormal heart rhythm leads to detailed cardiac evaluation. Routine cardiac screening in cases of various dysmorphic syndromes, chromosomal abnormalities or congenital abnormalities of the gastrointestinal tract also enables early diagnosis of asymptomatic heart disease. The initial evaluation should be aimed at the recognition of the cardiac problem and its severity, followed by stabilization of the neonate for safe and timely transfer to a specialist cardiac unit.

Cyanotic heart defects

Cyanosis refers to blue discoloration of the skin and the mucous membranes due to presence of more than 4–5 g/dl of reduced haemoglobin in circulation. Clinically it is usually apparent at oxygen saturations of 85% or below. It is one of the most significant signs of serious cardiac abnormality and hence prompt recognition and diagnostic evaluation is mandatory. Central cyanosis results from arterial desaturation or abnormal haemoglobin and affects the tongue, mucous membranes and peripheral skin. Peripheral cyanosis results from prolongation of the circulation time and an increase in tissue oxygen extraction and is confined to the extremities. It is typically seen in neonates with poor cardiac output, sepsis, polycythaemia or metabolic acidosis. The arterial oxygen saturation and PaO_2 is normal in peripheral cyanosis.

Differential cyanosis (lower limbs >> upper limbs) is seen in neonates with right-to-left ductal shunting associated with PPHN or an aortic arch obstruction. Reversed differential cyanosis (upper limbs >> lower limbs) is seen in the setting of ventriculoarterial discordance and right-to-left ductal shunting.

Features of cyanosis due to CHD
- Central cyanosis with minimal respiratory distress.
- Worsening of cyanosis with crying/agitation.
- Differential cyanosis.
- Arterial blood gas analysis: low PaO_2 with normal $PaCO_2$.
- No response to challenge with 100% inspired oxygen (hyperoxia test).
- Abnormalities on cardiovascular examination: precordial hyperactivity, heart murmur, unequal peripheral pulses.
- Chest radiograph: abnormal cardiac size/shape, abnormal pulmonary vascularity.

- Abnormal ECG (normal ECG does not exclude serious cardiac abnormality in neonates).

The most important differential of cardiac cyanosis is cyanosis due to respiratory disorders which is accompanied by signs of respiratory distress. It is also characterized by CO_2 retention on blood gas analysis. Typically in response to 100% inspired oxygen the saturations improve and PaO_2 is raised to >150 mmHg (20 kPa). In addition there is evidence of parenchymal lung disease on chest radiograph. Rarely, both the pulmonary and cardiac components may contribute to cyanosis, as seen in obstructed anomalous pulmonary venous connection, with pulmonary oedema making the distinction more difficult.

Initial evaluation

Investigations

- FBC – check haemoglobin, white cell count, platelets and markers of sepsis.
- Biochemistry – urea, creatinine, electrolytes, calcium, blood glucose.
- Chest radiograph – heart size/shape, pulmonary vascularity (N/↓/↑).
- ECG – note cardiac rhythm, QRS axis, ventricular hypertrophy (right/left/both).
- Blood gases – arterial sample from the right radial or temporal arteries to avoid the effect of right-to-left ductal shunt. Additional post-ductal arterial sample from lower limb in case of differential cyanosis. Capillary samples from a warmed heel can be reliably used for estimation of acidosis and $PaCO_2$.
- Hyperoxia test – measurement of arterial blood gas tensions and pH in room air and after administration of 100% oxygen for 5–10 min aids in the differential diagnosis of central cyanosis. Little or no change in oxygen tension is suggestive of cyanotic heart disease. PaO_2 >>20 kPa makes it less likely and PaO_2 >>30 kPa excludes cyanotic CHD.

Monitoring

Careful monitoring of the following parameters is mandatory during stabilization and transfer:

- Body temperature (toe–core differential).
- Respiratory rate and pattern.
- Heart rate and rhythm.
- Blood pressure.
- Oxygen saturation by pulse oxymetry.
- Blood gases with electrolytes, blood glucose.
- Urine output.

Stabilization

The **ABCD** of neonatal cardiopulmonary resuscitation is:

Airway. Secure airway; monitor for apnoeas if airway is not secured.
Breathing. Ventilatory support in presence of pulmonary oedema or persistent acidosis.
Circulation. Volume expansion (5–10 ml/kg of 4.5% human albumin) if hypovolaemic.
Drugs.

1. *To ensure ductal patency.* Prostaglandin E_1 or E_2 infusion. Recommended dilution: 500 µg in 500 ml of 5% dextrose, i.e. 1 µg/ml. Starting dose: 0.3 ml/kg/hour = 0.005 µg/kg/min. Double the dose in 20 min if SaO_2 is unchanged. Apnoea is a recognized side-effect.

2. *Correction of metabolic acidosis.* Sodium bicarbonate: half correction, dose guided by the base deficit.

3. *Inotropic support.* Dobutamine infusion (5–10 µg/kg/min) via peripheral i.v. canula.

4. *To improve renal perfusion.* Dopamine infusion (3–5 µg/kg/min) via central venous canula.

5. *Diuretics.* Frusemide 1 mg/kg i.v. if in cardiac failure (but not circulatory failure!) to reduce the increased extravascular fluid volume.

Differential diagnosis of cyanotic CHD in neonates

CHD with decreased pulmonary blood flow

Lesions characterized by obstruction to pulmonary blood flow (PBF) with right-to-left shunt at atrial or ventricular level (see *Figure 1*).

CHD with normal or increased pulmonary blood flow

Transposition of great arteries (TGA) is the commonest lesion of this type in neonates (see *Figure 2*).

Structurally normal hearts with right-to-left shunts

1. Persistent pulmonary hypertension of the newborn (PPHN). In this condition, the normal fall in pulmonary vascular resistance at birth is delayed. This results in persistence of pulmonary hypertension which leads to a right-to-left shunt through the patent ductus arteriosus and foramen ovale causing arterial desaturation. Right-to-left ductal shunt results in typical differential cyanosis (lower limbs >> upper limbs), whereas predominantly atrial shunt results in generalized central cyanosis, making distinction from structural heart disease more difficult. Association with precipitating conditions like meconium aspiration, perinatal asphyxia or sepsis, and increase

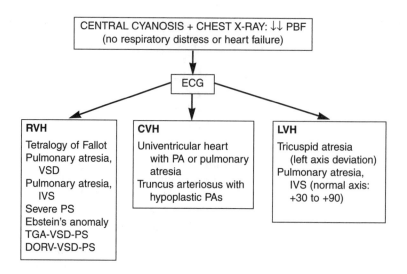

Figure 1. CHD with decreased pulmonary blood flow.

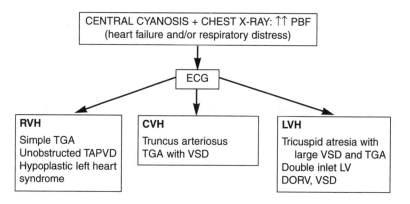

Figure 2. CHD with increased pulmonary blood flow.

in the post-ductal PaO$_2$ in response to hyperventilation causing hypocapnia and respiratory alkalosis, helps distinguish PPHN from structural heart defects. Echocardiographic evaluation is essential to confirm structurally normal heart with right-to-left ductal and/or atrial shunt.

2. Transient myocardial ischaemia (TMI). This condition is characterized by ischaemic myocardial dysfunction and presents either with cyanosis or with congestive cardiac failure and a low output state. Preceding history of perinatal hypoxia and/or hypoglycaemia is common. Right-to-left atrial shunt results in central cyanosis and global myocardial dysfunction causing heart failure. The condition may co-exist with PPHN. The ECG shows ischaemic S–T and T-wave changes (S–T depression and T-wave inversion) and at times anterior or inferior infarct patterns. Echocardiography reveals dilated poorly contractile left and right ventricles with right-to-left atrial shunt on colour Doppler. Treatment is supportive and aimed at controlling heart failure.

Further reading

Anderson R, Baker E, Rigby M, Shinebourne E, Tynan M (eds). *Pediatric Cardiology*, 2nd edn. Edinburgh: Churchill Livingstone, 1998.

Burton DA, Cabalka AK. Cardiac evaluation of infants. *Pediatric Clinics of North America,* 1994; **41**: 991–1011.

Freedom RM, Benson LN, Smallhorn JF. *Neonatal Heart Disease*. New York: Springer-Verlag, 1992.

Park MK. *Pediatric Cardiology for Practitioners*, 3rd edn. Chicago: Year Book Medical Publishers, 1996.

Silove ED. Assessment and management of congenital heart disease in the newborn by the district paediatrician. *Archives of Disease in Childhood*, 1994; **70**: F71–4.

Snider AR, Serwer GA. *Echocardiography in Pediatric Heart Disease*. St. Louis: Mosby Year Book, 1990.

Stark J, de Leval M (eds). *Surgery for Congenital Heart Defects*, 2nd edn. Philadelphia: W.B. Saunders, 1994.

Related topics of interest

Acute collapse (p. 6)
Cardiac arrhythmias (p. 43)
Congenital heart disease – congestive heart failure (p. 61)
Heart murmurs in neonates (p. 103)

CONGENITAL MALFORMATIONS AND BIRTH DEFECTS

The assessment of a dysmorphic newborn infant requires a systematic approach in order to make a correct diagnosis, implement appropriate management and provide the parents with an accurate prognosis and appropriate genetic counselling. Congenital malformations are present in approximately 2.5% of the general population. Most of these occur as single minor abnormalities but they occur with increased frequency in infants with other major malformations.

Certain definitions are important at the onset. A *birth defect* is a fault or disorder present or arising at birth. A *malformation* arises during embryonic life as an abnormal developmental process. A *deformation* is a mechanical alteration in the form or shape of a part of the body with previous normal development (e.g. talipes). A *disruption* is an interruption of normal development resulting in destruction of the body part (e.g. limb loss from amniotic band).

A single insult that results in a cascade of secondary consequences is a *malformation sequence*. If an insult causes multiple defects not causally related, the term *malformations syndrome* may be used. A *syndrome* is a pattern of malformations thought to be pathogenically related. An *association* is a non-random occurrence of several anomalies not known to be a syndrome or sequence. Malformation syndromes may be chromosomal, inherited or environmentally induced, whereas disruptions and deformations rarely have a genetic basis.

Clinical approach

Obtain a detailed history:

- Family history of malformations with a genetic basis.
- Parental consanguinity (autosomal recessive disorders).
- Multiple miscarriages/stillbirths.
- Elderly mother.
- Exposure to alcohol, drugs, radiation and infection during pregnancy.
- Oligo- or polyhydramnios.
- Prolonged premature rupture of membranes.
- Intrauterine growth restriction.
- Reduced fetal movements (? neuromuscular disorder).
- Breech presentation (? neuromuscular disorder).

Examination

This should be detailed with careful examination of any physical abnormalities.

- Describe abnormal signs accurately.
- Obtain photographic records if possible.
- Are the malformations present part of a recognized syndrome (e.g. Downs syndrome) or sequence (e.g. Pierre–Robin sequence)?

If immediate recognition is not possible, identify some well-defined unusual physical signs as 'handles' (e.g. ptosis, microcephaly, polydactyly, short limbs, hypogenitalia) and use the handle or a combination of them to scroll through the possible diagnoses. This process may be facilitated by the use of computerized databases.

Investigations
- Chromosome analysis.
- Specialized genetic techniques (e.g. DNA probes for Di George or Williams' syndromes).
- Cytogenetic analysis of specific tissue samples (e.g. skin fibroblast culture for the diagnosis of 12p tetrasomy – Killian–Pallister syndrome).
- Skeletal X-rays (e.g. osteogenesis imperfecta congenita).
- Ultrasound imaging (e.g. of head or abdomen).
- Haematological (e.g. TAR syndrome).
- Biochemical analysis (e.g. amino-aciduria, renal tubular acidosis in Lowe syndrome).

Management
- Depending on the malformations/deformations present, specialist teams may be required, e.g. ophthalmologist for ocular defects, ENT surgeon for ear and nose defects, maxillofacial and plastic surgeons for facial anomalies (e.g. cleft lip and palate), orthopaedic surgeons and physiotherapists for limb malformations and deformations.
- If the diagnosis remains uncertain always seek review by a clinical geneticist. Genetic counselling is vital in most cases (recurrence risks and possible future antenatal diagnosis).
- Infants with feeding difficulties may require input from dieticians, speech and language therapists and the assistance of community nurses.
- Neurodevelopmental follow-up will be required.
- Where appropriate, put the parents in touch with the appropriate parents' self-help organizations (e.g. Association for Spina Bifida and Hydrocephalus).

Further reading

Baraister M, Winter RM. *Colour Atlas of Congenital Malformation Syndromes*. London: Mosby-Wolfe, 1996.
Jones KL. *Smith's Recognizable Patterns of Human Malformation*, 5th edn. Philadelphia: W.B. Saunders, 1997.
Wiedemann H-R, Kunze J. *Clinical Syndromes*, 3rd edn. London: Mosby-Wolfe, 1997.

Related topics of interest

Chromosomal abnormalities (p. 49)
Neural tube defects (p. 203)

DEATH OF A BABY

The care of a dead or dying baby and his/her family has been called the neglected side of neonatal care. It is a daunting task that must be carried out sensitively and empathetically. Most parents need a lot of time to deal with the issues, and on a busy neonatal unit, staff must be careful not to rush them. In major neonatal units, 5–10% of all admissions die, including approximately 20% of those in intensive care. Common causes of death include extreme prematurity, lethal anatomical and biochemical abnormalities and birth asphyxia. In some, death will be completely unexpected: the parents may have never even contemplated it. For others, the congenital abnormality may have been diagnosed before birth, or the parents may have witnessed a heroic fight to save their very preterm baby against all odds. If time permits it is best to ask the parents if they want any religious blessing or naming of their baby when the critical nature of the illness is recognized, rather than waiting until death is imminent. It is also the time to take a first set of photographs.

Whatever the circumstances, most parents instinctively feel that their baby should not die 'alone' in a mass of tubes and wires. They want to cuddle their dying baby, even though they may be very afraid of this at first. In some circumstances, continuation of intensive care is to prolong death not to sustain life. Staff must therefore help parents recognize that nothing more can be done to save their baby. Parents then usually accept discontinuation of intensive care so long as full nursing care continues while they hold their baby and say goodbye. It is unethical to let the baby suffer in any way during this period – and parents are both acutely and persistently upset if their baby is distressed. It is a period of intensive nursing care – and doctors must be involved! The baby should be dressed in clothes of the parents' choice and taken to them in a quiet and entirely private room. At this point the baby is usually still alive.

While the parents are holding their baby, they should be asked if they wish to have photographs taken of the three of them together. Skilled carers can often point out some beautiful features of the baby – the hair, ears, face and hands – to help parents really look at and remember their baby whose face may have previously been hidden behind ventilator apparatus. Even very dysmorphic babies have fine features for parents to remember – wriggly toes and long fingers, perhaps! The moment of death – when the heart stops – cannot be recognized by parents as the baby quietly passes away after a period of apnoea. The heart may beat for 20–30 min after the final breath. Parents are comforted to be told that death will not be a cataclysm, but a quiet fading of life while their baby is unconscious and unaware of the change.

After the death the parents may wish to be alone with their baby. If so, they must be given as much time as they desire – sometimes several hours. They should have free access to a phone to contact relatives, and the extended family should be allowed to gather with the baby and parents if that is what they wish. Staff should pop in and out from time to time to ensure that they are coping and to offer support if needed. When they are ready to leave, they must go to an environment where on-going support is available. This may be a special bereavement suite on the postnatal ward where neonatal staff and midwife counsellors can help, or it may be home with the support of grandparents, relatives and other health professionals. The parents should know where their baby is going next, and should be advised that they can see him/her again at any time.

For the staff there are practical things to do and achieve. A most useful checklist published by the Royal College of Obstetricians and Gynaecologists is used in many units. A modified list of tasks (some of which have been covered above) based on that checklist includes:

- Mother and father informed of death.
- Parents given opportunity to handle baby.
- Consultant paediatrician and consultant obstetrician informed.
- General practitioner informed.
- Community midwives and/or health visitor informed.
- Consent for post-mortem (PM) requested – given/refused.
- Parents offered 'Guide to the Post-Mortem Examination'.
- PM form completed: date and time of PM confirmed.
- Preliminary results of PM explained to parents.
- Death/stillbirth certificate completed and given to parents.
- Information about funeral arrangements given to parents.
- Parents offered booklet 'Saying Goodbye to Your Baby'.
- Parents told about support groups and given contact telephone numbers.
- Parents seen by counsellor/social worker.
- Parents seen by consultant obstetrician/paediatrician.
- Religious adviser notified if parents wish.
- Religious service requested/arranged.
- Photographs taken of baby – with parents if wished.
- Footprints/handprints of baby taken.
- Other keepsakes collected: parents advised of book of remembrance.
- Follow-up visits arranged.

Some of the items on this list must be dealt with promptly – the family doctor and community midwife must know of the death before grieving relatives call them. If religious beliefs allow, discussion about the PM and funeral may be left to the following day, when the parents will be more able to absorb what is said to them.

Follow-up meetings must be arranged. The paediatrician should have clear goals for such visits. At a first meeting the tasks of the paediatrician include:

- Reviewing the baby's medical problems and answering all questions about them.
- Discussing the findings of the PM if one was performed.
- Ensuring that appropriate postnatal follow-up is in place, including an appointment with a consultant obstetrician if necessary.
- Assessing how the couple are grieving.
  Can they talk to each other about the baby, using his/her first name?
  Have they had a funeral and said goodbye?
  Are they grieving differently – is the father buried in work while the mother weeps at home?
  Are they eating and sleeping reasonably under the circumstances?
- Reminding them of support groups and encouraging contact if appropriate.
- Helping them to begin to look to the future.
- Considering if genetic counselling is needed.
- Asking if the parents are thinking about the next pregnancy. Could there be an unplanned early conception – would this be a problem if it happened?
- Explaining the risks of the same thing happening again.

- Counselling the parents that it is normal to feel sad for many months after such a loss, but that they should seek help if symptoms worsen or persist too long.

It is virtually impossible to achieve all this at one visit soon after the death. The paediatrician or a counsellor may need sessions with the parents over a period of several months, and these may be best held away from the hospital.

Last but not least is the question of caring for the carers. Junior nurses and doctors find perinatal deaths extremely distressing and must be given time to reflect on the issues surrounding an individual death, particularly if they feel guilt as part of their grief. Senior colleagues must support and counsel them. These same senior staff who may have been involved in very distressing conversations and procedures must learn to turn to each other for help, or be confident of strong support outside the neonatal unit. The stress of dealing with a neonatal death is one of the experiences known to contribute to psychological 'burn-out' of neonatologists. Its impact should not be dismissed lightly.

The Stillbirth and Neonatal Death Society can be contacted at:

Stillbirth and Neonatal Death Society
28 Portland Place
London W1N 4DE
Tel: 0171 436 5881 (Helpline)
     0171 436 7940 (Administration)

Further reading

Guide to the Post-Mortem Examination. London: Department of Health, 1994.
McIntosh N, Eldridge C. Neonatal death – the neglected side of neonatal care? *Archives of Disease in Childhood*, 1984; **59**: 585–7.
Royal College of Paediatrics and Child Health. *Withholding or Withdrawing Life Saving Treatment in Children*. Royal College of Paediatrics and Child Health, 1997.
Royal College of Obstetricians and Gynaecologists. *Report of the Working Party on Management of Perinatal Deaths*. London: Royal College of Obstetricians and Gynaecologists, 1985.
Saying Goodbye to Your Baby. London: Stillbirth and Neonatal Death Society, 1997.
Wigglesworth JS. *Perinatal Pathology*, 2nd edn. London: W.B. Saunders, 1996.

Related topics of interest

Congenital malformations and birth defects (p. 70)
Extreme prematurity (p. 80)
Hypoxic–ischaemic encephalopathy (p. 128)
Inherited metabolic disease – investigation and management (p. 156)

DISCHARGE PLANNING AND FOLLOW-UP

There are three main groups of infants to consider.

1. The otherwise well term or near-term newborn infant following a hospital delivery.
2. Term or near-term infants with proven or suspected disorders, e.g. congenital anomaly, which require medical intervention(s) in the perinatal period.
3. Preterm infants who have required varying periods of care on the neonatal unit.

The well term or near-term newborn infant

There is no consensus on the optimum post-partum length of stay for healthy term infants. There is a worldwide variation in policies and guidelines on the perinatal stay. Generally, the usual stay for a vaginal delivery in most countries is 1–3 days and up to 7 days after a Caesarean section. Discharges may, however, be done as early as 6–8 hours depending on, among other things, social and financial factors. The timing of each discharge is probably best individualized for each infant depending on the individual medical, social and economic aspects. Prior to discharge, however, the following important points should be noted:

- The infant is feeding well.
- The infant has voided urine and passed stools.
- The physical examination is normal.
- There is no evidence of clinical jaundice in the first 24 hours.
- The mother is well and capable of looking after her newborn infant(s).
- There are no adverse social, environmental or familial factors which would jeopardize the safety or wellbeing of the infant following discharge (e.g. history of domestic violence, child abuse or homelessness).
- Any necessary vaccinations (e.g. for hepatitis B or BCG have been administered).

The problematic term or near-term infant

These infants may be discharged once their problems have resolved (e.g. transient tachypnoea) or once appropriate investigations or therapies have been instituted (e.g. renal scan for antenatally diagnosed hydronephrosis) and follow-up appointment(s) have been made.

The ex-preterm infant

The discharge of infants who have required neonatal care for prematurity and related disorders requires more planning. Once it looks likely that the infant's discharge is imminent, the parent(s) should be notified so they can prepare themselves for their baby's homecoming. This enables the parents to receive a comprehensive training which reduces parental anxiety and increases their satisfaction. The following should be addressed.

1. *Social and environmental factors*
   - Assess adequacy of home environment and domestic arrangements and obtain a home visit by the health visitor if necessary.
   - If home oxygen therapy will be required, make arrangements for the appropriate equipment to be installed.
   - Check that there are no concerns regarding child protection matters (e.g. parental drug or alcohol abuse, maternal postnatal depression or other adverse factors) which would prejudice the infant's care.

2. *Parental factors*
   - Instruct parents on the special requirements of their infant (e.g. general routine infant care after discharge, positioning, avoidance of over-heating, risk of cot death, avoid smoking indoors especially with home oxygen therapy).
   - Inform parents of the common signs of ill-health and when to obtain assistance for their infant.
   - Assess adequacy of parenting skills and teach parents where appropriate (e.g. cardiopulmonary resuscitation training for infants on supplemental oxygen therapy).
   - The mother should be invited to 'room in' on the neonatal unit to familiarize herself with her infant's care requirements (especially first-time mothers) and this also gives the NICU staff an opportunity to assess parental skills and competency.

3. *Infant factors*
   - Temperature should be maintained in an open cot.
   - The infant should be feeding well with a steady weight gain (10–30 g/day).
   - There should be no recent apnoeas or bradycardias (5–8 days before discharge).
   - Infants at risk of retinopathy of prematurity (ROP) should have been screened for this and any outstanding follow-up appointments formalized.
   - High-risk infants (e.g. severe jaundice, neonatal meningitis, congenital rubella or cytomegalovirus (CMV), family history of deafness) should have a formal audiological examination.
   - No absolute discharge weight requirements exist, though most infants are >1800 g at discharge and >35–37 weeks gestation. Infants of birthweight <1000 g are generally older at discharge (>37 weeks gestation) due to associated problems of prematurity.
   - Earlier home discharges are possible in the presence of comprehensive support in the community by dedicated and skilled neonatal nurses and competent parents who have been adequately prepared prior to discharge.

4. On discharge home

- Ascertain that the parents are clear on how to administer any necessary medications and how to obtain further supplies.
- Document any immunizations given in the parent-held record.
- Give written records of any follow-up appointments or hospital visits.
- Send summary of hospital course, medications and follow-up plans to the general practitioner and any other relevant primary care workers (e.g. health visitor, community midwife) with copies to the relevant hospital records.

Who needs follow-up?   Conditions needing follow-up are numerous and partly depend on the available resources and expertise. While a complete list would be inappropriate for every setting, some of the common reasons include:

- Prolonged jaundice.
- Infants at risk from child abuse.
- Infants of drug abusing mothers.
- Congenital infections (e.g. CMV).
- Haematological disorders (e.g. thalassaemia).
- Infants who had severe sepsis (e.g. meningitis).
- Complications of neonatal intensive care (e.g. BPD, IVH, ROP).
- Infants with metabolic or endocrine disorders (e.g. suspected hypothyroidism).
- Congenital malformations and birth defects (e.g. renal and urinary tract disorders).
- Infants who experienced significant perinatal complications (e.g. birth injuries, asphyxia).

Further reading

Britton JR (ed). Early perinatal hospital discharge: issues and concerns. *Clinics in Perinatology*, 1998; **25** (2).

Powell PJ, Povell CV, Hollis S, Robinson MJ *et al*. When will my baby go home? *Archives of Disease in Childhood*, 1992; **67:** 1214–6.

Casiro OG, McKenzie ME, McFadyen L *et al*. Early discharge with community-based intervention for low birthweight infants: a randomized trial. *Pediatrics*, 1993; **92:** 128–34.

Rawlings J, Scott J. Post-conceptional age of surviving low birthweight preterm infants at hospital discharge. *Archives of Pediatrics and Adolescent Medicine*, 1996; **150:** 260–2.

Samuels MP, Southall DP. Home oxygen therapy. In: David TJ (ed). *Recent Advances in Paediatrics, No. 14*. Edinburgh: Churchill Livingstone, 1995; 37–51.

Related topics of interest

EXTRACORPOREAL MEMBRANE OXYGENATION

ECMO is a technique for treating severe respiratory failure from which the patient can be expected to recover within 1–2 weeks. One of its main applications is the treatment of term babies with meconium aspiration syndrome, CDH, PPHN or pneumonia. Contraindications to ECMO include major congenital abnormalities, IVH, irreversible cardiopulmonary disease, NEC and a period of asystole. Before starting ECMO, each baby should have echocardiography to exclude cyanotic CHD (particularly total anomalous pulmonary venous drainage) and an ultrasound scan of the brain. Prolonged high-pressure ventilation causes lung damage, so babies need to be transferred onto ECMO ideally after less than 7 to 10 days' conventional ventilation. It is used only in babies ≥ 35 weeks as the heparinization could cause severe intracranial haemorrhage in more immature infants.

The jugular vein is cannulated and blood flows into a primed heparinized circuit with a pump, membrane oxygenator and bubble trap before being returned to the baby, either via the carotid artery (veno-arterial ECMO) or right atrium (veno-venous ECMO). The latter is now the treatment of choice as it avoids the need to tie off the cannulated carotid artery and thence relying on anastomoses to maintain the circulation from the contralateral carotid artery. During treatment the baby is gently ventilated to maintain lung inflation, but the main source of gas exchange is the membrane oxygenator. Following promising reports of trials on small numbers of babies, over 75 ECMO centres opened in the US and submitted data to the ECMO Registry. Currently, over 12 000 infants have been treated, with an overall 80% survival, but 95% survival for meconium aspiration syndrome. These infants would have had expected mortality rates of approximately 80%.

In the UK, a more circumspect approach was taken as fewer term babies were seen with respiratory failure. In a multicentre, randomized trial of 185 term babies, 30 of 93 babies allocated to ECMO died, compared with 55 of the 92 allocated to conventional management (CM). The relative risk was 0.55 (95% CI, 0.39–0.77), equivalent to one extra survivor for every three to four babies allocated ECMO. However, outcome in those with diaphragmatic hernia was poor: all 17 in the CM group died, as did 14 of the 18 allocated ECMO. More data are needed to help understand the role of ECMO in infants with diaphragmatic herniae. When that group was excluded, the survival was 79% in the ECMO group, 51% in those allocated CM. Of the 124 initially followed to 1 year, 51% of those allocated to ECMO were alive with no signs of impairment (74% of survivors), compared with only 28% of those allocated CM (71% of survivors).

ECMO therefore has a clearly established role in the treatment of term babies with severe respiratory failure. Technical problems of cannulation make it difficult to use this technique in smaller babies. The development of tubing with heparin bonded onto the walls may enable a reduction in systemic heparinization. Treatment with inhaled NO in babies who would normally qualify for ECMO reduces the need for ECMO by about 60%. Pleasing as this is, it does mean that neonatal transport incubators will need NO circuits in the future to transfer babies who have become NO-dependent but still need to be transported to an ECMO centre.

There remains the question as to the threshold for starting ECMO in babies with meconium aspiration, pneumonia or PPHN (persistent fetal circulation), and indeed diaphragmatic hernia. The criterion that is usually considered is the oxygenation index (OI) which is calculated as:

Mean airway pressure (cmH_2O) $\times$ FiO_2 (%) $\div$ post-ductal PaO_2 (mmHg).

In the UK trial, the entry criterion was an OI of ≥ 40, or a $PaCO_2$ of $>12\,kPa$ for 3 hours. In view of the success of ECMO it may be best to lower the threshold to an OI of 30 or even 25, though there are no published data to support this. The UK trial clearly showed, however, that referral of very ill infants to ECMO centres resulted in some infants dying before ECMO could be instituted.

The collaborative UK ECMO trial 1-year follow-up data show that ECMO support reduces the risk of mortality, without a major concomitant rise in severe disability, by about 45%, regardless of the severity of the infant's condition. The results of the economic evaluation, carried out alongside the trial, based on the principal end-point of death or severe disability at age 1 year, found the additional cost of ECMO per additional survivor to be within the range of other life-extending technologies such as renal transplantation.

Further reading

Graziani LJ, Gringlas M, Baumgart S. Cerebrovascular complications and neurodevelopmental sequelae of neonatal ECMO. *Clinics in Perinatology*, 1997; **24**: 655–75.

Kanto WP, Bunyapen C. Extracorporeal membrane oxygenation: controversies in selection of patients and management. *Clinics in Perinatology*, 1998; **25**: 123–35.

Soll RF. Neonatal extracorporeal membrane oxygenation – a bridging technique. *Lancet*, 1996; **348**: 70–1.

UK Collaborative ECMO Trial Group. UK collaborative randomized trial of neonatal extracorporeal membrane oxygenation. *Lancet*, 1996; **348**: 75–82.

UK Collaborative ECMO Group. The Collaborative UK ECMO Trial: follow-up to 1 year of age. *Pediatrics*, 1998; **101(4)**.

Related topics of interest

EXTREME PREMATURITY

The last 30 years have witnessed remarkable improvements in the survival of small preterm infants. US data, for instance, shows a 70-fold increase in the number of survivors per 1000 live births between 1960 and 1983. The introduction of surfactant in the last 10 years has produced even further improvements in survival (but with no concomitant reduction in neurodevelopmental morbidity), particularly in the lowest birthweights where survival had previously been exceptionally low. Until recent years, 28 weeks was considered the edge of viability for a neonate. However, this 'edge' has been retreating to the currently perceived limit of extrauterine survival (22–23 weeks). Intact survival of a 280 g infant has been reported. The term extreme prematurity is now used in everyday parlance to refer to gestations at the lower margin of viability, particularly those of 22–25 weeks (and not the strict definition of <28 weeks).

- Extremely preterm babies make heavy demands on health resources.
- They have a high mortality rate and a high risk of neurological or respiratory morbidity should they survive.
- Gestational age is a better predictor of neonatal mortality than birthweight.
- The great concern felt for individual babies and for the group as a whole has led to careful analysis of outcomes. The hope is that such information will enable appropriate decision-making that will in turn improve survival and the quality of survival.

Survival

- Many valuable data are emerging from the UK EPICure study which was a population-based study on the outcomes for babies born at 20–25 weeks gestation in the UK and Ireland during 9 months in 1995.
- 803 of 3781 such babies were admitted to NNUs. Data were available on 94% of the admissions.

Table 1 summarizes some outcomes at the expected date of delivery (EDD) of the babies. Survival and neurological data will be collected again after a further 2 years. The table also shows data collated by Rennie of reports on survival from 1977 to 1993, although the collection of denominator data (i.e. the total number of babies born at a given gestation) probably varied between reports.

Table 1. Survival by gestation

Gestation (weeks)	Admission rates to NNU (%)	Survival (%) to EDD of those admitted to NNU	Survival (%) as reported by Rennie with 95% CI
23	22	28	16 (12–19)
24	50	35	35 (31–38)
25	61	54	48 (45–50)
26			57 (55–60)

Neurodevelopmental disability and handicap

The issue is not just of survival but of intact survival. By the time of their EDD:

- 50% of survivors in the EPICure study were still in oxygen.
- 17% had parenchymal cysts and/or hydrocephalus on their last scan.
- 13% had needed treatment for retinopathy of prematurity.

Normality has proved hard to define: initial studies concentrated upon major handicaps – cerebral palsy, deafness, blindness and major learning difficulties. It is now recognized that subtle effects upon behaviour with reduced attention span and increased distractibility contribute to learning difficulties and school failure in some ex-premature babies. Many of these children need extra help to fulfil their potential. The incidence of chronic lung disease varies inversely with gestation and adds to the morbidity of the most preterm babies.

Table 2 shows some published data on handicap rates amongst survivors of extreme prematurity. Rates vary between centres because outcomes may genuinely be different, or because definitions and the age of assessment vary. Furthermore, the 95% confidence intervals for these proportions of handicapped children are very wide – in excess of 20% at the lowest gestations, where the numbers of survivors are small. Nevertheless, about 25% of surviving babies of 26 weeks gestation have severe disability: most centres have higher rates of handicap below 26 weeks.

Management at birth

- Two experienced paediatricians should attend the birth of an extremely preterm baby.
- If time allows, they should see the parents beforehand, discuss the possible outcomes and draft a plan of management. However, it may be very difficult to communicate effectively with a distressed couple or mother once preterm labour has started.
- Prior to birth, the chances of normal and/or handicapped survival should be assessed and discussed. The purpose of

Table 2. Disability by gestation

Gestation (weeks)	Handicapped survivors (%) Data from Rennie's review[a]:	Severe disability in survivors at 4 years (%) Babies born 1984–6 Data from Oxford region	Severe disability in survivors at 1 year (%) Babies born 1983–94 Data from Northern region
23	62	50 (≤ 25 weeks)	24 (≤ 25 weeks)
24	38		
25	31		
26	24	21	27 (26 and 27 weeks)

[a] Rennie's review included the Oxford data.

resuscitation and neonatal intensive care is to achieve a healthy outcome, but this goal is not always reached. Doctors need to be realistic and help parents accept the very real difficulties. This is particularly hard for those who have waited many years and perhaps had multiple courses of infertility treatment.

Individual units and paediatricians reach their own ethical decisions. In the light of published survival and morbidity rates, few paediatricians encourage active resuscitation below 23 weeks. At 25 weeks and above, full resuscitation and intensive care should be started, remembering that to start intensive care is not to continue it unconditionally. If the likelihood of severe neurological handicap becomes very high, there is the option of discontinuing intensive care and offering palliative nursing care. The greatest dilemmas lie at 23 and 24 weeks. A personal approach is to discuss the issues jointly with parents and obstetricians, and to offer resuscitation and then early assessment – with a view to stopping or continuing intensive care. If risk factors such as prolonged oligohydramnios or reversed EDF in the fetus have been recognized and the chances of viability are lowered even further, then resuscitation may be reasonably withheld if all agree. When circumstances do not permit a full discussion and assessment before birth, resuscitation is the rule. The baby could be several weeks older than the mother thinks!

Special notes

- The 3-year survival for infants of birthweight ≤500 g is extremely poor (3.4%).
- In infants of birthweight ≤500 g, 90% of all deaths occur within the first 3 days of life.
- World literature reports very few survivors at 22 weeks (mostly from Japan, but none were free of neurological sequelae).
- Some degree of impairment is found in up to 70% of survivors at 23 weeks gestation.
- Female infants have a survival advantage equivalent to almost one additional gestational week.
- In extremely preterm infants, morbidity is inversely related to birthweight and gestational age.

Further reading

Bregman J. Developmental outcome in very low birthweight infants: current status and future trends. *Pediatric Clinics of North America*, 1998; **45:** 673–90.

Johnson A, Townshend P, Yudkin P, Bull D, Wilkinson AR. Functional abilities at age 4 years of children born before 29 weeks of gestation. *British Medical Journal*, 1993; **306:** 1715–8.

Rennie JM. Perinatal management at the lower margin of viability. *Archives of Disease in Childhood*, 1996; **74:** F214–8.

Royal College of Paediatrics and Child Health. *Withholding or Withdrawing Life-saving Treatment in Children*. London: Royal College of Paediatrics and Child Health, 1997.

Tin W, Wariyar U, Hey N (Northern Neonatal Network). Changing prognosis for babies of less than 28 weeks gestation in the north of England between 1983 and 1994. *British Medical Journal*, 1997; **314:** 107–11

Wilkinson AR, EPICure Study Steering Group. The extremely preterm baby – a population-based study of outcomes of babies born before 26 weeks gestation in the UK and Ireland. *Pediatric Research*, 1997; **42:** 402 (Abs. 103).

Related topics of interest

Bronchopulmonary dysplasia (p. 38)
Death of a baby (p. 72)
Multiple pregnancy (p. 192)
Pregnancy complications and fetal health (p. 247)
Resuscitation (p. 282)

FEEDING DIFFICULTIES

Feeding difficulties are extremely common in the newborn period. These may be categorized as transient or persistent. Transient feeding difficulties invariably are related to perinatal factors and commonly resolve within the first few days or weeks of life. Persistent feeding difficulties suggest an underlying organic cause and require careful evaluation to determine the correct aetiology and therefore appropriate management. For transient feeding difficulties, both maternal and infant factors can be identified.

Transient feeding difficulties

Maternal factors

- Inexperienced first-time mother(s).
- Pregnancy-related maternal illness (e.g. severe pre-eclampsia, eclampsia, delivery complications, postnatal depression).
- Pre-existing chronic maternal illness (e.g. rheumatoid arthritis, multiple sclerosis).
- Breast abnormalities in breast-feeding mothers (e.g. inverted nipples, previous breast surgery or injury).
- Maternal medication – drugs taken during pregnancy and/or delivery may adversely affect the infant, e.g. benzodiazepines (drowsy infant) and methadone (neonatal drug withdrawal syndrome).
- Maternal anxiety.

Infant factors

- Prematurity (immature suck and swallow reflex).
- Traumatic delivery (instrumental delivery with facial injury).
- Hypoglycaemia.
- Birth asphyxia.
- Cold stress.
- Intrauterine growth restriction (IUGR).
- Sepsis.

With appropriate support from the midwifery and neonatal staff, most mothers and their infants can be successfully supported through the initial transitional period to feed their infants by their preferred method. If feeding is particularly poor, capillary blood sugars should be monitored regularly (until they are persistently ≥ 4 mmol/l). Nasogastric tube feeds may be required in the preterm, small for gestational age, or large infants of diabetic mothers.

Persistent feeding difficulties

A careful search often reveals a cause in most of these infants. The possible causes are numerous.

Neurological abnormalities	• Local (e.g. facial nerve palsy, bulbar and suprabulbar palsy, vocal cord palsy). • Central (e.g. CNS malformations, severe intracranial haemorrhage, severe hydrocephalus, seizures).
Neuromuscular disorders	• Spinal muscular atrophy. • Myotonic dystrophy and other muscular dystrophies. • Prader–Willi syndrome. • Myasthenia gravis.
Syndromic disorders	• Down's syndrome. • Moebias syndrome. • Pierre–Robin sequence. • Roberts' syndrome. • Beckwith–Wiedemann syndrome.
Anatomical defects	• Cleft lip and palate. • Submucous cleft. • Choanal atresia/stenosis. • Oesophageal atresia (associated polyhydramnios). • Tracheoesophageal fistula. • Laryngeal webs and clefts. • Oesophageal compression (e.g. vascular rings). • Gut malrotation. • Oropharyngeal vascular malformations (e.g. carvenous haemangioma). • Tumours.
Metabolic disorders	• Galactosaemia. • Hypothyroidism. • Organic and amino acidopathies (e.g. propionic acidaemia, non-ketotic hyperglycinaemia). • Urea cycle defects. • Other inherited metabolic disorders.
Miscellaneous disorders	• Isolated swallowing disorders with pharyngeal and cricopharyngeal incoordination. • Chalasia or achalasia of oesophagus. • Stomatitis. • Oesophagitis.
Investigations	• pH monitoring (reflux oesophagitis). • Endoscopy (reflux oesophagitis). • Barium swallow and follow through (haitus hernia, malrotation). • Chromosomes (dysmorphic infants). • Laryngoscopy. • Video fluoroscopy. • Cranial ultrasound. • Cranial CT/MRI.

Management

- Oropharyngeal stimulation (non-nutritive sucking).
- Use of special teats and bottle (cleft lip/palate).
- Orthodontic devices (cleft lip/palate).
- Nasogastric tube feeding.
- Gastrostomy (persistent difficulties especially in the neurologically impaired).
- Nissen fundoplication (especially in neurologically impaired infants).

Multidisciplinary teams are often required in managing these infants. Infants with anatomical defects (e.g. cleft lip and palate, oesophageal atresia) may require the input of plastic surgeons, orthodontists, faciomaxillary surgeons, speech therapists and dietitians. Even in the absence of anatomical defects requiring surgery, speech and language therapists and dietitians are often required to optimize the calorie intake of such infants. Similarly, a paediatric neurologist and clinical geneticist may offer valuable advice in infants with suspected neurological disorders and dysmorphic features, respectively. Remember to exclude feed intolerance, especially with a family history of atopy, cow's milk protein intolerance, or other rarer metabolic disorders.

Further reading

Arvedson JC, Brodsky L. *Paediatric Swallowing and Feeding Assessment and Management*. London: Wharr Publishers, 1993.

Cooper PJ, Stein A (eds). *Feeding Problems and Eating Disorders in Children and Adolescence*. Reading: Harwood Academic Publishers, 1992.

Gisel EG, Birnbaum R, Schwartz S. Helping the feeding impaired child. In: David TJ (ed). *Recent Advances in Paediatrics, Number 16*. Edinburgh: Churchill Livingstone, 1997; 59–71.

Hyman P. Gastroesophageal reflux: one reason why baby won't eat. *Journal of Pediatrics*, 1994; **125**: S103–9.

Related topics of interest

FLUID AND ELECTROLYTE THERAPY

The management of fluid and electrolyte administration is vital in the management of sick newborn infants. The handling of water and solute by the immature kidneys is impaired and this is often compounded by large water losses through the highly permeable immature skin. To maintain normal fluid and electrolyte balance it is therefore necessary to accurately control their administration.

Water balance

Approximately 75% of the total bodyweight is water, half of which is extracellular fluid. A reduction of the extracellular space occurs during the first week of life, accounting for most of the 10–15% reduction in bodyweight; inadequate calorie intake accounts for the remainder of the weight loss. Respiratory distress syndrome (RDS) is associated with a delayed contraction of the extracellular fluid volume which occurs with resolution of RDS.

Factors associated with increased water loss

- Use of radiant warmers.
- Phototherapy.
- Preterm thin skin.
- Poor humidification of respiratory gases.
- Watery stools.
- High ileostomy losses.
- Osmotic diuresis (e.g. glycosuria).
- Low ambient humidity.

Factors associated with water overload

- Excess fluid administration.
- Inappropriate sodium administration.
- Conditions associated with inappropriate antidiuretic hormone (ADH) secretion (e.g. pneumonia, RDS).

Remedial steps to maintain optimal water balance

- Avoid nursing very preterm infants under radiant warmers.
- Cover infants with plastic sheeting to reduce fluid losses.
- Nurse newborn infants in humid environment.
- Humidify respiratory gases adequately for infants receiving respiratory support.

Adverse effects of fluid overload

- Persistence of ductus arteriosus.
- Chronic lung disease.
- Increased mortality.

Electrolyte balance

The main extracellular and intracellular cations are sodium and potassium, respectively. Sodium absorption is under the influence of renin–angiotensin–aldosterone, while potassium absorption is influenced by mineralocorticoids with potassium being exchanged for hydrogen in the kidneys. Potassium excretion is greatly reduced in renal failure. Sodium supplementation is not required until after the reduction of extracellular fluid space (24–48 hours), but thereafter sodium may be supplemented at 4 mmol/kg/day (or more depending on serum sodium) in preterm infants and 2 mmol/kg/day in term infants. Aim to keep sodium between 135–140 mmol/l. Potassium is supplemented at 2 mmol/kg/day if urine output is satisfactory.

While calcium is predominantly stored in bone, 40% of that in the extracellular fluid is bound to albumin, the rest (approximately 1.25 mmol/l) being free ionized calcium (ionized calcium falls with rising pH). For every 10 g fall in albumin below 40 g/l, the total calcium is reduced by 0.05 mmol/l.

Calcium homeostasis is under the influence of calcitonin, parathormone and vitamin D (1,25-dihydroxyvitamin D). Parathormone increases calcium absorption from the gut and kidneys. Intravenous supplementation should provide 2 mmol/kg/day and oral supplementation 1.75–3.5 mmol/kg/day (with a calcium phosphate ratio of 1.4–2:1). Avoid rapid i.v. administration of calcium (as calcium gluconate) as this causes bradycardia, and beware of extravasation (produces unsightly scars).

Phosphate, like calcium, is a major constituent of bone and its absorption from the gut and kidneys is influenced by vitamin D and parathormone. Intravenous supplements of 1 mmol/kg/day are appropriate with oral supplements of 1.6 mmol per 100 kilocalories. Human milk contains low phosphorus levels (0.4 mmol/l), making it mandatory to supplement preterm infants fed on breast milk.

Magnesium is mainly an intracellular ion excreted by kidneys and absorbed from the gut. Always check serum magnesium when hypocalcaemia is present. For urgent replacement, give a slow infusion of 25% magnesium sulphate at 0.5 mmol/kg or intramuscularly as 0.1 ml/kg of 50% magnesium sulphate. For oral supplementation, give as 10% magnesium chloride once daily. Diuretics may cause hypomagnesaemia.

Chloride is an extracellular ion whose requirements are usually met from the normal dietary chloride.

Monitoring fluid and electrolyte therapy

Changes in weight relate well to total body water in newborns. Daily weights are a valuable aid in fluid management. Similarly, urine output should be monitored (minimum 1 ml/kg/hour and maximum 7 ml/kg/hour).

- Measure serum sodium, potassium, urea, creatinine and calcium daily in sick infants.
- With abnormal electrolytes and/or large fluid requirements, 6-hourly electrolyte determinations may be required.
- Paired measurements of plasma and urine osmolarity are helpful in diagnosing inappropriate ADH secretion.

Plasma osmolarity = $(2 \times \text{sodium}) + (2 \times \text{potassium})$ + glucose + urea (all values in mmol/l).

Suspect inappropriate ADH if the urine is not maximally dilute (>100 mosmol/l) with serum osmolarity of <270 mosmol/l.

Normal values

Sodium	132–145 mmol/l
Potassium	3.6–5.9 mmol/l
Urea	1–5 mmol/l
Creatinine	<20–150 μmol/l
Chloride	90–110 mmol/l
Calcium	
Total	1.9–2.85 mmol/l
Ionized	1.12–1.52 mmol/l
Magnesium	0.71–1.1 mmol/l
Phosphate	1.4–3.0 mmol/l
Plasma osmolarity	280–300 mosmol/l
Urine osmolarity	100–700 mosmol/l

Further reading

Modi N. Development of renal function. *British Medical Bulletin*, 1988; **44**: 925–56.

Modi N. Sodium intake and preterm babies. *Archives of Disease in Childhood*, 1995; **69**: 87–91.

Sedin G. Fluid management in the extremely preterm infant. In: Hansen TN, McIntosh N (eds). *Current Topics in Neonatology, No. 1*. London: W.B. Saunders, 1996; 50–66.

Shaffer SG, Weisman DN. Fluid requirements in the preterm infant. *Clinics in Perinatology*, 1992; **19**: 233–46.

Sinclair JC, Bracken MB (eds). *Effective Care of the Newborn Infant*. Oxford: Oxford University Press, 1992.

Spitzer AR (ed). *Intensive Care of the Fetus and Neonate*. St. Louis: C.V. Mosby, 1996.

Tsang RC, Lucas A, Uauy R, Zlotkin S (eds). *Nutritional Needs of the Preterm Infant: Scientific Basis and Practical Guidelines*. Baltimore: Williams & Wilkins, 1993.

Related topics of interest

GASTRO-OESOPHAGEAL REFLUX

Gastro-oesophageal reflux (GOR) is one of the commonest symptomatic clinical disorders affecting the gastrointestinal tract of infants and children. In recent years, GOR has been recognized more frequently because of the increased awareness of the condition and more sophisticated diagnostic techniques that have been developed for both identifying and quantifying the disorder. It must be appreciated, however, that virtually all infants have some degree of GOR, though the severity of symptoms varies from the occasional posset to persistent vomiting. In the vast majority of infants with GOR, symptoms improve spontaneously between the ages of 9 and 24 months. Most infants with GOR are healthy and thriving and require no diagnostic or therapeutic interventions, other than a careful history and examination with appropriate reassurance being given to the parents.

Aetiology

GOR is commonly due to a weakness of the gastro-oesophageal junction sphincter. In addition, there may be an associated hiatus hernia. Chronic respiratory disorders, particularly bronchopulmonary dysplasia, are associated with an increased incidence of GOR, as are some neuromuscular disorders. It is also more common following some forms of thoraco-abdominal surgery (e.g. repair of oesophageal atresia and congenital diaphragmatic hernia). Conditions which delay gastric emptying encourage GOR. Methylxanthines may also promote GOR as they reduce the lower oesophageal sphincter tone. Overfeeding may also encourage reflux.

Clinical features

- Frequent small vomits to severe vomiting after feeds.
- Persistent small or large vomits which continue long after feeds.
- Difficulty with feeds and crying during feeds from associated oesophagitis.
- 'Unexplained' deteriorations in respiratory status.
- Repeated aspirations and aspiration pneumonias.
- Reflex apnoeas refractory to other therapies.

Some infants with GOR exhibit abnormal behaviour and posturing with tilting of the head to one side and bizarre contortions of the trunk, which has been labelled the Sandifer's syndrome.

Investigation

1. Chest X-ray. Look for the radiographic changes of aspiration.

2. Barium swallow. Look for oesophageal anomalies, reflux, malrotation and hiatus hernia.

3. pH monitoring. Oesophageal pH monitoring for 12–24 hours is the most sensitive investigation for detecting, quantifying and monitoring GOR. The pH should be less than 4.0 for <5% of the study time. Values of ≥15% denote severe GOR.

4. Endoscopy. The availability of small fibreoptic endoscopes in recent years has made it possible for small infants and children with GOR to undergo endoscopy in order to directly visualize the oesophageal mucosa and take biopsies to determine the severity of reflux oesophagitis.

Management

1. Postural. Keep the infant prone with head elevated (anti-Trendelenberg position). Do *not* nurse the infant sitting at an angle of 60° as this is associated with worse reflux. The right lateral position is associated with more reflux than positioning the infant in the prone or left lateral positions.

2. Feeding. Give small frequent feeds. Nasogastric feeds may also be helpful as may food thickening agents, e.g. Carobel (Cow & Gate) or Nestargel (Nestlé). Food thickeners, however, are not suitable for small preterm infants, and although they may produce symptomatic relief, they do not improve reflux. Thickeners may also increase episodic coughing.

3. Drugs
- Antacids such as Gaviscon may be beneficial.
- H_2-antagonists (e.g. cimetidine or ranitidine) may relieve associated oesophagitis.
- Gastrokinetic agents (e.g. cisapride and domperidone) are agents which improve gastro-oesophageal motility and gastric emptying. Cisapride is thought to enhance the physiological release of acetylcholine at the myenteric plexus of the intestine. Gastric emptying is accelerated by an increase in gastric and duodenal contractility. Gastric reflux into the oesophagus is decreased through a mechanism of increasing oesophageal peristaltic activity and enhancing oesophageal sphincter tone. Studies report decreased gastric residuals, decreased incidence of vomiting, a decrease in all reflux parameters measured and improved weight gain in infants with vomiting. The average dose used in most studies is 200 μg/kg 6–8-hourly.
- Proton pump inhibitors (e.g. omeprazole) are relatively new agents which inhibit the final step (H^+/K^+ ATPase) in gastric acid release from the parietal cell. They not only increase the pH of the refluxate, but also decrease total gastric secretion volume, thereby facilitating gastric emptying. Omeprazole is effective therapy for histamine receptor type 2 antagonist-resistant peptic oesophagitis and relieves most symptoms and signs of GOR, including those who have failed surgery. It is safe for short-term use (3–6 months) at doses of 20–40 mg/m^2/day (0.5 mg/kg once daily = 20 mg/m^2/day).

4. Surgery. When medical therapy has failed in infants with severe symptoms, especially in the presence of severe chronic lung disease, Nissen fundoplication may be required. It is worth remembering, however, that antireflux surgery has a significant failure and complication rate and occasional mortality, particularly in the neurologically impaired. In one study, >30% of neurologically impaired children had major complications or died within 30 days of surgery; within a mean follow-up of 3.5 years, 25% had documented operative failure, and overall 71% had return of one or more pre-operative symptoms of GOR. Increasing use of proton pump inhibitors may decrease the need for surgery.

Special note The Committee on Safety of Medicines has recently advised against the use of Cisapride in preterm infants (<36 weeks' gestation) for up to 3 months after birth, due to the risk of arrhythmias. (CSM/MCA. *Current Problems in Pharmacovigilance*, 1998; **24**: 11.)

Further reading

Alliet P, Raes M, Bruneel E, Gillis P. Omeprazole in infants with cimetidine-resistant peptic oesophagitis. *Journal of Pediatrics*, 1998; **132**: 352–4.

Ashcraft KW. Gastroesophageal reflux. In: Ashcraft KW, Holder TM (eds). *Pediatric Surgery*, 2nd edn. Philadelphia: W.B. Saunders, 1993; 270–88.

Gunasekaran TS, Hassall E. Efficacy and safety of omeprazole for severe gastroesophageal reflux in children. *Journal of Pediatrics*, 1993; **124**: 148–54.

Hassall E. Wrap session: is the Nissen slipping? Can medical treatment replace surgery for severe gastroesophageal reflux in children? *American Journal of Gastroenterology*, 1995; **90**: 1212–20.

Hillemeier AC. Gastroesophageal reflux: diagnosis and therapeutic approaches. *Pediatric Clinics of North America*, 1996; **43**: 197–212.

Hyams JS, Ricci A, Leighkner AM. Clinical and laboratory correlates of oesophagitis in young children. *Journal of Paediatric Gastroenterology and Nutrition*, 1988; **7**: 52–6.

Hyman P. Gastroesophageal reflux: one reason why baby won't eat. *Journal of Pediatrics*, 1994; **125**: S103–9.

Newell SJ, Booth IW, Morgan MEI, Durbin GM, McNeish AS. Gastro-oesophageal reflux in preterm infants. *Archives of Disease in Childhood*, 1989; **6**: 780–6.

Related topics of interest

GERMINAL MATRIX-INTRAVENTRICULAR HAEMORRHAGE

The last two decades have witnessed a striking improvement in the survival of very premature infants due mainly to the major improvements in perinatal medicine. There has also been a reassuring fall in the incidence of germinal matrix-intraventricular haemorrhage (IVH) from 40–50% to 20% in infants of birthweights less than 1500 g. However, IVH remains very common in the extremely preterm infant. The two major sequelae of IVH are post-haemorrhagic hydrocephalus (PHH) and periventricular haemorrhagic infarction. In contrast to the declining incidence of IVH, recent studies suggest that the prevalence of PHH has remained constant or may in fact be increasing.

Incidence

IVH occurs primarily in the preterm infant requiring mechanical ventilation for RDS. The incidence of IVH is inversely related to gestation, being approximately 40% in infants of 30 weeks gestation but rising to ~70–80% in extremely preterm infants (<26 weeks gestation). Ultrasound studies suggest that it may occur asymptomatically in ~5% of term infants.

Aetiology

The germinal matrix is a transient zone of the brain found in various periventricular sites, but most abundant in the caudate nucleus where only a single layer of ependymal cells separates it from the lateral ventricles. In the germinal matrix, mitosis is active and neurones then migrate out to their final position within the brain. At the end of the second trimester, it is one of the most metabolically active areas of the brain, and has a rich vascular network. The vessels have thin epithelial cell walls and no muscular layer; it is hard to distinguish arterioles, capillaries and veins, and they are particularly prone to bleeding. The germinal matrix slowly involutes until 33 to 34 weeks gestation.

Bleeding from the germinal matrix is thought of as an initial bleed which is then followed by its extension. IVH is essentially a postnatal event, although prenatal haemorrhage is well documented though uncommon. Approximately 30% of IVH has occurred by 6 hours of age and more than 50% occurs during the first 24 hours of life. Onset after 72 hours of age is unusual. This high incidence of bleeds in the early hours of life in unstable preterm babies with respiratory distress has led to the view that haemodynamic instability and vessel wall immaturity are the major risk factors for IVH. Thus the aetiology of the bleeding is considered under:

- Changes in cerebral haemodynamics.
- The wall of the blood vessels.
- Coagulation abnormalities.

The cerebral blood flow (CBF) of preterm babies is pressure dependent; that is, if the blood pressure rises or falls, so does the CBF including that through the germinal matrix. Increases in CBF may lead to vessel rupture and hence IVH. Situations known to cause rises in blood pressure include pneumothoraces, breathing against (fighting) the ventilator, painful procedures, endotracheal suction and rapid infusions of blood or plasma. Hypercapnia – such as seen during a pneumothorax – is a potent cerebral vasodilator and an independent risk factor for IVH.

The thin capillary endothelial cell wall may be at risk from free-radical damage. If so, administering a free-radical scavenger, such as vitamin E, should reduce the risk of haemorrhage. Conflicting evidence exists as to whether this is so. If IVH is a very early postnatal phenomenon, it may be hard to give therapeutic doses of free-radical scavengers prior to the onset of bleeding.

Once vessel rupture has occurred, bleeding is more likely to continue or recur if coagulation abnormalities exist. Conflicting evidence exists as to whether the administration of clotting factors in fresh frozen plasma (FFP) is beneficial in preventing or reducing the extent of haemorrhages. Studies looking at clotting factor status at birth as a predictor of IVH have also produced conflicting evidence.

Classification

The extent of the bleeding has been classified by a number of authors. One frequently used in the UK is that of Papile:

Grade I: isolated germinal matrix haemorrhage.
Grade II: rupture of the haemorrhage into the ventricle but without ventricular dilatation.
Grade III: rupture of the haemorrhage into the ventricle with ventricular dilatation.
Grade IV: IVH with parenchymal extension.

Prevention

If a preterm delivery cannot be avoided, then the single most effective intervention is antenatal dexamethasone, which benefits the infant both by reducing RDS and, by an independent effect, reducing IVH, probably by improving capillary wall stability. Postnatal prevention of IVH is based on the recognition of the associated risk factors. Meticulous attention should be paid to rapid but gentle stabilization of the sick preterm baby with RDS. Ventilation to achieve desired $PaCO_2$ should be achieved early with low peak pressures, with the baby not fighting the ventilator. Surfactant should be administered early, preferably during resuscitation on the labour ward for the extremely premature baby at greatest risk. Humidification of the airway reduces the risk of tube blockage and associated hypercapnia. If the baby is hypotensive, blood pressure should be raised slowly and smoothly. Although the role of prophylactic FFP in reducing haemorrhage is unproven, many neonatologists use FFP 'prophylactically' if colloid is needed for volume expansion. Severe thrombocytopenia or coagulopathy should be treated without causing rapid volume overload.

A number of drug treatments have been attempted (e.g. phenobarbitone). As yet none have consistently shown benefit in both reducing the extent of haemorrhage and preventing later handicap.

Consequences

1. Periventricular haemorrhagic infarction. This is thought to occur when a clot distending the lateral ventricle obstructs the medullary veins draining into the subependymal veins. This stasis leads to haemorrhage and infarction. Extension of sonographic echodensities from an IVH into the parenchyma is difficult to interpret. They may represent direct extension, venous infarction, or bleeding into an ischaemic infarction of periventricular leucomalacia.

2. Post-haemorrhagic hydrocephalus. Defined as a ventricular index above the 97th centile, this occurs in 20–40% of babies after IVH. The ventricular index is the distance from the midline to the most lateral point of the ventricle in the coronal plane at the level of the hippocampal gyrus. Such dilatation is usually transient and only 15–20% go on to need shunting for progressive hydrocephalus.

3. Death. Occurs in over 50% of babies with parenchymal extension of their IVH. These babies usually have the worst respiratory problems, and the IVH is not always the principal cause of death.

4. Neurodevelopmental handicap. Most common in those with parenchymal involvement. The most potent predictor of handicap is ultrasonographic abnormalities of the white matter. Two-thirds of babies left with periventricular cysts after grade IV IVH or periventricular leucomalacia develop cerebral palsy. PHH also increases the risk of severe neurological sequelae to 50–60%. This may be related more to cerebral atrophy after parenchymal infarction and/or haemorrhage rather than to the hydrocephalus *per se*. Preterm babies with only grade I or II IVHs have handicap rates of 4–5%, little different from the risk of about 2% for babies of the same gestation with normal scans.

Further reading

Govaert P. Cranial haemorrhage in the term newborn infant. In: *Clinics in Developmental Medicine, No. 129*. London: MacKeith Press, 1994.

Levene MI, Liford RJ, Bennett MJ, Punt J (eds). *Fetal and Neonatal Neurology and Neurosurgery 2nd edn.* Edinburgh: Churchill Livingstone, 1995.

Paneth N, Rudelli R, Kazam E, Monte W. Brain damage in the preterm infant. In: *Clinics in Developmental Medicine, No. 131.* London: MacKeith Press, 1994.

Papile L-A, Burstein J, Burstein R, Koffler H. Incidence and evolution of sub-ependymal and intraventricular haemorrhage: a study of infants with a birthweight less than 1500 g. *Journal of Pediatrics*, 1978; **92**: 529–534.

Rennie JM. *Neonatal Cerebral Ultrasound.* Cambridge: Cambridge University Press, 1997.

Volpe JJ. Intracranial hemorrhage: germinal matrix-intraventricular hemorrhage of the premature infant. In: *Neurology of the Newborn*, 3rd edn. Philadelphia: W.B. Saunders, 1995.

Related topics of interest

HAEMOLYTIC DISEASE

Haemolytic disease may have adverse but transient effects on the developing fetus and the newborn infant but also has the potential to cause permanent adverse sequelae. Timely antenatal diagnosis and appropriate treatment may prevent many of these unfavourable effects.

In the fetus

In haemolytic disease, antibodies acquired trans-placentally from a sensitized mother destroy fetal red cells. Several blood group antigens can cause problems in pregnancy, but rhesus incompatibility still accounts for the majority of severe disease. It is diagnosed antenatally by rising maternal antibody titres, and is then monitored at three levels of increasing complexity and risk:

1. Antibody titres in maternal serum in pregnancy.
2. Optical density of the amniotic fluid.
3. Cordocentesis to measure fetal haemoglobin.

Most affected pregnancies are managed expectantly and monitored by serum antibody levels alone. Unfortunately, these have a poor predictive value for fetal disease, and when severe fetal disease is suspected, invasive monitoring and treatment is indicated. Liley's curves of optical density at 450 nm, the absorption wavelength of bilirubin, are used to predict the severity of the disease from 27 weeks onwards. They have been extended and modified by others. If very severe disease is present, then either delivery – if the baby is definitely viable – or cordocentesis and intrauterine transfusion is indicated. The transfused cells must be compatible with maternal serum. This does not stop the haemolysis of fetal cells, but maintains an adequate haemoglobin level until delivery is possible.

Rhesus haemolytic disease can develop only after maternal exposure to fetal cells at birth, an abortion, antepartum haemorrhage (APH), amniocentesis, etc., or after an incompatible transfusion. About 90% of rhesus-incompatible pregnancies cause no reaction, either because the inoculum is small, or because ABO incompatibility protects the fetus. Usually, first pregnancies are unaffected, and the disease worsens in second and later pregnancies after recurrent exposure of the mother's immune system to foreign red cell proteins. The risk of rhesus sensitization and hence disease is greatly reduced by the administration of anti-D Ig to affected mothers at 28 weeks and again within 24 hours of delivery. Overall, the incidence of severe disease has now fallen to about 1 per 1000 births.

Other red cell antigen incompatibilities, notably ABO, can cause haemolysis. ABO incompatibilities can occur in a first pregnancy, as the AB red cell markers are strongly antigenic.

Early severe jaundice can result, but haemolysis and anaemia are generally mild. Haemolysis in babies can also result from:

- Hereditary spherocytosis.
- Deficiencies of enzymes such as glucose-6-phosphate dehydrogenase (G6PD) and pyruvate kinase.
- Infection.
- Vitamin E deficiency in preterm babies some weeks after birth.

The first two groups may result in anaemia and prolonged jaundice starting soon after birth.

In the neonate

Many babies will have only mild disease, needing either no treatment or only phototherapy and tests to exclude anaemia. When a neonate is at risk of severe disease, early assessment and treatment are essential.

Assessment at birth

1. History. Check previous pregnancies and their outcome. In the present pregnancy, check the antibody titres, amniotic fluid optical density, and if necessary perform cordocentesis. Monitor biophysical profile for fetal wellbeing, and if preterm delivery is likely give dexamethasone.

2. Physical examination. The main features are:

- Pallor.
- Jaundice.
- Tachycardia.
- Hepatosplenomegaly.
- Oedema, ascites, effusions.
- Respiratory distress.

3. Laboratory tests on the cord blood

- Blood group and Coombs' test.
- FBC.
- Clotting screen.
- Serum bilirubin.
- Serum albumin.
- Liver function tests.
- U&E.
- Blood glucose and blood gases.

Treatment at birth

Prompt cardiorespiratory resuscitation and stabilization may be necessary if severe rhesus disease and hydrops fetalis are expected. Intubation, ventilation, insertion of an umbilical venous catheter (UVC) and drainage of effusions and ascites may be necessary on the labour ward. If there is heart failure, the UVC can facilitate central venous pressure measurement.

If necessary, a negative-balance partial exchange with mother-compatible cytomegalovirus (CMV)-negative O-negative blood performed within minutes of birth can reduce the circulating volume and begin to correct the anaemia. Other complications such as hypoglycaemia, thrombocytopenia (± DIC), hypoalbuminaemia and surfactant deficiency may also require prompt attention.

1. Early treatment. After initial stabilization, the major concerns are to control hyperbilirubinaemia and prevent kernicterus, and to correct the anaemia further if necessary. Cord haemoglobin and bilirubin have been suggested as a guide to when early exchange transfusion (i.e. one initiated within an hour or so of birth solely on the basis of cord blood values) should be performed. There is poor correlation between these single cord blood values and the need for early exchange. The advent of more effective phototherapy has further undermined these old criteria. However, a rise in bilirubin of >8 µmol/dl/hour is indicative of a need for an early exchange transfusion, particularly if the cord bilirubin is >95 µmol/l. These crude guidelines need to be interpreted against a knowledge of the output and effectiveness of the phototherapy unit used on an individual baby.

The criteria for later exchange transfusions in haemolytic disease have been debated, but most authorities still consider a total bilirubin level of >340 µmol/l to be the threshold. Exchange transfusions and phototherapy are considered further in the topic 'Jaundice'.

2. Later treatment. Late anaemia, at 3–8 weeks of age, is a frequent complication of haemolytic disease. Top-up transfusion should be considered if the infant is lethargic or feeding poorly rather than on a specific haemoglobin concentration, though if the latter falls below 6 g/dl, most would then transfuse. Erythropoietin is currently being researched as an adjunct to therapy, but it cannot yet be recommended on a routine basis.

Outcome for rhesus haemolytic disease is good. More research is needed to establish whether paediatricians should remain 'vigintiphobic', i.e. afraid of letting the bilirubin level rise above 20 mg/dl (340 µmol/l), or if higher levels in well term babies with haemolysis can be tolerated without fear of long-term neurological sequelae.

Further reading

Fanaroff AA, Martin RJ. *Neonatal–Perinatal Medicine: Diseases of the Fetus and Neonate*, 6th edn. St Louis: Mosby, 1997.

Gollin YG, Copel JA. Management of the Rh-sensitized mother. *Clinics in Perinatology*, 1995; **22**: 545–59.

Hann IM, Gibson BES, Letsky EA (eds). *Fetal and Neonatal Haematology*. London: Baillière Tindall, 1991.

Peterec SM. Management of neonatal Rh disease. *Clinics in Perinatology*, 1995; **22**: 561–92.

Reed GB, Claireaux AE, Cockburn F (eds). *Diseases of the Fetus and Newborn: Pathology, Imaging, Genetics and Managing*, 2nd edn. London: Chapman & Hall Medical, 1995.

Related topics of interest

Anaemia (p. 9)
Hydrops fetalis (p. 122)
Jaundice (p. 173)
Prenatal diagnosis (p. 253)

HEAD SIZE

The size of the head in the newborn infant is an important physical sign, as a small or large head may be indicative of an underlying malformation, antenatal infection, or metabolic or chromosomal disorder, often with resultant cerebral damage. An occipito-frontal head circumference above the 90th centile or below the 10th centile (especially if unduly disproportionate compared to the birthweight) should make the doctor consider possible pathological causes for the discrepant head size. The infant may otherwise look normal or have a number of malformations which might be recognizable as a specific disorder or syndrome. It is therefore important to carefully evaluate any dysmorphic features in an infant with an abnormally sized head as this will help achieve the correct diagnosis and management plans.

Large head

Aetiology

1. *Hydrocephalus*
   - Post-haemorrhagic (e.g. alloimmune thrombocytopenia).
   - Post-infection (e.g. TORCH – toxoplasmosis, rubella, cytomegalovirus and herpes – infections).
   - Malformations (e.g. spina bifida, Dandy–Walker cyst).
   - X-linked.
   - Syndromic (e.g. neurofibromatosis).

2. *Hydranencephaly*

3. *Megalencephaly.* (For example, Soto's syndrome or familial megalencephaly.)

Clinical features

- Obviously large head with large anterior fontanelle, widely separated sutures and open posterior fontanelle at term.
- Head circumference greater than 97th centile by ≥2 cm.
- Sunsetting.
- Head freely transilluminates (hydranencephaly or severe hydrocephalus).
- Accompanying dysmorphic features or malformations when part of a syndrome or malformation sequence (e.g. myelomeningocele).
- Depressible 'springy' membranous bones of the cranial vault (craniolacunae).

Investigations

- Cranial ultrasound.
- CT scan.
- MRI scan (best resolution).
- Coagulation studies (unusual haemorrhages).
- Search for congenital infections (signs of prenatal infection evident).

Management

- Hydrocephalus is treated by insertion of ventriculo-peritoneal shunt.

- Acetazolamide (100 mg/kg/day) may suffice for moderate hydrocephalus or as a temporary measure in an infant not fit for surgery.
- Repeated lumbar or ventricular punctures are not appropriate for congenital hydrocephalus.
- Rectify coagulation defect(s) where appropriate.
- If syndromic – address accompanying problems appropriately.
- Congenital infections – treat if appropriate (e.g. toxoplasmosis).
- Provide genetic counselling where indicated.

Small head

Aetiology
- Syndromic.
- Chromosomal abnormalities.
- Hereditary – autosomal recessive and X-linked.
- Antenatal developmental malformations.
- Metabolic disorder (phenylketonuria – late).
- Intrauterine infections, e.g. TORCH infections.

Clinical features
- Head circumference below 2nd centile.
- Forehead slopes backwards.
- Dysmorphic features or malformations if syndromic.
- Other signs of congenital infection (e.g. chorioretinitis).

Investigations
- Ultrasound scan.
- CT scan (intracranial calcification).
- MRI scan (for congenital malformations).
- Chromosomal analysis.
- Obtain a family history.
- Review by clinical geneticist/syndromologist.
- Audiology assessment (exclude deafness).
- Ophthalmology assessment (congenital infection).

Management
- Isolate infants with congenital infection (e.g. CMV).
- Counsel parents on prognosis and recurrence.
- Arrange appropriate developmental follow-up.
- Treat congenital infections if appropriate.

Further reading

Levene MI, Liford RJ, Bennett MJ, Punt J (eds). *Fetal and Neonatal Neurology and Neurosurgery*, 2nd edn. Edinburgh: Churchill Livingstone, 1995.
Volpe JJ. *Neurology of the Newborn*, 3nd edn. Philadelphia: W.B. Saunders, 1995.

Related topics of interest

Infection – prenatal (p. 151)   Neural tube defects (p. 203)

HEART MURMURS IN NEONATES

Neonatal heart murmurs are extremely variable due to the postnatal cardiopulmonary adaptations. The intensity and the character of the murmur may not bear any relation to the severity of the underlying cardiac malformation, and distinction between innocent and pathological murmurs is often difficult on clinical grounds only.

Innocent cardiac murmurs in neonates

Transient murmurs are common in the neonatal period. Two-thirds of normal neonates will have an innocent murmur in the first few days of life. These neonates are entirely asymptomatic from a cardiac viewpoint and there are no abnormal physical findings on examination. The ECG and chest X-ray are normal. The commonest innocent murmurs in neonates are:

Pulmonary flow murmur of the newborn	This is common in preterm and small-for-gestational-age infants. The murmur is soft, grade 2/6 or less in intensity. This is best heard in the pulmonary area and may radiate over both lung fields, the axillae and the back. This murmur is thought to be largely due to a physiological pulmonary branch stenosis which resolves in two-thirds of newborns by 6 weeks and in almost all infants by 6 months.
Transient systolic murmur of the patent ductus arteriosus (PDA)	This murmur presents due to delayed closure of the PDA and is best heard beneath the left infraclavicular area. The murmur is soft, systolic, grade 2/6 or less in intensity and usually disappears in the few days after birth as the PDA is closed. PDA murmurs may be detected in up to 60% of healthy infants at term within the first 48 hours of life. By 6 weeks of age, however, most if not all PDAs should have closed.
Transient systolic murmur of tricuspid regurgitation	This soft systolic murmur localized to the left sternal edge is due to mild tricuspid regurgitation in the presence of high pulmonary vascular resistance (PVR). It disappears in the first few days of life as PVR falls to normal values.

Murmurs persisting beyond the neonatal period require further cardiac evaluation.

Pathological heart murmurs in neonates

In contrast to innocent murmurs, pathological heart murmurs are louder in intensity (grade 3/6 or more), longer in duration and are less variable. Presence of a diastolic component points to the pathological nature of the murmur. In general, murmurs audible soon after birth are due to obstructive lesions, for example pulmonary stenosis, aortic stenosis, coarctation of aorta and other lesions, whereas murmurs due to left-to-right shunts are audible a few days later when PVR is sufficiently lowered. Evaluation in an asymptomatic and otherwise well neonate should include detailed cardiac examination with recording of four-limb blood pressure, pulse oximetry, ECG and chest radiograph. Echocardiogram is essential for anatomical diagnosis and also to plan subsequent therapy and follow-up. A neonate with cardiac symptoms and associated dysmorphic features or congenital anomalies of other organ systems requires a complete evaluation by a paediatric cardiologist.

Further reading

Arlettaz R, Archer N, Wilkinson AR. Natural history of innocent heart murmurs in newborn babies: controlled echocardiographic study. *Archives of Disease in Childhood, Fetal and Neonatal Edition*, 1998; **78**: F166–70.

Burton DA, Cabalka AK. Cardiac evaluation of infants. *Pediatric Clinics of North America*, 1994; **41**: 991–1011.

Freedom RM, Benson LN, Smallhorn JF. *Neonatal Heart Disease*. Springer-Verlag, 1992.

Park MK. *Pediatric Cardiology for Practitioners*, 3rd edn. Chicago: Year Book Medical Publishers, 1996.

Silove ED. Assessment and management of congenital heart disease in the newborn by the district paediatrician. *Archives of Disease in Childhood*, 1994; **70**: F71–4.

Related topics of interest

HEPATITIS B

Hepatitis B infection is a significant global public health problem, with the total number of asymptomatic carriers worldwide being greater than the combined population of Europe. The majority of carriers reside in the developing countries. Prevalence of hepatitis B surface antigen (HBsAg) varies from 0.1% in parts of Europe to 20% in the Far East.

Hepatitis B is transmitted parenterally (blood to blood contact, injury with contaminated sharp instruments), by perinatal transmission from mother to child, or sexually. Transplacental infection is uncommon and most infants acquire the infection at birth from their carrier mothers or later during childhood. Susceptibility to infection and perinatal transmission varies with ethnicity, being highest in the Chinese. Expression of 'e' antigen (HBeAg) markedly increases the risk of infection in the baby. The risk is low when the mother is e-antibody positive (anti-HBe positive) and e-antigen negative, and intermediate when neither the e-antigen nor antibody are detectable. Transfusion-associated infection is now rare in the UK.

Following infection, the HBsAg appears in the infant's blood after 6–16 weeks, with most infants (90%) becoming chronic asymptomatic carriers in contrast to 2–10% of those infected as adults. A few may develop a severe and fatal hepatitis. Currently, the carrier status, once developed, is permanent and is significantly associated with a fatal chronic liver disease and carcinoma in adulthood. Prevention of hepatitis B by immunization is therefore particularly important. All medical and nursing staff should be immunized against hepatitis B.

Risk factors

- Maternal hepatitis B carriage (HBsAg positive) especially HBeAg positivity.
- Parent(s) originating from a region with high prevalence of hepatitis B.
- Parent(s) been resident in certain high-risk institutions (e.g. prison and mental institutions).
- Parent(s) is an i.v. drug abuser.
- Parent(s) with recent hepatitis infection or chronic liver disease.
- Parent(s) frequent traveller(s) to areas of high hepatitis B prevalence.
- Parent(s) changes sexual partners frequently.
- Parent(s) is a haemophiliac.

Treat all patients as potential hepatitis B carriers!

Investigations

Screen all mothers or those in at-risk groups for the presence of serological markers of hepatitis B virus (HBV) infection (HBsAg and HBeAg). Offer human immunodeficiency virus (HIV) screening for HBsAg-positive drug abusers.

Prevention

Take appropriate precautions at the delivery and resuscitation of all infants but especially where mothers are known hepatitis B carriers or one of the parents has the risk factors above. Breast-feeding by hepatitis B carrier mothers is discouraged because of a small risk of infecting the infant, but in developing countries the dangers of not breast-feeding may be greater than the risks of continuing breast-feeding.

Immunization

There are two types of immunization product: a vaccine which produces an immune response, and a specific hepatitis B immunoglobulin (HBIG) which provides passive immunity conferring immediate but temporary protection after accidental inoculation or contamination with antigen-positive blood.

Infants of hepatitis B carriers or at a high risk of infection should be immunized against hepatitis B as follows: hepatitis B vaccine 0.5 ml (10 μg) Engerix B (SmithKline Beecham) or 0.5 ml (5 μg) H-B-Vax II (Pasteur Merieux MSD) i.m. at birth, then 1 month and 6 months after the first. An accelerated schedule may be used where the third dose is given at 2 months after the initial dose with a booster dose at 12 months. If the mother is e-antigen positive but e-antibody negative, or had acute hepatitis B during pregnancy, HBIG 200 mg (200 IU) is also given i.m. (deep thigh injection) within 48 hours of birth. Use anterolateral thigh and not the buttock, as vaccine efficacy may be reduced.

Check for evidence of adequate immunity at 1 year. Individuals producing antibodies to HBsAg (anti-HBs) at levels of ≥100 mIU/ml are considered immune; poor responders (anti-HBs 10–100 mIU/ml) should receive a booster dose and non-responders (anti-HBs <10 mIU/ml) should receive a repeat course of vaccine. The duration of antibody persistence is variable but generally a booster dose is required after 5 years.

The above schedule of active/passive immunization is highly effective at conferring immunity (9 out of 10 immune at 1 year).

Post-exposure prophylaxis

Active/passive immunization is recommended for all staff who accidentally inoculate themselves or contaminate their eye(s), mouth, fresh cuts or skin abrasions with blood from a known HBsAg-positive person. The affected area should be washed well with soap and warm water and HBIG (500 IU adults, 200 IU infants) administered with simultaneous administration of hepatitis B vaccine at a different site. In the previously adequately immunized, only a single booster dose of hepatitis B vaccine is required, whereas an accelerated complete course of hepatitis B vaccine should be used in the non-immunized. If, however, infection has already occurred at the time of immunization, severe illness and the development of the carrier state may still be prevented.

Further reading

Beasley RP, Hwang L-Y, Lee GC-Y *et al.* Prevention of perinatally transmitted hepatitis B virus infections with hepatitis B immune globulin and hepatitis B vaccine. *Lancet*, 1983; **ii**: 1099–102.

Mazel JA, Schalm SW, de Gast BC *et al.* Passive active immunisation of neonates of HBsAg-positive carrier mothers: preliminary observations. *British Medical Journal*, 1984; **288**: 513–15.

Polakoff S, Vandervelde EM. Immunisation of neonates at high risk of hepatitis B in England and Wales. A national surveillance. *British Medical Journal*, 1988; **297**: 249–53.

Salisbury DM, Begg NT (eds). *Immunisation against Infectious Disease*. London: HMSO Publications, 1996.

Related topics of interest

HIV and AIDS (p. 114)
Immunization (p. 132)
Infection – perinatal (p. 147)

HERNIAE

Inguinal hernia

A patent processus vaginalis left in the wake of the descending testes predisposes the infant to develop an inguinal hernia. Inguinal herniae are therefore six times more common in boys than girls. The right side is more commonly affected (60%) than the left (30%), with 1 in 10 being bilateral. The more premature the infant, the greater the incidence and the more likely are the complications. As the risks of strangulation are highest during the first few months of life, aim to repair herniae before discharge from hospital.

Presentation
- Persistent or intermittent mass in the groin.
- Constant crying or irritability.
- Abdominal distension.
- Bilious vomiting.
- Apnoeic spells.

Diagnosis
- This is made on clinical grounds when a mass is felt overlying the inguinal ring, in the scrotum, or labia majora on the affected side.
- Mass enlarges when infant strains or cries.
- A tender discoloured swelling which does not reduce is a surgical emergency.

The differential diagnosis includes an encysted hydrocele of the cord (cyst is non-tender, moves with cord and is translucent), torsion of the testis (testis is swollen and tender), superficial inguinal lymphadenitis and localized inguinal abscess (located below and lateral to the external inguinal ring).

Management
- Herniae should be repaired when the respiratory status is optimal – usually before discharge from hospital.
- Spinal anaesthesia reduces respiratory morbidity.
- Exploring the contralateral side may be beneficial as the processus may be patent in up to 50%.
- In female patients, the surgeon should ascertain that the hernia does not contain male gonads.

Oxygen requirements frequently decrease following inguinal hernia repair in infants with BPD who are oxygen-dependent.

Umbilical hernia

Umbilical herniae are fairly common and result from failure of the umbilical ring to obliterate. In infants, the hernia may be quite large giving the skin a blue hue. They are always reducible and cause no symptoms, although they may be blamed for 'colic'. Even large herniae tend to resolve spontaneously as the umbilical cicatrix contracts over the first few years of life, so repair should be delayed for at least 1 year and probably up to the age of 3 years. The main indication for surgery is cosmetic appearance, as strangulation is almost unknown in children.

Epigastric hernia

An epigastric hernia occurs when extraperitoneal fat bulges through a small defect in the linea alba, commonly mid-way between the xiphisternum and umbilicus. The fat arises from within the falciform ligament and the hernia presents as a midline small lump between the xiphisternum and umbilicus. The lump is usually irreducible but rarely causes symptoms (discomfort after meals). Bowel or peritoneum never protrudes through the defect (commonly only 1–2 mm diameter). Surgery is only required if they cause discomfort or for cosmetic reasons.

Further reading

Beasley SW, Hutson JM, Auldist AW. *Essential Paediatric Surgery*. London: Arnold, 1996.
Black JA, Whitfield MF. *Neonatal Emergencies: Early Detection and Management*, 2nd edn. Oxford: Butterworth-Heinemann, 1991.
Liebert PS. *Color Atlas of Pediatric Surgery*, 2nd edn. Philadelphia: W.B. Saunders, 1997.
Puri P (ed). *Newborn Surgery*. London: Butterworth-Heinemann, 1995.
Vidyasagar D, Reyes H. Neonatal surgery. *Clinics in Perinatology*, 1989; **61**: 1.

Related topics of interest

Abdominal distension (p. 1)
Neonatal surgery (p. 200)
Surgical emergencies (p. 312)
Vomiting (p. 331)

HIRSCHSPRUNG'S DISEASE

Hirschsprung's disease, or congenital aganglionic megacolon, was first accurately described by Harald Hirschsprung of Copenhagen in 1886, although this disorder had been recognized almost some 200 years earlier. It is the commonest cause of intestinal obstruction in the neonate (80–90% of patients present in the neonatal period), with an incidence of 1 in 5000 births. Seventy-five percent of patients have short-segment disease confined to the rectosigmoid, 14% have involvement of the transverse and descending colon (long-segment disease), and in 5–10% of patients the entire colon is affected (Zuelzer–Wilson syndrome).

There is a male to female preponderance in both the more common short-segment disease (4:1) and the long-segment disease (2:1). There is an increased familial incidence with a family risk of 9–12.5% in the long-segment disease and 2% in the short-segment disease, and a genetic influence giving a risk of 7.6% for siblings of a female patient and 2.5–6% for siblings of a male patient. Approximately 4% of patients with Hirschsprung's disease have associated genitourinary abnormalities, 5–9% have trisomy 21, and an association with Waardenburgh, Laurence–Moon–Bardet–Biedl and congenital central hypoventilation syndrome (Ondine's curse) has also been noted. Five to ten percent of infants with Hirschsprung's disease are preterm.

Pathophysiology

Hirschsprung's disease is due to an arrest of neuroblast migration from the proximal bowel (oesophagus) to the distal hindgut resulting in abnormal innervation of the affected distal segment. There is a total absence of ganglion cells in the affected segment of the intestine and an overgrowth of large nerve trunks in the intermuscular and submucosal zones. The distal rectum is always affected and this extends to variable lengths of the more proximal gut.

The classical gross pathological picture is one of a narrow contracted aganglionic segment which extends proximally into a markedly dilated, thickened, hypertrophied and normally innervated but functionally obstructed colon. A cone-shaped 'transitional' zone is noted between the dilated and contracted intestine. Histologically, hypertrophied nerve bundles with a high concentration of acetylcholinesterase between the muscle layers and in the submucosal are noted, with an absence of ganglion cells in the submucosal plexus of Meissner and hypoganglionosis or aganglionosis in the intermyenteric plexus of Auerbach. More recently, there have been some new insights into the aetiology of Hirschsprung's disease. It appears that a loss of neural cell adhesion molecules could be the cause of neuroblasts failing to migrate to aganglionic segments and a lack of neuronal NO synthase (and therefore NO) in nerve fibres of aganglionic intestine may contribute to the inability of the smooth muscle to relax and the absence of peristalsis in the aganglionic segment. Some forms of Hirschsprung's disease have also been found to be associated with gene deletions.

- Delayed passage of meconium (i.e. >24 hours after birth) in >90% of cases. Ninety-nine percent of term infants pass meconium within 48 hours of birth.
- Bilious vomiting, marked abdominal distension and complete intestinal obstruction.
- Chronic constipation following normal passage of meconium.
- Rectal examination shows normal anal tone and is followed by explosive foul-smelling stools and gas.
- Meconium plug syndrome: 10–20% of infants with this disorder may have Hirschsprung's disease.
- Enterocolitis (which is most common in the first 2–4 weeks of life). This is the main cause of mortality in Hirschsprung's disease and is a consequence of delayed diagnosis. Inability to pass stools leads to massive abdominal distension, increased intraluminal pressure, decreased intestinal blood flow and a breach of the mucosal integrity. The stasis also encourages bacterial proliferation (*Clostridium difficile*, anaerobes, coliforms) and sepsis. The infant presents with profuse mucusy and bloody diarrhoea, abdominal distension, bilious vomiting, hypotension (large fluid losses) and occasionally shock. Left untreated, 33% of infants with Hirschsprung's disease develop enterocolitis within the first 3 months of life and a third of these develop it within 30 days of birth. Once an infant has developed enterocolitis he/she remains at increased risk of further bouts of enterocolitis, even after a successful pull-through procedure.

Diagnosis

1. Radiology. Plain abdominal films show gas-filled bowel loops throughout the abdomen except for the pelvis which is devoid of gas. A barium contrast enema in a previously *unprepared* colon shows a small calibre aganglionic segment followed by a funnel-shaped 'cone' or 'transitional zone' leading into a normal but dilated proximal colon. However, a barium enema is less accurate in the neonatal period than at any other time, as a transitional zone may not be seen before the age of 2 weeks and a megacolon may not be present. Delayed films (after 24 hours) show retention of contrast material. A barium enema may, however, reveal other disorders which cause neonatal lower bowel obstruction.

2. Manometry. Failure of the internal anal sphincter to exhibit a relaxation wave in response to inflation of a balloon inserted into the rectum is diagnostic of Hirschsprung's disease (>90% accuracy) but it cannot be performed in infants of <3 kg in weight (39 weeks post-conceptual age) as the anal relaxation reflex may be physiologically absent. Diagnosis of ultrashort-segment Hirschsprung's disease can only be made with manometry which shows failure of the internal sphincter to relax, with a seemingly normal suction biopsy.

3. Biopsy. Suction, punch or open rectal biopsy is the gold standard for diagnosis. The submucosa must be included in the biopsy specimen to determine the presence or absence of ganglion cells. Absence of ganglion cells or elevated acetylcholinesterase staining is diagnostic of Hirschsprung's disease (91% accuracy). In ultrashort-segment disease, the aganglionic segment is limited to the internal sphincter so ganglion cells may be present on rectal suction biopsy. Excision of a strip of rectal muscle including the internal sphincter is diagnostic and therapeutic.

Management

1. Obstruction. This is relieved by gentle rectal washouts using warm saline till various investigations are completed. A defunctioning colostomy sited in the ganglionic bowel is commonly performed initially. Definitive repair is performed between 2–6 months of age by one of five techniques, namely: Swenson's operation (rectosigmoidectomy), Duhamel procedure (retrorectal pull-through), Soave procedure (endorectal pull-through), Rehbein's procedure (resection of rectum and aganglionic bowel and dilatation of anal sphincter) and rectal myomectomy. Duhamel's procedure is probably the best technique when the entire colon is affected.

2. Enterocolitis. These infants may be critically ill from massive fluid and electrolyte losses. Resuscitate with fluid expansion (e.g. 20 ml/kg of FFP or albumin), correct acid–base imbalance, replace fluid and electrolytes, and commence broad-spectrum antibiotics (including vancomycin and metronidazole). Emergency colostomy is contraindicated.

Long-term outcome

In the majority (85%), the outcome for surgically treated Hirschsprung's disease is satisfactory. Complications include disturbances of micturition (4%), anastomotic leaks (2%), anal stenosis (5–14%), prolapse, perianal abscesses, incontinence and soiling. Once enterocolitis occurs, the patient is at increased risk of recurrence, even years after a successful definitive repair operation. The current mortality rate is 1–3%. Note, however, that Hirschsprung's disease is only one of several disorders with abnormalities of the neuronal intestinal network. In neuronal intestinal dysplasia, ganglion cells are present but in an ectopic site. The submucosal and intermyenteric plexuses are also hypertrophied. Approximately 25% of patients with Hirschsprung's disease may have concomitant neuronal intestinal dysplasia.

Further reading

Doody DP, Donahoe PK. Hirschsprung's disease. In: Morris PJ, Malt RA (eds). *Oxford Textbook of Surgery*. Oxford: Oxford University Press, 1994; 2048–52.

Holschneider AM (ed). *Hirschsprung's Disease*. New York: Thieme-Stratton, 1982.

Joseph V, Sim C. Problems and pitfalls in the management of Hirschsprung's disease. *Journal of Pediatric Surgery*, 1988; **23**: 398.

Kusafuka T, Puri P. Altered mRNA expression of the neuronal nitric oxide synthase gene in Hirschsprung's disease. *Journal of Pediatric Surgery*, 1997; **32**: 1054–8.

Teitelbaum DH. Hirschsprung's disease in children. *Current Opinion in Pediatrics*, 1995; **7**: 316–22.

Tomita R, Munakata K, Kurosu Y, Tanjoh K. A role of nitric oxide in Hirschsprung's disease. *Journal of Pediatric Surgery*, 1995; **30**: 437–40.

Related topics of interest

HIV AND AIDS

It is estimated that over 18 million adults and 1.5 million children worldwide have been infected with HIV, and by the year 2000 over 40 million individuals (4 million children) will be infected. The HIV/AIDS epidemic now represents a formidable public health burden, particularly for developing countries. The prevalence of HIV infection among pregnant women varies from below 1.5 cases per 1000 in developed nations to an excess of 1 in 10 in some developing nations. The rate of mother-to-child (vertical) transmission of HIV is also lower in industrialized countries (14–33%) than in developing countries (22–40%).

Based on some of the most recent epidemiological data (data to end-July, 1997), the prevalence of HIV infection among pregnant women in the UK was 0.19% (1 in 520) in Greater London, and 0.02% (1 in 5700) elsewhere in the UK. Approximately 300 infants are born to HIV-infected mothers each year in the UK. However, over 75% of HIV infections in pregnant women remain undiagnosed at the time of birth, and often women only discover they are HIV-positive when their child develops AIDS. Vertical transmission accounts for approximately 85% of cases of paediatric AIDS in the UK. These statistics and the fact that transmission of HIV from an infected mother to her child can be greatly reduced by interventions in pregnancy and in the perinatal period were recently highlighted in the recommendations of the Intercollegiate Working Party for Enhancing Voluntary Confidential HIV Testing in Pregnancy (Royal College of Paediatrics and Child Health, April 1998).

Risk factors for HIV transmission

1. Maternal disease status
- Advanced maternal disease (e.g. development of clinical symptoms).
- Decreased CD4+ count.
- Increased viral load (e.g. p24 antigenaemia, positive HIV blood culture).

2. Obstetric determinants
- Prolonged rupture of membranes.
- Chorioamnionitis.
- Vaginal delivery.
- Preterm delivery.
- Post-term delivery.
- Invasive intrapartum procedures.

3. Maternal immune response
- Neutralizing antibody.
- Cigarette smoking.
- Multiple sexual partners.
- Breast-feeding.

Timing of HIV transmission
- Intrauterine (24–50%).
- Intrapartum (~66% in developed countries, in the absence of breast-feeding). Ingestion of blood or maternal secretion and also maternal–fetal transmission.
- Postnatal (14%), mainly via breast-feeding. HIV is present in the cell-free and cellular portions of human milk with

highest concentration in colostrum. Breast-feeding doubles the rate of transmission. Transmission to infants occurs at a higher rate if the mother has a primary HIV infection during breast-feeding. In industrialized countries, HIV-exposed infants should be formula-fed but breast-feeding may still be safer in some developing countries.

Prevention of perinatal transmission

- Zidovudine therapy from early pregnancy through labour and for the newborn infant in HIV-infected women can reduce perinatal transmission by up to 67% to around 5%. Other potentially useful anti-retrovirals as single agents or as combination therapy are currently undergoing evaluation.
- Intact fetal membranes may decrease the risk of vertical transmission.
- Avoid invasive procedures (e.g. scalp sampling, operative vaginal delivery) in HIV-seropositive labouring women.
- Passive immunization of mother and infant with HIV hyperimmune i.v. immunoglobulin (ACTG 185).
- Maternal vitamin A supplementation.
- HIV-seropositive mothers should not breast-feed.
- Ongoing trials of reverse-transcriptase inhibitors (e.g. didanosine) and active immunization of mother and infant are awaited.

Clinical manifestations of HIV infection

Signs and symptoms are rarely present in the newborn period or first few weeks of life.

1. General. IUGR, hepatosplenomegaly, lymphadenopathy, failure to thrive.

2. Respiratory. Pneumocytis carinii pneumonia (PCP), lymphoid interstitial pneumonia/pulmonary lymphoid hyperplasia (LIP/PLH).

3. Dermatological. Fungal, bacterial and viral skin infections, severe seborrhoeic dermatitis, vasculitis, drug eruptions.

4. Gastrointestinal. Oral candidiasis, aphthous ulcers, parotid gland swellings, diarrhoea.

5. Cardiovascular. Myocarditis, cardiac dysrhythmias, pericardial effusions, cardiomyopathy.

6. Neurological. Developmental delay or regression, spastic weakness of extremities, microcephaly, cerebral atrophy, basal ganglia calcification, HIV encephalopathy, seizures.

7. Renal. Proteinuria, renal failure, nephrotic syndrome.

8. Haematological. Thrombocytopenia, anaemia, leucopenia.

9. Infection. Recurrent bacterial infections, especially *Streptococcus pneumonia*, *Salmonella* sp., *Staphylococcus aureus*, *Haemophilus influenzae* type b.

Diagnosis of HIV infection

Early diagnosis is important for the family's peace of mind and has implications for decisions concerning prophylaxis for opportunistic infections, intercurrent illnesses and therapeutic medications including anti-retroviral agents. However, standard HIV serological tests are not useful during the first 18 months because of the presence of transplacentally passed maternal IgG. Infection in infancy can be diagnosed by either direct (detecting virus or viral products) or indirect assays (detecting host response to virus). Direct tests include HIV culture (gold standard), polymerase chain reaction (PCR) for detection of HIV proviral DNA and p24 antigen detection after immune complex dissociation (p24–ICD) – a technique of freeing p24 antigen from immune complexes. Indirect assays detect intrinsically produced anti-HIV antibodies (e.g. anti-HIV IgA). The sensitivity of anti-HIV IgA and IgM for diagnosing HIV infection during infancy is debatable. Direct assays are more widely used. However, in the first week of life these assays have a sensitivity of only 50%, but by the age of ≥1 month HIV culture or PCR have a sensitivity and a specificity greater than 90%.

Practical approach to an HIV-exposed neonate

Perform HIV culture or PCR at 1–2 months and repeat before 6 months, but obtain a repeat sample if either test is positive. However, combining two tests does not increase sensitivity.

An infant <18 months old may be considered HIV-infected if he/she is HIV-seropositive, or was born to an HIV-infected mother *and* has positive results on two separate direct tests performed on separate blood samples (not cord blood).

An infant is also considered HIV-infected if he/she meets the US Centers for Disease Control and Prevention (CDC) surveillance case definition for AIDS. AIDS-defining conditions include PCP, LIP/PLH, CMV, HIV encephalopathy, recurrent bacterial infections, wasting syndrome, candida oesophagitis, pulmonary candidiasis, cryptosporidiosis, herpes simplex disease and mycobacterium avium–intracellulare complex infection.

Commence PCP prophylaxis at 4–6 weeks of age until at least 12 months of age unless HIV infection has been excluded (two or more negative direct tests performed at ≥1 month of age, one of which is performed at ≥4 months of age). Continue prophylaxis after 1 year in the presence of severe immunosuppression. Following PCP, maintain life-long prophylaxis. Prophylaxis consists of daily (or alternate day, i.e. 3 days a week) trimethoprim-sulphamethoxazole. Alternatively, oral dapsone and monthly i.v. pentamidine may be given.

Monthly i.v. immunoglobulin may reduce infectious complications in some HIV-infected children, though mortality is unaffected.

Treatment

Symptomatic HIV infection or asymptomatic infection with significant HIV-related immunosuppression is an indication for anti-retroviral therapy (currently nucleoside analogues that inhibit viral nucleic acid synthesis by binding to the reverse transcriptase enzyme). The largest experience is with zidovudine (ZDV, AZT). Didanosine (ddI) is an alternative agent for children with advanced HIV disease and ZDV intolerance or deterioration during ZDV therapy.

Prognosis

Approximately one in five infants contracting HIV develop AIDS or die in the first year of life. Without anti-retroviral therapy and PCP prophylaxis, median survival times for infants with vertically acquired HIV infection is 2–3 years. By age 6 years, 25% of the children will have died or developed some illness because of HIV infection. PCP, especially in the first year of life, candidal oesophagitis or severe encephalopathy indicate a poor prognosis, while low CD4+ lymphocyte counts, poor lymphocyte proliferative responses to mitogens and antigens and lack of anti-HIV neutralizing antibodies indicate rapid disease progression. Survival has improved, however, with anti-retrovirals and prophylaxis. While the long-term outcome is not yet known, most infected infants will die from AIDS or AIDS-related illnesses with only a few surviving until adulthood.

Further reading

Intercollegiate Working Party for Enhancing Voluntary Confidential HIV Testing in Pregnancy. *Reducing Mother-to-Child Transmission of HIV Infection in the United Kingdom*. London: Royal College of Paediatrics and Child Health, 1998.

Kline MW. Vertical human immunodeficiency virus infection. In: Hansen TN, McIntosh N (eds). *Current Topics in Neonatology, Number 1*. London: W.B. Saunders, 1996; 195–223.

Lindsay MK, Nesheim SR. Human immunodeficiency virus infection in pregnant women and their newborns. *Clinics in Perinatology*, 1997; **24**: 161–80.

Related topics of interest

Hepatitis B (p. 105)
Infection – perinatal (p. 147)
Maternal drug abuse (p. 182)

HOME OXYGEN THERAPY

Home oxygen therapy enables ex-preterm babies with chronic lung disease to go home from hospital weeks or months before they would if all oxygen therapy was hospital-based and they had to wait until they were in air all the time. Such babies should have been stable on low-flow nasal oxygen for some weeks, and show no sign of coming out of oxygen in the immediate future.

There are advantages to the baby, the family and the health service. The baby no longer has multiple caregivers, who can offer attention only when their other charges are well or sleeping. Instead the baby gets to know his/her parents really well for the first time, as they become his/her regular providers. The home environment is more friendly and stimulating, and the baby starts to develop the normal diurnal rhythm missing in the ever-bright lights and noise of a neonatal unit. The parents feel that their baby is truly theirs to care for and bring up in their own fashion, without the 'supervision' of hospital staff. Home oxygen therapy is cost-effective care for the health service, saving considerable sums of money by taking the oxygen-dependent baby out of a hospital cot that then becomes available for another patient.

Concerns about home oxygen therapy focus on the ability of the parents to cope with the 24-hours-a-day therapy, and in particular on their responses to sudden respiratory illnesses or life-threatening events. Babies with bronchopulmonary dysplasia are at increased risk of sudden infant death. Before they agree to take their baby home, an experienced doctor must have discussed these issues openly and honestly. Usually the parents will have seen their baby have a series of critical episodes, and be all too aware of what they are taking on. Discharge home should only be with the full support of the family doctor, health visitor, district paediatric nurse and/or neonatal liaison nurse. A planning meeting to which the parents and these support workers are invited is useful.

The following has to be achieved once it is agreed that the baby should go home in oxygen:

- A home assessment visit is undertaken to ensure the baby can be kept warm, bathed and cared for while on oxygen therapy.
- The family doctor has to prescribe oxygen via nasal prongs at a specific flow rate.
- An oxygen concentrator with a low flow meter has to be installed in the home with a number of outlets to enable the baby to be cared for in two or three rooms. This equipment can only be installed once the home oxygen has been prescribed.
- Small portable oxygen cylinders (at least two) with low flow heads are provided. These are to enable brief outings to the shops, relatives and clinics! Clear arrangements should exist for their replacement when empty, and the supplier must always have some full cylinders.
- Both parents must be shown an ABC of neonatal resuscitation. Simple mucus extractors can be provided to help the parents clear the airway (no risk of HIV transmission here). The parents must practise mouth to mouth and nose breathing and know how to check air is entering the lungs. They should also practise external cardiac massage with intermittent breaths. Baby mannequins provide excellent material for teaching these skills. The only thing they need do with their own baby is to learn how to find a radial or brachial pulse – rapidly, repeatedly and reliably.
- A decision must be made as to whether the family should have an apnoea alarm at home (most choose to do so). This would be more for parental reassurance than any proven efficacy at preventing death, and this should be made clear to the parents.

- The family must have a telephone.
- The possibility of qualifying for an attendance allowance should be explored.
- The family must have open access to the children's ward.
- Planned follow-up by health visitors and nurses is coordinated so as to avoid conflicting advice over therapy, feeding and other issues.
- Regular clinic follow-up and assessment is planned.

Home oxygen therapy should be continued until placing the carefully monitored baby in air for periods of 30 to 60 min no longer leads to an early desaturation. If the baby's saturations in air remain in the mid-90s in this situation, oxygen therapy should be continued until an overnight oximetry sleep study in air has been performed. Only if this is satisfactory can the continuous oxygen be stopped. The oxygen concentrator and small cylinders should be retained for a few weeks after that in case of a transient deterioration with a viral infection.

Further reading

Angell C. Equipment requirements for community-based paediatric oxygen treatment. *Archives of Disease in Childhood*, 1991; **66**: 755.

Samuels MP, Southall DP. Home oxygen therapy. In: David TJ (ed). *Recent Advances in Paediatrics, No. 14*. Edinburgh: Churchill Livingstone, 1995; 37–51.

Sauve RS, McMillan DD, Mitchell I, Creighton D, Hindle NW, Young L. Home oxygen therapy. Outcome of infants discharged from NICU on continuous treatment. *Clinical Pediatrics*, 1989; **28**: 113–8.

Related topics of interest

Bronchopulmonary dysplasia (p. 38)
Discharge planning and follow-up (p. 75)

HYDROCEPHALUS

Hydrocephalus may be evident at birth (congenital hydrocephalus) or result from complications in the perinatal or postnatal period. Hydrocephalus is commonly due to obstruction to the CSF pathways (and rarely CSF over-production) leading to dilatation of the ventricles and back pressure proximal to the site of obstruction. The most common sites of obstruction are the aqueduct of Sylvius (between the third and fourth ventricles) and the exit foramina of the fourth ventricle (the central foramen of Magendie and the two lateral foramina of Luschka). In communicating hydrocephalus, CSF can flow out of the ventricular system reaching the subarachnoid space. Communication is easily confirmed clinically by the rise and fall of lumbar CSF pressure on jugular venous compression (Quecken–Stedt's test).

Aetiology

1. Congenital hydrocephalus. This may be a single abnormality or associated with other congenital malformations within or outside the central nervous system (CNS).

- Arnold–Chiari malformation (commonly associated with myelomeningocele) obstructs the fourth ventricle foramina and occasionally the aqueduct of Sylvius.
- Dandy–Walker malformation (cystic dilatation of the fourth ventricle) obstructs the fourth ventricle foramina and occasionally the aqueduct of Sylvius.
- Sex-linked aqueductal stenosis confined to males (associated with flexion and adduction defects of the thumbs).
- Post-infection (toxoplasma, rubella, CMV) – cerebral atrophy may also contribute to hydrocephaly.
- Cerebral tumours and arterio-venous malformations.
- Choroid plexus papilloma (hydrocephalus from CSF over-production not obstruction – rare).

2. Secondary hydrocephalus
- Post-haemorrhagic (following intraventricular haemorrhage especially in preterm infants), usually communicating, but with obstruction of the fourth ventricle foramina may become non-communicating.
- Post-infection (meningitis) due to obstruction of the aqueduct of Sylvius and the fourth ventricle foramina as well as cerebral atrophy.

Clinical features

The anterior fontanelle is large or bulging with widely separated sutures and open posterior fontanelle in newborn period. Other features are down-turning eyeballs (sunsetting), a head circumference exceeding the 97th centile by ≥2 cm, and the head may transilluminate.

Investigations

- Cranial ultrasonography (most useful first-line investigation) – serial scans may be necessary.

- CT scan or MRI may be required for more detailed imaging.
- Congenital infection screen (TORCH titres if intrauterine infection suspected).
- For post-haemorrhagic hydrocephalus in newborn term infants, exclude a bleeding disorder (clotting studies and platelet count) and alloimmune thrombocytopenia (mother produces immunoglobulin G (IgG) antibodies to Pl^{A1} antigen or infant's platelets).

Management

This partly depends on the aetiology. Congenital hydrocephalus is probably best treated surgically by insertion of a ventriculoperitoneal or ventriculoatrial shunt. As a temporary measure if the infant is not fit for surgery, medical therapy (e.g. acetazolamide 100 mg/kg/day) may be of value. Repeated lumbar or ventricular taps are not beneficial and are associated with a high risk of infection. However, following post-haemorrhagic hydrocephalus, serial CSF drainage (lumbar or ventricular taps) may be required to control rapid head growth or symptoms (apnoeas, fits) until CSF protein level is below 1 g/l, when a shunt may then be inserted.

Shunt complications include CSF over-drainage, blockage, infection with low-grade septicaemia (*Staphylococcus albus*). Long-term neurodevelopmental follow-up is required.

Further reading

Bayston R. *Hydrocephalus Shunt Infections*. London: Chapman and Hall, 1989.

Levene MI, Liford RJ, Bennett MJ, Punt J (eds). *Fetal and Neonatal Neurology and Neurosurgery, s*. Edinburgh: Churchill Livingstone, 1995.

Reed GB, Claireaux AE, Cockburn F (eds). *Diseases of the Fetus and Newborn: Pathology, Imaging and Managing,* 2nd edn. London: Chapman and Hall, 1995.

Volpe JJ. *Neurology of the Newborn*, 3rd edn. Philadelphia: W.B. Saunders, 1995.

Related topics of interest

Bleeding disorders (p. 25)
Germinal matrix-intraventricular haemorrhage (p. 93)
Head size (p. 101)
Neural tube defects (p. 203)

HYDROPS FETALIS

Hydrops is a generalized hypoalbuminaemic oedema of the fetus and neonate. Ascites and pleural and pericardial effusions occur, and heart failure is common. It is diagnosed antenatally by ultrasound scanning with characteristic appearances – a halo of oedema, thickened subcutaneous tissues, ascites, effusions and hepatosplenomegaly. There are many causes, grouped into 'immune' and 'non-immune'.

Immunological hydrops

This is secondary to haemolytic disease from rhesus or other isoimmunization. It is now rare, in fewer than 1 in 10 000 deliveries because of improved antenatal care. Treatment is as for severe rhesus haemolytic disease, but with the added issues discussed below under emergency treatment at birth.

Non-immunological hydrops (known associations)

Chromosomal
- Trisomies (13, 15, 18, 21).
- 45XO (Turner's).
- XX/XY.
- Triploidy.

Cardiac

1. *Structural*
- Septal defects.
- Hypoplastic left heart.
- Truncus arteriosus.
- Pulmonary atresia.
- Cardiac rhabdomyoma.
- Premature closure of ductus arteriosus.
- Pericardial teratoma.
- Subaortic stenosis with fibroelastosis.
- Right atrial haemangioma.

2. *Dysrhythmias*
- Supraventricular tachycardia.
- Heart block.

3. *Other cardiac*
- Myocarditis.
- Cardiomyopathy.
- Calcification of arteries or myocardium.
- Asplenia syndrome.
- Causes of cardiac failure (e.g. arterio-venous malformation or haemangioma).

Pulmonary
- Diaphragmatic hernia.
- Cystadenomatoid malformation.

* Tracheo-oesophageal fistula (TOF).
* Sequestered lung.

Infective
* Parvovirus B19.
* Cytomegalovirus.
* Toxoplasmosis.
* Syphilis.
* Hepatitis.
* Chagas' disease.

Maternal/placental
* Multiple births (especially twin–twin transfusion).
* Diabetes.
* Toxaemia.
* True knot in cord/umbilical vein thrombosis.
* Vascular malformation of the cord or placenta.

Gastrointestinal
* Biliary atresia.
* Jejunal atresia.
* Volvulus.

Renal
* Congenital nephrotic syndrome.
* Urethral obstruction (posterior urethral valves).
* Polycystic kidneys.
* Renal vein thrombosis.

Haematological
* Twin–twin transfusion.
* Alpha thalassaemia.
* Fetomaternal haemorrhage.
* G6PD deficiency.
* Any fetal anaemia.

Neurological
* Encephalocoele.
* Tuberous sclerosis.
* Agenesis of corpus callosum.
* Holoprosencephaly.
* Intracranial haemorrhage.

Skeletal
* Osteogenesis imperfecta.
* Some dwarfisms.

Congenital tumours
* Teratoma.
* Neuroblastoma.
* Choriocarcinoma.
* Hepatoblastoma.

Storage disorders
* Gaucher's disease.
* Niemann–Pick disease.
* Mucopolysaccharidoses.

Miscellaneous
* Beckwith–Wiedemann syndrome.
* Prune belly syndrome.
* Myotonic dystrophy.

- Neu–Laxova syndrome.
- Infant of a diabetic mother.
- Idiopathic.

It is important to remember these are some of the associations with non-immune hydrops, and that they are not necessarily the cause.

Antenatal investigation and management

Isoimmunization and rhesus disease must be excluded first by investigating ABO, rhesus and other blood group antigens and haemolysins. If negative, detailed ultrasound scanning is essential, as is karyotyping and TORCH, parvovirus and venereal disease research laboratory (VDRL) screening. If samples are taken by cordocentesis, the presence of fetal anaemia and abnormal haemoglobin can be detected in addition to the other tests. Treatment as appropriate with maternal anti-dysrhythmic drugs, supportive transfusions to the fetus and possibly procedures to drain fetal ascites and pleural effusions should be considered.

Postnatal investigations and management

1. *Emergency treatment at birth*
- Intubate and ventilate with high pressures (up to $30\,cmH_2O$).
- Drain pleural effusions and ascites (diagnosed antenatally): keep aspirates for analysis.
- Insert umbilical venous lines to secure vascular access.
- Transfer ventilated to the neonatal unit.

2. *On the neonatal unit*
- Insert UAC and obtain blood for baseline observations including gases, glucose, albumin, electrolytes, FBC, clotting screen, blood group and Coombs' test.
- If a pericardial effusion is suspected, perform cardiac echocardiography to confirm and then perform pericardiocentesis under ultrasonic guidance.
- Get a chest and abdominal X-ray.
- Assess the baby for congenital abnormalities: plan second-line investigations for diagnoses listed above.
- As first results come back, adjust ventilation to achieve satisfactory gases, maintain blood pressure and circulation, bring central venous pressure down to 6 mmHg, if necessary by withdrawing further aliquots of blood 10 ml at a time, and treat any metabolic acidosis as necessary. Colloid can be given slowly later, when hypoalbuminaemia has been confirmed.

Long-term management

If the baby survives, long-term management begins with the stabilization of the baby on the ventilator. Once haematological and biochemical abnormalities have been corrected, and heart failure, pleural effusions and ascites resolved, intensive care is discontinued. If still undiagnosed, further investigations may be necessary, and the parents should be supported and referred to a clinical geneticist. In 50% of cases, no cause is found. Mortality is also 50% or more. If the baby is stillborn or dies later, request a post-mortem examination. The parents should be counselled and referred to a clinical geneticist.

Further reading

Fanaroff AA, Martin RJ. *Neonatal–Perinatal Medicine: Diseases of the Fetus and Neonate*, 6th edn. St Louis: Mosby, 1997.

Hann IM, Gibson BES, Letsky EA (eds). *Fetal and Neonatal Haematology*. London: Baillière Tindall, 1991.

Phibbs RH. Hydrops fetalis and other causes of neonatal edema and ascites. In: Polin RA, Fox WW (eds). *Fetal and Neonatal Physiology*, 2nd edn. Philadelphia: W.B. Saunders, 1998; 1730–6.

Reed GB, Claireaux AE, Cockburn F (eds). *Diseases of the Fetus and Newborn: Pathology, Imaging, Genetics and Managing*, 2nd edn. London: Chapman & Hall Medical, 1995.

Stephenson T, Zuccollo J, Hohajer M. Diagnosis and management of non-immune hydrops in the newborn. *Archives of Disease in Childhood*, 1994; **70**: F151–4.

Related topics of interest

Anaemia (p. 9)
Cardiac arrhythmias (p. 43)
Haemolytic disease (p. 97)
Respiratory distress (p. 275)
Resuscitation (p. 282)

HYPOTONIA

Most floppy babies do not have a persistent neuromuscular disorder. They may have benign neonatal hypotonia – characterized by a floppiness with normal strength – or a transient hypotonia related to conditions such as prematurity or mild birth asphyxia (stage 1 hypoxic–ischaemic encephalopathy). Hypotonia is classified 'anatomically' in a centrifugal fashion: that is, as central in origin, or from the spinal cord, the peripheral nerves, the neuromuscular junction or the muscles themselves.

Central hypotonia

1. Primary
- Down's syndrome.
- Prader–Willi syndrome.
- Peroxisomal disorders.
- Cerebral palsy – the hypertonia develops later.
- Brain malformations.

2. Secondary
- Anaesthesia.
- Drugs, e.g. maternal benzodiazepines.
- Sepsis.
- Respiratory distress.
- Hypoglycaemia.
- Metabolic disorders.

Spinal cord disorders
- Birth injuries to the cervical spine and cord.
- Spinal muscular atrophy – type 1 (Werdnig–Hoffman).

Peripheral nerve abnormalities
- A generalized peripheral neuropathy is very rare in neonates.
- Local palsies secondary to trauma are easily recognized.

Neuromuscular junction disorders
- Transient neonatal myasthenia – anti-acetylcholine receptor antibodies cross the placenta.
- Feeding and respiratory difficulties – usually respond to neostigmine, ventilation occasionally needed. Improvement after days/weeks.
- Congenital myasthenic syndromes.

Muscle disease

1. Congenital muscular dystrophy. Weak, with contractures/ arthrogryposis. Many improve slowly. Several subgroups are now recognized (see 'Neuromuscular disorders – muscular').

2. Myotonic dystrophy. The mother is always affected. Symptoms are polyhydramnios secondary to swallowing difficulties *in utero*; immobile face, triangular mouth, respiratory difficulties; not myotonic as a baby. Many have learning difficulties and some have gut, and later CNS and endocrine involvement.

3. Congenital myopathies. Symptoms include hypotonia, respiratory difficulties and later learning difficulties. Biochemical abnormality has yet to be clarified in many types, and diagnosis is usually by muscle biopsy.

Investigation and management

As is evident from the above lists, the causes of neonatal hypotonia are legion. The approach to investigating hypotonia is determined to a large part by the clinical impression of the suspected underlying cause(s). The investigation and management of the various disorders are outlined under the relevant topics. Detailed accounts on neuromuscular investigations have been set out under 'Neuromuscular disorders'.

Further reading

Crawford TO. Clinical evaluation of the floppy infant. *Pediatric Annals*, 1992; **21**: 348.

Curran A, Jardine P. The floppy infant. *Current Paediatrics*, 1998; **8**: 37–42.

Dubowitz V. *The Floppy Infant*, 2nd edn. Clinics in Developmental Medicine No. 76. Cambridge: Cambridge University Press, 1980.

Dubowitz V. *Muscle Disorders in Childhood*, 2nd edn. London: W.B. Saunders, 1995.

Roper HP. Neuromuscular diseases in children. *British Journal of Hospital Medicine*, 1993; **49**: 537–45.

Related topics of interest

HYPOXIC–ISCHAEMIC ENCEPHALOPATHY

The term birth asphyxia is poorly defined, but includes decreased oxygen delivery to, and perfusion of, vital organs, particularly the brain. It is associated with metabolic acidosis, low Apgar scores and end organ damage. Many authorities feel the term should no longer be used and more objective measures should be recorded (e.g. umbilical cord blood gases). Although birth asphyxia is a multi-system disorder, it is the effect on the brain – the post-asphyxial encephalopathy – which is of prime importance in the outcome. Post-asphyxial or hypoxic–ischaemic encephalopathy (HIE) is a variable constellation of symptoms and signs, including alterations in consciousness and behaviour, feeding difficulties, abnormal tone, convulsions and failure to maintain regular respiration. About 1 in 500 term babies has HIE severe enough to cause fits or coma.

Prognostic evaluation Early prediction of prognosis in each case of perinatal asphyxia and HIE is important. Accurate information should be given to parents, for starting resuscitation or withdrawing therapy, and in the future, the possibility of offering effective neuroprotective therapy. Prognostic statements for infants with HIE are best made from the level of severity of the clinical syndrome. Two main classifications are in use and their features are summarized in *Tables 1* and *2*.

Table 1. Sarnat and Sarnat classification of HIE

	Stage 1	Stage 2	Stage 3
Consciousness	Hyperalert	Lethargic	Stuporose
Seizures	None	Common: focal or multifocal	Uncommon: excluding decerebration
Muscle tone	Normal	Mild hypotonia	Flaccid
Duration	<24 hours	2–14 days	Hours to weeks
EEG	Normal	Variable changes: seizures <1–1.5 Hz spike and wave	Periodic pattern with isopotential phases, later totally isopotential

Table 2. Levene *et al.* classification of HIE

	Mild	Moderate	Severe
Consciousness	Hyperalert	Lethargy	Comatose and fails to maintain ventilation
Seizures	Absent	Present	Present
Muscle tone	Minor disturbances	Abnormal	Profound hypotonia
Duration	Recovering by 48 hours	Recovering by 7 days	

Both groups reported on the outcome, albeit in slightly different ways.

- All babies with mild or stage 1 HIE did well; 75% of those with moderate or stage 2 HIE also did well, but with more severe asphyxia (stage 3 HIE) some 60% died, and a high proportion of the survivors were handicapped.
- In one large American study, neonates with clinically recognized seizures, a 5 min Apgar score ≤5 and at least one sign compatible with HIE had a 33% risk of death in the first year, and 55% of the survivors had a motor disability.
- At age 1 year, infants with mild (stage 1) or moderate (stage 2) HIE for less than 5 days had developed normally. Severe (stage 3) HIE or the persistence of moderate encephalopathy was associated with seizures, motor and cognitive delay.
- At age 8 years, infants who had mild HIE as neonates were free of handicap in motor, cognitive and school performance. However, infants who had experienced moderate or severe HIE had greater impairment of performance in each of these developmental spheres.
- The likelihood of long-term neurological sequelae after HIE was increased by the presence of neonatal seizures. Interictal background EEG abnormalities, such as persistently low voltage, isoelectric activity and burst-suppression, correlated with poor outcome.

Management

1. *Immediate*
(a) Establish effective ventilation and oxygenation. If intrapartum asphyxia is suspected, an experienced resuscitator should be at the delivery with the aims of:
- Clearing the airways of meconium if present.
- Establishing effective ventilation.
(b) Circulatory support if necessary
- External cardiac massage.
- Adrenaline.
- Glucose 200 mg/kg as a bolus if there is profound hypoglycaemia (the myocardial glycogen stores are depleted in severe asphyxia).
(c) Correct hypoglycaemia, but marked hyperglycaemia may exacerbate brain damage

2. *Ongoing management*
- Restrict fluids by 20–25% . This protects against cerebral oedema and reduces the risk of fluid overload if there is renal failure.
- Monitor urine output and electrolytes.
- Monitor and support blood pressure and perfusion with inotropes. If, after initial resuscitation, hypotension persists

then the asphyxiated myocardium may be more contractile on an inotrope such as dopamine (initially $10 \mu g/kg/min$), and if thought to be hypovolaemic, an infusion of 10–20 ml/kg of albumin (but hazard of fluid overload).

- Ventilate if $PaCO_2$ rises above 7 kPa with spontaneous respiration. A raised $PaCO_2$ causes cerebral vasodilatation and may contribute to raised intracranial pressure and may also indicate impending coma.
- If ventilated, maintain $PaCO_2$ at 4.5–5 kPa. This will reduce cerebral oedema. Lower $PaCO_2$ may cause cerebral vasoconstriction to the point of causing further ischaemic damage to compromised parts of the brain. Hyperventilation for HIE is associated with a high risk of pneumothoraces.
- Cerebral oedema. Following perinatal hypoxic–ischaemic cerebral injury, intracranial pressure may be elevated due to cytotoxic cerebral oedema. However, cerebral perfusion pressure (mean arterial blood pressure minus intracranial pressure) remains within the normal range throughout the postnatal course, unless intracranial pressure becomes markedly increased. Trials performed to protect the neonatal brain by reducing this oedema, by mannitol, steroids, frusemide or elective intubation followed by hyperventilation, all lack effect on eventual outcome.
- Give anticonvulsants if recurrent or prolonged convulsions occur. Anticonvulsants are generally given to babies with hypoxic–ischaemic fits though they have not been shown to improve outcome. Fits develop in the first 48 hours (75% in the first 24 hours) and often settle within another 2–3 days. The concern is that under-perfusion or under-oxygenation of excited cells will lead to further damage. Reducing cellular metabolism with membrane stabilizing anticonvulsant drugs should be beneficial, but this has yet to be confirmed.

  Phenobarbitone, given as a loading dose of 20 mg/kg and then 5– 6 mg/kg/day is the first line anticonvulsant.

  Phenytoin, with a loading dose of 20 mg/kg then 8 mg/kg/day, is also used.

  Clonazepam is also effective (loading dose of $100 \mu g/kg$, then 'titrated' as an infusion starting at $10 \mu g/kg/hour$ and increasing in $10 \mu g$ increments until fits are controlled).

Withdrawal of intensive care

- As up to 93% of infants with severe HIE die or are severely handicapped, withdrawal of life support should be an option.
- Doppler studies and EEG are of value in evaluating severity of brain injury.

- Severe EEG abnormalities include burst suppresion, low-voltage or isoelectric EEGs, and moderate EEG abnormalities include slow-wave activity.
- The overall risk of death or handicap for a severely abnormal early EEG is up to 95%, 64% for a moderately abnormal EEG, and 3.3% for a mildly abnormal EEG.
- After the first 24 hours of life, abnormal Doppler signals from the anterior cerebral artery accurately predict very poor outcome. A low Pourcelot resistance index (<0.55) predicts adverse outcome with a sensitivity of 100% and a specificity of 81%.
- Discussions with the parents should always be frank, truthful and to the point to allow them to come to terms with the situation and be prepared for the eventuality of withdrawing life support (see 'Death of a baby').

Birth asphyxia and cerebral palsy

Only about 8% of cases of cerebral palsy (CP) are caused by perinatal factors. The vast majority of CP is of uncertain antenatal origin.

Further reading

Blennow M, Lagercrantz H. Management of the asphyxiated infant. In: Hansen TN, McIntosh N (eds). *Current Topics in Neonatology, No. 2.* London: W.B. Saunders, 1997; 39–64.

Levene MI. Management of the asphyxiated full-term infant. *Archives of Disease in Childhood*, 1993; **68:** 612–6.

Peliowski A, Finer NN. Birth asphyxia in the term infant. In: Sinclair JC, Bracken MB (eds). *Effective Care of the Newborn Infant.* Oxford: Oxford University Press, 1992; 249–79.

Volpe JJ. Hypoxic–ischaemic encephalopathy: clinical aspects. In: *Neurology of the Newborn*, 3rd edn. Philadelphia: W.B. Saunders, 1995; 314–69.

Related topics of interest

IMMUNIZATION

Immunity can be conferred by passive transfer (for short-term) or actively (long-term). Passive immunity results from the injection of human immunoglobulin and affords immediate but short-lived (few weeks) protection. There are two types of human immunoglobulin: human normal immunoglobulin (HNIG) and specific immunoglobulins (e.g. for varicella-zoster or tetanus). Active immunity is induced by using attenuated live organisms (e.g. oral poliomyelitis vaccine (OPV) and BCG vaccine) or their products (e.g. tetanus and diptheria) or inactivated organisms (e.g. pertussis and inactivated poliomyelitis virus (IPV)). Vaccines produce their protective effect by inducing cell-mediated immunity and serum antibodies which can be demonstrated by their detection in the serum.

All infants should receive their full complement of immunizations unless valid medical contraindications exist. The date of each immunization, type of vaccine, batch number and, for BCG, the site of injection, should always be recorded on the recipient's record. Where two vaccines are given concurrently, the relevant sites should be recorded to facilitate identification of any untoward reactions. Expired vaccines should not be used and the expiry date should be noted. The specified routes of administration should be adhered to. With the exception of BCG (given intradermally), OPV and oral typhoid vaccine, all vaccines should be given by deep i.m. or s.c. injection (antero-lateral thigh or upper arm, avoid buttocks). Allow skin-cleaning agents to dry *before* injecting vaccines as live vaccines may be inactivated by the disinfecting agents. Live vaccines should not be given within 3 months of an immunoglobulin injection as the immune response may be suboptimal. When two or more live vaccines have to be administered at the same time, they should be given at different sites concurrently (unless using a combined preparation) or be separated by a 3-week interval. There is no need for an interval between the administration of inactivated and live vaccines.

Contraindications for immunizations

- Immunizations should be postponed during an acute febrile illness, but minor infections without fever or systemic disturbance are not a contraindication.
- A clear history of a general reaction or a severe local reaction is a contraindication.
- Infants receiving prednisolone at doses of 2 mg/kg/day for ≥ 1 month are effectively immunosuppressed and should *not* receive live vaccines until 3 months after stopping therapy. Replacement corticosteroids are not a contraindication.
- Infants with impaired cell-mediated immunity commonly receive immunoglobulin preparations as part of their therapy which make most live vaccines ineffective.
- HIV-positive infants should not be given BCG (risk of dissemination of BCG). In the UK, where the risk of tuberculosis is low, withhold BCG to all infants *suspected* of being HIV-positive (e.g. infants of HIV-positive mothers). HIV-positive infants (with or without symptoms) may receive measles, mumps and rubella live vaccines. IPV may be safer. They can receive the usual inactivated vaccines (diptheria, pertussis, tetanus, Hib, hepatitis B).

- OPV should not be given to immunosuppressed infants, their siblings or other household contacts. Instead IPV should be given.
- Stable neurological conditions (e.g. previous IVH or cerebral palsy) are not a contraindication to immunization.

Schedule for primary immunizations

Preterm infants should be immunized according to the recommended schedule from the age of 2 months *irrespective* of their prematurity. The efficacy and safety of the vaccines are similar in term and preterm infants using the recommended schedule. Infants remaining on the NNU should receive IPV, or OPV on discharge.

Additional vaccinations

1. BCG vaccine. This was introduced for general use in the UK in 1953. It has an efficacy of 70–80% in protecting against tuberculosis when given to British school children. This protection lasts 15 years. It is a live attenuated form of *Mycobacterium bovis*, of which there are two types, one for percutaneous use (for infants only, using multiple puncture technique), and one for intradermal injection. Neonatal immunization policies vary widely but generally they aim to target those at higher risk of tuberculosis. In the UK, this generally means the following:

- Infants born to immigrants from countries with a high prevalence of tuberculosis (e.g. Indian subcontinent, Africa, infants of refugees).
- Infants born to parents with a recent family history of tuberculosis.
- Newborns whose parents request BCG immunization.
- Infants who will be taken on travel into countries/regions with high prevalence of tuberculosis.

BCG vaccine should be administered strictly intradermally (0.05 ml for those <3 months), using a separate tuberculin syringe and needle for each subject (not by jet injectors); alternatively the percutaneous route may be used (same site), using a multiple puncture technique (and appropriate vaccine!). Use the insertion of the deltoid muscle near the middle of the left arm as the main site of injection (keloid formation is more common if higher sites are used). Alternatively, use the upper and lateral thigh (but clearly record this in the records).

2. Hepatitis B. This should be performed on infants born to mothers who are chronic carriers of HBV or to mothers developing acute hepatitis B during pregnancy (see 'Hepatitis B').

3. Varicella (chickenpox). Varicella is an acute, highly infectious disease transmitted directly by droplet spread and personal contact and indirectly via articles (e.g. towels, clothing) which have been in contact with an affected individual. The disease can be life-threatening in neonates and immunosuppressed infants. Herpes zoster is a reactivation of the patient's varicella virus. Infants in the following groups are particularly at risk of developing severe disseminated or haemorrhagic varicella if exposed to varicella-zoster and should be given human varicella-zoster immunoglobulin (VZIG):

- Infants with evidence of impaired cell-mediated immunity (e.g. severe combined immunodeficiency (SCID) or Di George syndrome).
- Infants with evidence of immunosuppression (e.g. immunosuppressive treatment).
- Infants with symptomatic HIV infection.
- Neonates whose mothers develop chickenpox within 7 days before delivery to 28 days after delivery.
- Neonates exposed to chickenpox or herpes zoster in the first 28 days of life and who are varicella-zoster antibody negative.
- Preterm infants born before 28 weeks gestation or weighing <1000 g at birth but whose mothers have a positive history of chickenpox (inadequate transfer of maternal antibody).

VZIG (1 vial, 250 mg) is given by i.m. injection as soon as possible but within 10 days after exposure. Immunocompromised infants at long-term risk should be immunized with varicella vaccine (e.g. Varivax™, Oka/Merck, USA). Currently a live attenuated varicella vaccine is available on a named patient basis only in the UK.

4. Respiratory syncytial virus. RSV is a highly contagious and potentially fatal disease in high-risk infants (young infants, preterm infants, infants with BPD and CHD). RSVIG provides passive immunity against RSV infections. It decreases the occurrence and duration of moderate to severe RSV infection in infants under 24 months of age who were born <35 weeks gestation or with BPD. Currently this is the only effective means of preventing severe RSV lower respiratory tract infection in high-risk preterm infants. However, prophylactic RSVIG has to be administered i.v. each month at a cost of £2000–£3000 per infant per season.

Further reading

Campbell AGM. Immunization for the immunosuppressed child. *Archives of Disease in Childhood*, 1988; **63:** 113–4.
Groothuis JR, Simoes EA, Hemming VG. Respiratory syncytial virus (RSV) infection in preterm infants and the protective effects of RSV immune globulin (RSVIG). Respiratory syncytial virus immune globulin study group. *Pediatrics*, 1995; **95:** 463–7.

Plotkin SA, Edward A. *Vaccines*, 2nd edn. Philadelphia: W.B. Saunders, 1994.

Salisbury DM, Begg NT (eds). *Immunization against Infectious Disease*. London: HMSO Publications, 1996.

Simpson N, Lenton S, Randall R. Parent refusal to have children immunised: extent and reasons. *British Medical Journal*, 1995; **310**: 227.

WHO/UNICEF. Global Programme on AIDS and Expanded Programme on Immunization. Joint WHO/UNICEF statement on early immunization for HIV-infected children. *Weekly Epidemiology Records,* 1989; **7** (Feb 17): 48–9.

Related topics of interest

Bronchopulmonary dysplasia (p. 38)
Discharge planning and follow-up (p. 75)
Hepatitis B (p. 105)
HIV and AIDS (p. 114)

INFANTS OF DIABETIC MOTHERS

The term IDM is used here to describe infants of insulin-dependent diabetics. Babies born to mothers with gestational diabetes are less severely affected, particularly with regard to congenital abnormalities. During the 77 years since the discovery of insulin, the outcome of pregnancies complicated by diabetes mellitus has continued to improve. Currently, except for those deaths due to major malformations, perinatal mortality in the pregnancies of women with insulin-dependent diabetes mellitus who receive excellent medical care approaches that of the general population.

Problems in pregnancy
- Polyhydramnios.
- IUGR especially in mothers with a diabetic nephropathy (characterized by macroproteinuria, hypertension, retinopathy, declining glomerular filtration, and uraemia). IUGR may be three to seven times more common in a diabetic pregnancy as compared with non-diabetic pregnancies.
- Sudden unexpected fetal death in the third trimester associated with maternal keto-acidosis, pre-eclampsia and maternal vascular disease, although many deaths are unexplained. It is the fear of this that results in many IDMs being delivered at 38 to 39 weeks. Delivery earlier than that is contraindicated because of pulmonary immaturity.

Problems for the neonate Many of the problems are secondary to fetal hyper-insulinism. They can therefore be reduced or prevented by good diabetic control before and throughout the pregnancy. Pre-pregnancy counselling of the parents helps them to understand the importance of tight control.

1. Congenital abnormalities. These are two to eight times more common in IDMs than in other babies, though this may be reduced by tight preconceptual diabetic control. The incidence of major congenital malformations remains at 6–9%, accounting for 40% of perinatal deaths among IDMs. The caudal regression syndrome (sacral agenesis) is particularly common (600 times more common compared with non-diabetic mothers). Other CNS anomalies include microcephaly, anencephaly and other neural tube defects (3- to 20-fold risk of normals). Others reported include situs inversus, arthrogryposis, skeletal abnormalities, renal and genital anomalies (hydronephrosis, renal agenesis, ureteral duplication), gastrointestinal (duplex livers, duodenal atresia, anorectal atresia and small left colon syndrome), cardiac anomalies (VSDs, single ventricle, hypoplastic left heart syndrome, pulmonary valve stenosis and atresia, transposition of the great arteries with or without VSD, coarctation of the aorta with or without VSD, PDA, or atrial septal defect (ASD)) and single umbilical artery. Current evidence supports the notion that hypergly-caemia and its resulting metabolic derangements are terato-gens, and that strict metabolic control in the preconceptual period may reduce the overall incidence of diabetes-related malformations.

2. Macrosomia. A birthweight of >90th centile or birth-weight ≥4000 g, is secondary to fetal hyper-insulinism in the poorly controlled diabetic. The incidence of infants with birth-weights of ≥4000 g is 8% in non-diabetic women and 26% in diabetic women. Insulin is a growth factor causing hypertro-phy of organs and deposition of fat. Macrosomia is associated with protracted labour, birth asphyxia, shoulder dystocia, and nerve and skeletal injuries. Consequently, up to 47% of such infants are delivered by Caesarean section. The macrosomic neonate is especially at risk of other complications seen in IDMs.

3. Hypoglycaemia. Most common in macrosomic babies – 'diabetic cherubs' – with an onset immediately after birth. Approximately 47% of macrosomic infants and 20% of non-macrosomic IDMs become hypoglycaemic. The neonate is hyper-insulinaemic as a result of the hyperglycaemic intra-uterine environment, and rapidly becomes hypoglycaemic once delivered. IDMs who develop hypoglycaemia have ele-vated cord C-peptide and free insulin levels at birth. Some IUGR babies will have inadequate glycogen stores and become hypoglycaemic some hours later. Maternal blood glucose con-trol in the later part of pregnancy, including during labour and delivery, significantly influences the frequency and severity of neonatal hypoglycaemia.

4. Respiratory distress. This is more common as IDMs have delayed lung maturation. Delivery at 30 to 37 weeks gestation is associated with much higher respiratory morbidity than in normal babies.

5. Hypocalcaemia. Also common (seen in ~50%), possibly caused by a delay in the usual postnatal rise of parathyroid hor-mone. In most infants, this will resolve spontaneously within a few days, but in some it may be prolonged and require a slow infusion of i.v. 10% calcium gluconate or added vitamin D to enhance calcium absorption.

6. Hypomagnesaemia. Often co-exists with hypocalcaemia and may present with jitteriness, irritability, apnoeas and sometimes frank seizures. Symptomatic infants with a normal serum calcium level but a magnesium level of <0.7 mmol/l should receive a single i.m. injection of 0.1–0.3 ml/kg of 50% magnesium sulphate solution.

7. *Polycythaemia*. Most common in IDMs who have suffered placental insufficiency. Reduced oxygen delivery secondary to elevated glycosylated haemoglobin may also contribute. Renal vein thrombosis and other complications may occur. Hyperbilirubinaemia is more common.

8. *Myocardial dysfunction*. Ventricular septal hypertrophy secondary to hyper-insulinism is common. It can cause subaortic obstruction and lead to cardiac failure. Once the insulin levels are normal, the hypertrophy resolves over 8 to 12 weeks. Other cardiac abnormalities may occur.

9. *Intrapartum asphyxia*. There is an increased incidence of asphyxia in pregnancies complicated by diabetic nephropathy. There may be an accompanying vasculopathy of the placental bed leading to fetal compromise. The macrosomic infant may also be more prone to delivery complications, which predispose to birth trauma and asphyxia, for example failure to progress, fetal distress and instrumental delivery.

Long-term complications Long-term complications associated with diabetic pregnancies include childhood obesity (which correlates with maternal prepregnant weight), neuropsychological deficits and an increased tendency (risk of up to 20-fold compared with offspring of non-diabetic mothers) to develop diabetes mellitus. Infants of gestational diabetic mothers and infants of diabetic fathers also have an increased incidence of diabetes. It remains unclear whether maternal diabetes predisposes the offspring to subtle developmental problems.

Further reading

Cordero L, Landon MB. Infant of the diabetic mother. *Clinics in Perinatology*, 1993; **20**: 635–48.
Fanaroff AA, Martin RJ. *Neonatal–Perinatal Medicine: Diseases of the Fetus and Neonate*, 6th edn. St Louis: Mosby, 1997.
Taeusch HW, Ballard RA (eds). *Avery's Diseases of the Newborn*, 7th edn. Philadelphia: W.B. Saunders, 1998.

Related topics of interest

INFECTION – GENERAL

Newborn infants, and in particular preterm infants, are especially vulnerable to infections due to an immaturity of their host defence systems. Their impaired immunological competence is partly due to an opsonization defect and a functional immaturity of their white blood cells. Consequently, sepsis remains a major cause of morbidity and mortality in the neonatal period.

Aetiology

Infections presenting in the neonatal period may antedate delivery by several days or weeks (congenital infections), or be acquired during delivery (perinatal infections) or later in the postnatal period (postnatal infections). Causative organisms are varied, ranging from common bacteria and viruses, through fungi to unusual protozoa.

Clinical features

These vary from non-specific signs to obvious signs of sepsis with pallor and shock.

1. General
- Fever.
- Hypothermia.
- Temperature instability.
- Poor colour.
- Lethargy.
- Irritable or unresponsive.
- Acute collapse.
- Being just 'not right'.

2. Respiratory
- Tachypnoea.
- Grunting.
- Recession.
- Cyanosis.
- Apnoeas.

3. Cardiovascular
- Tachycardia >160/min.
- Hypotension.
- Poor peripheral perfusion and prolonged capillary refill time (>3 s).
- Cold and clammy.
- Shock.

4. Gastrointestinal
- Vomiting.
- Abdominal distension.
- Ileus.
- Loose and/or bloody stools.
- Hepatosplenomegaly.
- Jaundice.
- Abdominal redness and induration.

- Periumbilical staining.
- Poor weight gain.

5. *Metabolic*
- Hyperglycaemia ($\pm$ glycosuria).
- Hypoglycaemia.

6. *Haematological*
- Petechiae.
- Purpura or bleeding from puncture sites, gut or renal tract.

7. *Neurological*
- Hypotonia.
- High-pitched cry.
- Bulging fontanelle.
- Retracted head.
- Seizures.
- Coma.

8. *Musculoskeletal*
- Swollen and tender limb(s) or joint(s).
- Pseudoparalysis and crying when moved (arthritis or osteomyelitis).

9. *Skin*
- Pallor.
- Mottled skin (cutis marmorata).
- Septic spots.
- Erythema.
- Paronychia.
- Omphalitis.
- Discharging umbilicus.

Investigations

For suspected serious infection in a symptomatic infant, carry out a full septic infection screen. Lumbar puncture may be omitted in symptomatic but less unwell patients. The following investigations should be included:

- FBC, differential and film. WBC <5 or >20 $\times$ 10^3/mm^3, neutrophils <2 or >10 $\times$ 10^3/mm^3 or immature leucocytes (band cells) with toxic granulation and thrombocytopenia suggest sepsis.
- Blood cultures.
- Urine culture suprapubic aspirate or clean catch specimen (on microscopy, eight organisms per high power field suggests infection).
- Surface swabs of ear, nose, throat and umbilicus. Microscopy and Gram stain, culture and virology ($\pm$ electron microscopy for virus particles).
- Stools for bacteriology and virology.

- CSF for microscopy and Gram stain, culture and sensitivity, virology and biochemistry (protein >1.5–2.0 g/l in term infants and >3.7 g/l in preterm infants, CSF glucose <50% of blood glucose or <1.0 mmol/l, with >1 white cell per 500 red cells (traumatic samples) or >20–30 polymorphonuclear leucocytes/mm^3 (atraumatic samples), all suggest meningitis). CSF serology for group B streptococcal or *E. coli* antigen.
- Clotting screen (when bleeding present or serious infection suspected).
- Blood gases, glucose, U&E, C-reactive protein (CRP).
- Chest radiograph(s) and abdominal radiograph(s), in the presence of abdominal signs.
- Abdominal ultrasound (intra-abdominal masses and sepsis, renal and urinary tract infection, ascites).

Management

- Commence broad-spectrum i.v. antibiotics immediately. In general, if cultures are negative and the infant is well, antibiotics may be discontinued after 48–72 hours. Where cultures are negative but a temporal improvement in the infant's condition is noted with antimicrobial therapy, therapy is continued for 5–7 days. If sepsis is confirmed by positive culture(s), therapy is continued for at least 10 days and occasionally longer depending on the focus of infection (e.g. brain or bone) and the isolated pathogen.
- In sick infants, commence continuous monitoring of physiological parameters including transcutaneous oxygen saturations by pulse oximetry.
- Commence assisted ventilation for recurrent apnoeas and respiratory failure.
- Monitor arterial blood gases 4–6-hourly in infants with respiratory distress or receiving assisted ventilation.
- Monitor BP by an indwelling arterial device or non-invasively regularly (1–4-hourly) in all ill and unstable infants, more frequently in sicker infants.
- Correct hypotension with FFP (10–15 ml/kg) and add inotropes (dopamine/dobutamine at 10–20 µg/kg/min) if BP still suboptimal.
- Administer i.v. dextrose solutions to maintain normal blood glucose and electrolytes (check U&E).
- Monitor the core–peripheral temperature gap in sick infants as a guide to the adequacy of tissue perfusion.
- Modify drug therapy according to the evolution of the illness, taking into account reports from bacteriology (pathogens isolated and their sensitivity).

Further reading

Gerdes JS. Clinicopathologic approach to the diagnosis of neonatal sepsis. *Clinics in Perinatology*, 1991; **18**: 361–81.

Isaacs D, Moxon ER. *Neonatal Infections*. Oxford: Butterworth-Heinemann, 1991.

Klein JO, Remington JS. Current concepts of infections of the fetus and newborn infant. In: Remington JS, Klein JO (eds). *Infectious Diseases of the Fetus and Newborn Infant*, 4th edn. Philadelphia: W.B. Saunders, 1995; 1–19.

Lewis DB, Wilson CB. Developmental immunology and role of host defenses in neonatal susceptibility to infection. In: Remington JS, Klein JO (eds). *Infectious Diseases of the Fetus and Newborn Infant*, 4th edn. Philadelphia: W.B. Saunders, 1995; 20–98.

Powell KR, Marcy SM. Laboratory aids for diagnosis of neonatal sepsis. In: Remington JS, Klein JO (eds). *Infectious Diseases of the Fetus and Newborn Infant*, 4th edn. Philadelphia: W.B. Saunders, 1995; 1223–40.

Related topics of interest

INFECTION – NEONATAL

Neonatal infections may be acquired at birth but with a late presentation (after 3 days), or be acquired postnatally as nosocomial infections. This section covers the traditional 'late-onset' infections, i.e. those occurring after the first week of life. Untreated, infections in newborns can become life-threatening. It is important, therefore, that infections in newborn infants be identified and treated promptly. The global burden of neonatal infections is substantial. Worldwide, some 30 million infants develop an infection in the neonatal period and five infants die from neonatal infection every minute. The organisms associated with neonatal infections vary significantly in different geographical areas. Thus while group B streptococcus (GBS) continues to be the most important bacterial pathogen associated with early-onset sepsis in many developed countries, for reasons which remain unclear, neonates in some developing nations are rarely infected with GBS, which only accounts for 1–8% of neonatal infection. Neonatal infections in the developing nations are dominated by Gram-negative (e.g. *Klebsiella* sp.) and Gram-positive organisms (e.g. *Staphylococcus aureus*). It is therefore essential that antibiotic therapy be tailored to the specific microbial needs of a particular geographical region.

General infections

Common causative organisms

1. *Bacterial infections*
   - *Staphylococcus epidermidis.*
   - *Escherichia coli.*
   - *Streptococcus.*
   - *Staphylococcus aureus.*
   - *Pseudomonas aeruginosa.*
   - *Enterobacter cloacae.*
   - *Klebsiella.*
   - *Proteus.*

2. *Viral infections*
   - Respiratory syncytial virus (RSV).
   - Enterovirus.
   - Echo virus.

3. *Other*
   - *Candida.*
   - *Chlamydia trachomatis.*

Risk factors

- Prematurity.
- Intubation.
- Central intravascular access.
- Recent surgery (including drains *in situ*).
- Indwelling peripheral arterial and umbilical catheters.
- Congenital anomalies (urinary tract, gastrointestinal, spinal).
- Presence of infectious organism in other patients, parents or staff.

Clinical presentation	Commonly presents as:

- Septicaemia.
- Oral and perineal thrush.
- Snuffles, sticky eyes and coughing.
- Pneumonia (intubated infants, aspiration).
- Meningitis (apnoeas, seizures).
- Diarrhoea.
- Urinary tract infection (vomiting, feeding intolerance).
- Osteomyelitis (immobile, oedematous inflamed and tender limbs or joints).
- Cardiac failure (myocarditis with cyanosis, poor cardiac output, hepatosplenomegaly).

Investigations

1. General
- A full septic screen.
- Always culture urine – clean catch or suprapubic aspirate.
- ECG – suspected myocarditis (low voltage complexes and arrhythmias).
- Renal and bladder ultrasound scan – UTI.
- For suspected osteomyelitis aspirate fluid from infected bone or joint and obtain radiographs.

2. Special
- Cranial CT or MRI scans (CNS sepsis).
- Bone isotope scans.
- Labelled leucocyte scans.

Management

Antibiotic choice for pneumonia, septicaemia, or meningitis depends on the local microbiological flora. Commonly a combination of penicillin or ampicillin with an aminoglycoside (usually gentamicin) will suffice until microbial culture reports are available. The antibiotic choice may be modified depending on the sensitivities of the isolated organisms.

Specific infections

Staphylococcal infections

Staphylococci belong to the family Micrococcaceae and can be differentiated into two large groups on the basis of their ability to ferment mannitol and produce the extracellular enzyme coagulase. Organisms able to ferment mannitol and produce coagulase are called coagulase-positive organisms or *Staphylococcus aureus*. Organisms negative for these products are called coagulase-negative staphylococci, the most important being *Staphylococcus epidermidis* and *Staphylococcus saprophyticus*. Gram stain shows Gram-positive cocci. In recent years coagulase-negative staphylococci have assumed predominance as NICU pathogens. Infants are colonized by coagulase-negative staphylococci and *S. aureus* soon after birth and mostly by staff contact. Hand washing is one of the most effective means of reducing colonization. The virulence of *S. aureus* is related to the production of coagulase, alpha-haemolysin and leucocidin whereas coagulase-negative staphylococci produce a polysaccharide mucoid (slime) which facilitates their adherence to foreign bodies (e.g. catheters) and hinders phagocytosis.

S. aureus causes the following infections:

- Impetigo.
- Staphylococcal scalded skin syndrome.
- Chronic recurrent furunculosis.
- Eye, ear, nose and throat infections.
- Breast abscesses.
- Septicaemia.
- Pneumonia.
- Osteomyelitis.
- Septic arthritis.
- Endocarditis (rare, more likely with coagulase-negative staphylococci and intravascular catheters).

Coagulase-negative staphylococci are an important cause of nosocomial infection, especially in VLBW infants, and risk of infection is increased in the presence of indwelling medical devices (e.g. venous catheters or central nervous system shunts).

- *S. epidermidis* is the most frequent bacterial species isolated from blood.
- *S. aureus* and coagulase-negative staphylococci are now widely resistant to penicillin G due to ß-lactamase production.
- In recent years resistance to semisynthetic ß-lactamase resistant penicillins (e.g. methicillin) has produced problematic infections with methicillin-resistant *S. aureus* (MRSA) and methicillin-resistant coagulase-negative staphylococci.
- Once introduced into a hospital, MRSA are difficult to eliminate.

Treatment. First-line agents for methicillin-susceptible strains of *S. aureus* include flucloxacillin, oxacillin, and some 'first generation' cephalosporins (e.g. cephalexin). Glycopeptide antimicrobials (e.g. vancomycin, teicoplanin) are the agents of choice for methicillin-resistant staphylococcal infections, and coagulase-negative staphylococci infections resistant to the common first-line drugs.

Respiratory syncytial virus (RSV)

RSV is a pneumovirus of the family Paramyxoviridae of which two types (A and B) exist. It causes annual outbreaks of infection (bronchiolitis) during the winter months. The incubation period is 2–8 days with viral shedding lasting 3–4 weeks. Spread is by aerosol or direct contact with infected secretions.

- Clinical features include upper respiratory tract symptoms (cough and rhinitis) followed by lower respiratory tract symptoms (tachypnoea, recessions and cyanosis).
- Symptoms and disease severity are age-dependent. The very young (<4 weeks) may present apnoeas and non-specific signs of infection (lethargy, poor feeding, irritability, fever). Disease is more severe in preterm infants >12 weeks, especially preterm infants with chronic lung disease who are more likely to require assisted ventilation.
- Infants with congenital heart disease (CHD) are also at high risk for severe disease (more likely to require supplemental oxygen (83%), intensive care (30%), assisted ventilation (19%) and die (3.4%)).
- Diagnosis is by direct fluorescent antibody detection of virus and enzyme-linked immunosorbent assays of nasopharyngeal aspirates.
- Therapy is mainly supportive (fluids, supplemental oxygen, antibiotics for pneumonia) with ribavirin being given early to the high-risk groups (BPD, CHD).
- Hyperimmune RSV immunoglobulin, e.g. RespiGam™ (Medimmune Inc, Gaithersburg, MD, USA), is effective prophylaxis for preterm infants (<36 weeks' gestation and age <6 months) or those with BPD (reduces the incidence and severity of RSV infection). No benefit is reported for infants with CHD.

Further reading

Greenough A, Osborne J, Sutherland S (eds). *Congenital, Perinatal and Neonatal Infections.* Edinburgh: Churchill Livingstone, 1992.

Isaacs D, Moxon ER. *Neonatal Infections.* Oxford: Butterworth-Heinemann, 1991.

Remington JS, Klein JO (eds). *Infectious Disease of the Fetus and Newborn Infant,* 4th edn. Philadelphia: W.B. Saunders, 1995.

Stoll BJ, Weisman LE (eds). Infections in Perinatology. In: *Clinics in Perinatology,* 1997; **24:** 1.

Related topics of interest

Infection – general (p. 139)   Infection – prenatal (p. 151)
Infection – perinatal (p. 147)

INFECTION – PERINATAL

Infections presenting in the immediate postnatal period are likely to have been acquired during the delivery or *in utero*. Such infections often mimic respiratory distress syndrome (RDS) and if untreated may rapidly progress to a fulminant and fatal illness. Therefore where there are risk factors for sepsis, appropriate antibiotic therapy should be started immediately with recourse to full intensive care support if required. The traditional 'early-onset' infections, i.e. occurring during the first week of life, are covered in this section.

General infections

Common causative organisms

1. *Bacterial infections*
   - Group B streptococcus (GBS).
   - *Haemophilus influenzae.*
   - *Escherichia coli.*
   - *Listeria monocytogenes.*
   - *Neisseria gonorrhoea.*

2. *Viral infections*
   - Herpes simplex.
   - Varicella-zoster.
   - Hepatitis B.
   - HIV.

Common risk factors for perinatal infections
- Maternal infection or intrapartum pyrexia.
- Prolonged (>24 hours) rupture of membranes.
- Cloudy or foul-smelling liquor.
- Instrumental delivery.
- Premature labour.
- Long labour.

Clinical features
These vary from non-specific signs to obvious signs of sepsis with pallor and shock. See 'Infection – general'.

Investigations
- FBC.
- CRP.
- Chest X-ray.
- Blood and CSF culture.
- GBS antigen in urine and CSF.
- Coagulation studies in severe sepsis.
- Virus identification by electron microscopy in vesicle fluid, PCR, or serology.
- Chlamydia – direct immunofluourescence test and specific IgM.

Management
- For symptomatic infants perform a full septic screen and commence broad-spectrum antibiotics (commonly ampicillin/penicillin and an aminoglycoside).

- For asymptomatic infants perform a septic screen (omitting lumbar puncture) followed by broad-spectrum antibiotics.
- Discontinue antibiotics if bacteriology shows no growth at 48 hours and the infant is well. However, continue antibiotics for at least 5 days if the mother received antibiotics intrapartum.

Specific infections

Group B streptococcus

In the developed nations, GBS disease is the commonest cause of fatal bacterial infection in newborns. A quarter to a third of all adults carry GBS. It is found primarily in the gastrointestinal tract but also in the genital tract where it is usually asymptomatic. At birth ~25% of mothers have GBS in their genital tract. Early onset infection (which constitutes 60% of all GBS infection) is largely acquired from the maternal genital tract. The US average incidence is ~1.4 per 1000 births, while in the UK it is 0.5–0.7 per 1000 births. The majority of early onset infections occur *in utero* and are therefore not influenced by mode of delivery.

1. Risk factors for GBS infection
- Prolonged rupture of membranes.
- Intrapartum pyrexia (>37.8°C).
- Preterm rupture of membranes (PROM).
- Preterm labour (<37 weeks gestation).
- Maternal GBS carriage.
- GBS UTI during the pregnancy.
- Previous birth of an infant with GBS.

2. Clinical features
- Apnoeas.
- Grunting.
- Respiratory distress.
- Acute collapse and/or shock.

GBS mimics RDS, but left untreated, GBS is rapidly fatal. The infant may develop pneumonia, septicaemia or meningitis which carry a high mortality. Even with full therapeutic support, mortality still remains around 10%. Most infections can be prevented by the intrapartum administration of penicillin (or clindamycin) to the high-risk group. Antibiotic administration during pregnancy does not eradicate GBS carriage. Infants born to mothers who have received antibiotics during labour should still receive antibiotics (5-day course) if they were to receive therapy in any case (i.e. preterm infants, infants with PROM), but after first performing an infection screen. The treatment of choice is penicillin and gentamicin (10 days for septicaemia and 14–21 days for meningitis). Term infants admitted to the postnatal ward do not require antibiotics, but parents should be advised to look out for signs of infection in those given early discharges from hospital (who therefore have not been monitored while in hospital).

Listeriosis

Neonatal listeriosis accounts for the largest recognizable group of infections caused by *L. monocytogenes*. The incidence of neonatal listeriosis in Europe and the USA is 13 per 100 000 live births. Early onset listeriosis has similarities to GBS with respiratory symptoms which mimic RDS. Classically it develops within the first 48 hours of life. Most cases are clinically apparent at delivery with meconium staining, cyanosis, respiratory distress and pneumonia. A transient pink papular rash may be seen over the trunk. The chest radiograph may resemble RDS or an aspiration pneumonitis. Disseminated disease is often fatal. Mothers acquire listeria from refrigerated dairy products (soft cheeses, milk, paté), may have a fever pre-labour and have a discoloured amniotic fluid. Diagnosis is by cultivation of *L. monocytogenes* (a Gram-positive motile bacterium) from blood and other tissues. High-dose ampicillin with an aminoglyside is the treatment of choice. The long-term morbidity is unclear but if meningitis is not present outcome may be generally good.

Varicella-zoster

Severity of neonatal disease is dependent on the timing of maternal illness. Maternal rash soon after delivery or within 5 days before delivery greatly increases the risk of a severe perinatal infection. Zoster immunoglobulin (VZIG) (one vial, 125 units) should be administered as soon as possible after birth to infants whose mothers are diagnosed with chickenpox with lesions from 5 days before to 2 days after delivery. VZIG will ameliorate or prevent disease, but 50% will still develop chickenpox. Acyclovir should be administered to symptomatic infants (10–15 mg/kg, reduced in renal failure).

Herpes simplex

Herpes simplex virus (HSV) exists in two forms, types 1 and 2 (HSV-1 and HSV-2, respectively). HSV-2 accounts for 60–70% of neonatal HSV infection. The incidence of neonatal HSV infection in the UK is 0.03–0.05 per 1000 live births and 0.1–0.3 per 1000 in the USA (where the incidence is rising). Most HSV infection in neonates occurs intrapartum. The attack rate is ~33% in women with a primary infection, but only ~3% in women having a reactivation. Less commonly, HSV can be acquired in the post-partum period (mostly due to HSV-1). Skin vesicles may be diagnostic. Clinical signs may initially be mild and non-specific but may progress to a severe illness with pneumonitis, encephalitis or myocarditis. Note however, presentation may be delayed for up to 8 weeks. Diagnosis is by virus culture (urine, stool, blood, CSF, vesicle fluid, conjunctival scrapings, and swabs of the eye, throat and rectum), light microscopy (intranuclear inclusions) or electron microscopy of conjunctival scrapings, and PCR to detect HSV DNA (e.g. in CSF and serum). EEG may show localizing signs of high-voltage low-frequency activity, and CT or MRI scans may show temporal lobe necrosis or haemorrhage. Treatment is with acyclovir (or vidarabine) with full intensive care support. Mortality is 15% with CNS involvement, and 57% with disseminated disease. Risk of death is increased in infants in coma, DIC, seizures, and HSV–2. If in doubt, treat and review later!

Chlamydia trachomatis Conjunctivitis is the commonest early manifestion of an intrapartum chlamydial infection. Chlamydia (inclusion conjunctivitis) requires 1% tetracycline drops and a full course of oral erythromycin.

Further reading

Remington JS, Klein JO (eds). *Infectious Disease of the Fetus and Newborn Infant*, 4th edn. Philadelphia: W.B. Saunders, 1995.
Stoll BJ, Weisman LE (eds). Infections in Perinatology. *Clinics in Perinatology*, 1997; **24:** 1.
Greenough A, Osborne J, Sutherland S (eds). *Congenital, Perinatal and Neonatal Infections*. Edinburgh: Churchill Livingstone, 1992.

Related topics of interest

INFECTION – PRENATAL

TORCH infections

Several maternal infections during pregnancy may have permanent or long-lasting effects in the fetus. The outcome following such intrauterine infections may depend on the maturity of the fetus when the infection is contracted. The commonest congenital infections of significance constitute the 'TORCH' infections – namely Toxoplasmosis, Other (particularly syphilis), Rubella, Cytomegalovirus and Herpes simplex.

Toxoplasmosis

Infection with *Toxoplasma gondii* results in toxoplasmosis, one of the commonest infections in the world, with a marked variation in prevalence from <50% to 90% (e.g. France). The incidence of toxoplasmosis during pregnancy varies from 3–6 per 1000 to 1–2 per 1000 in low-risk countries (e.g. UK, USA). The mother can be infected by an infected cat, or by eating raw or inadequately cooked meat or contaminated vegetables. Most individuals will have either no or minimal signs of acute infection. The risk of fetal infection increases from the first trimester to the third trimester, while the risk of serious infection in the fetus decreases from 75% in the first trimester to being negligible in the third trimester. Congenital toxoplasmosis with clinical manifestation of disease in the newborn occurs when the fetus is infected before 26 weeks gestation. The incidence of congenital toxoplasmosis in the UK is approximately 1:10000. Approximately 60% of all infants born to infected mothers escape infection, 25% have subclinical infection without sequelae, and only 5–10% develop clinical infection. The classic tetrad of congenital toxoplasmosis is chorioretinitis, intracranial calcification, epilepsy and hydrocephalus. Affected infants may also be growth restricted and present with petechiae, jaundice and hepatosplenomegaly. Diagnosis is based on serological tests for toxoplasmosis, particularly of the CSF. Antenatal diagnosis is possible. Treatment with spiramycin, pyrimethamine and sulphonamides may improve fetal outcome for mothers who seroconvert during pregnancy. Infected neonates receive a year's therapy with spiramycin, sulphadiazine and pyrimethamine. Prognosis for mild or subclinical cases is good, but 25% of those with neonatal symptoms die. Infection in the first 20 weeks of pregnancy may be an indication for termination.

Rubella

Congenital rubella is rare in the UK with ≤10 cases reported each year. Rubella was made notifiable in the UK in 1988, the same year the MMR vaccine was introduced. In 1995 there were only eight confirmed rubella infections in pregnant women reported to the Communicable Disease Surveillance Centre.

Currently approximately five cases of congenital rubella syndrome (CRS) are reported annually to the National Congenital Rubella Surveillance Programme. The risk of fetal infection decreases with advancing gestation. In 90% of cases, maternal rubella infection in the first 8–10 weeks of pregnancy results in serious fetal infection and damage, whereas by 16 weeks the risk declines to 10–20% and thereafter fetal damage is rare. The clinical features of extended CRS include petechiae, jaundice, hepatosplenomegaly, eye and bone anomalies, a murmur and, in 33%, birthweight below third centile. Multiple fetal defects are common: eyes (cataract, glaucoma, microphthalmia), CNS (microcephaly, mental retardation, cerebral palsy), deafness (bilateral and sensorineural), cardiovascular (PDA, peripheral artery stenosis), liver (hepatitis and prolonged jaundice), bone (osteitis), haematological (anaemia, thrombocytopenia). Diagnosis is by culturing the virus from a throat swab or urine and demonstrating rubella-specific IgM in the infant's blood. Antiviral treatment is not available and infants remain very infectious during the first months of life (hazard to female staff). Glaucoma and cataracts require ophthalmological intervention and hearing should be formally assessed.

Cytomegalovirus (CMV)

Occurring at an incidence of 0.2–2.5% of all live births (UK 0.3–0.4%, USA ~1%), congenital CMV is the commonest disease of newborns with a significant morbidity. Both primary and recurrent maternal infections during pregnancy can result in fetal infection but the rate of fetal transmission is higher (24–75%) with a primary maternal infection than with a reactivation of infection (<1%). Approximately 90% of congenitally infected infants born to mothers who had their primary infection during pregnancy are asymptomatic at birth, but they are more likely to develop adverse sequelae than those infants born to mothers with reactivation of infection. The characteristic features include petechiae, hepatosplenomegaly, sensorineural hearing impairment, microcephaly, intracranial calcification, chorioretinitis, jaundice, growth restriction and thrombocytopenia. The standard diagnostic test is viral culture (the most sensitive and specific test) of urine, saliva, or other bodily secretions/tissues obtained within the first 3 weeks of life so as to distinguish congenital from perinatal and postnatal infection. Other tests include serology for CMV-specific IgM antibody, detection of CMV DNA by PCR, and urine electron microscopy for viral particles. These infants shed the virus for long periods (hazard to female staff). Therapy with ganciclovir and CMV-immunoglobulin should be considered in severe disease, though efficacy has not been proven.

Prognosis is generally good with most infants developing normally. Approximately 10% of asymptomatic neonates develop deafness in later life. Of those with CNS signs in the neonatal period, 73% develop long-term sequelae, while 30% will have neurological sequelae in the absence of signs in the neonatal period.

Herpes simplex virus (HSV)

HSV exists in two forms, types 1 and 2 (HSV-1 and HSV-2, respectively). HSV-2 causes ~85% of genital herpes, while HSV-1 causes mainly ophthalmic, orolabial and CNS disease. HSV-2 accounts for 60–70% of neonatal HSV infection. The incidence of neonatal HSV infection in the UK is 0.03–0.05 per 1000 live births and 0.1–0.3 per 1000 in the USA (where the incidence is rising). Most HSV infection in neonates occurs intrapartum but true congenital infection occurs in ~5% of cases as a result of both primary infection and (rarely) recurrent maternal infection. Congenital HSV is defined as the presence of vesicles or scarring at birth; abnormal brain CT scan within the first week of life; microcephaly, microphthalmia, or chorioretinitis. Congenital HSV has a different presentation from intrapartum HSV. The major clinical findings are cutaneous lesions (94%), CNS lesions (79%) (microcephaly, hydranencephaly, cerebral atrophy, intracranial calcification), prematurity (59%), ocular lesions (42%) (chorioretinitis, microphthalmia), organomegaly (hepatitis). HSV-2 causes >90% of congenital infection. The congenitally infected infant may be mildly affected with eye involvement only, or severely affected with skin lesions, chorioretinitis and microcephaly (or hydranencephaly). Diagnosis is by virus culture (urine, stool, blood, CSF, vesicle fluid, conjunctival scrapings, and swabs of the eye, throat and rectum), light microscopy (intranuclear inclusions) or electron microscopy of conjunctival scrapings, and PCR to detect HSV DNA (e.g. in CSF and serum). EEG may show localizing signs of high-voltage low-frequency activity, and CT or MRI scans may show temporal lobe necrosis or haemorrhage. Treatment is with acyclovir (or vidarabine) with full intensive care support. Mortality is 15% with CNS involvement, and 57% with disseminated disease. Rarely, infants with congenital HSV develop normally.

Other infections

Syphilis

Infected newborn infants may appear normal or be severely affected with extensive skin eruptions through to marked hydrops fetalis. All pregnant mothers should be screened (VDRL, TPHA or ELISA) for syphilis. False positives may occur after *Treponema pertenue* infection (yaws). Maternal infection leads to intrauterine infection in up to half of all pregnancies with increased fetal loss from abortions or stillbirths.

1. Clinical features
- Infant may initially appear normal, with signs only appearing weeks to months later.
- Extensive mucocutaneous lesions in the absence of systemic disturbance but with hepatosplenomegaly and lymphadenopathy.
- Severe systemic disturbance but without the typical skin rashes.
- Cutaneous manifestations (maculopapular rash with circinate lesions involving palms and soles of feet).
- Rhinitis followed by mucopurulent blood-stained nasal discharge.
- Destruction of nasal cartilage and bone produces flattened nasal bridge and saddle nose.
- Fissures and bleeding from lesions at mucocutaneous junctions.
- Rhagades.
- Condylomata around anus and female genitalia.
- Osteochondritis, especially wrists, elbows and knees.
- Periostitis, especially in limb bones and skull.
- Meningitis and hydrocephalus.

2. Investigations
- FBC.
- Liver function tests.
- Syphilis serology (VDRL, TPHA or ELISA with rising or persistently high titres).
- Dark-field microscopy of fluid from skin lesions and nasal discharge.
- Radiography of long bones (periostitis and osteochondritis).
- CSF examination (lymphocytosis, raised protein, normal glucose level, syphilis serology positive).

3. Management. Take precautions as skin lesions are infectious. Procaine penicillin 30 mg/kg/day i.m. for 10 days or single i.m. injection of long-acting benzathine penicillin 60 mg/kg. Treat mother and partner(s)!

Varicella-zoster

Varicella-zoster virus (VZV) infection during pregnancy (incidence ~0.7 in 1000), particularly during the first 20 weeks, may result in fetal loss or congenital varicella-zoster syndrome, with cutaneous lesions (scars) (70%), ocular abnormalities (chorioretinitis, microphthalmia, cataracts, Horner's syndrome), CNS lesions (50%) (cortical atrophy, calcifications, mental retardation), and abnormal limb development (hypoplasia, abnormal or absent digits). Administration of varicella-zoster immunoglobulin (VZIG) post-exposure may prevent fetal infection, and acyclovir therapy during pregnancy may be safe.

Parvovirus B19

Parvovirus B19, the causative agent of erythema infectiosum (Fifth's disease), has a predilection for bone marrow erythroid precursors. Lysis of the erythroid precursors is responsible for decreased red cell production. The incidence of B19 infection during pregnancy is reported as 3.7% with a vertical transmission of 16% during the first 20 weeks and 35% after 20 weeks gestation. Infection-related fetal loss is low at 0.6 per 1000 women. The commonest symptomatic presentation of prenatal infection is non-immune hydrops secondary to severe fetal anaemia, but this only occurs in ~1% of infected infants. Most infants with prenatal B19 infection are normal. No studies support a correlation between maternal infection and an increased risk of birth defects. Diagnosis is by electron microscopy of virions in tissue specimens, detection of viral DNA by PCR or serology (IgM and IgG antibodies). Negative IgM assay at birth does not rule out congenital infection.

HIV infection

Approximately 8% to 24–50% of the total HIV vertical transmission is estimated to occur *in utero*. Vertical transmission is reduced by prenatal, perinatal and early neonatal zidovudine therapy. No HIV-associated dysmorphic syndrome exists.

Further reading

Greenough A, Osborne J, Sutherland S (eds). *Congenital, Perinatal and Neonatal Infections*. Edinburgh: Churchill Livingstone, 1992.

Remington JS, Klein JO (eds). *Infectious Disease of the Fetus and Newborn Infant*, 4th edn. Philadelphia: W.B. Saunders, 1995.

Stoll BJ, Weisman LE (eds). Infections in Perinatology. In: *Clinics in Perinatology*, 1997; **24(1)**.

Related topics of interest

INHERITED METABOLIC DISEASE – INVESTIGATION AND MANAGEMENT

As over a hundred inherited metabolic diseases (IMDs) can present in newborn infants, it would be impractical to cover these disorders in any detail in a brief synopsis. A summary of an approach to the investigation and management of IMDs may be more useful. The diagnosis of IMD has implications for future pregnancies, as prenatal diagnosis is now possible for many of these conditions. Although IMDs may present in a myriad of ways, certain details offer important clues to the possibility of IMD, namely unexplained neonatal deaths, a previously affected sibling or close relative, and consanguinity. A history of sudden illness in a previously well infant (particularly when vomiting, acidosis and circulatory disturbance are followed by depressed consciousness and convulsions or neurological features out of proportion to the perceived insult) are also highly suggestive of IMD.

For simplicity, IMDs may be divided into three groups.

Group 1	These disorders lead to toxicity from accumulation of compounds proximal to the metabolic block, for example aminoacidopathies, organic acidurias, urea cycle defects and sugar intolerances. There is a symptom-free period followed by signs of acute intoxication (e.g. vomiting, lethargy, coma, etc.). Metabolic disturbances are common (hypoglycaemia, ketosis, acidosis, hyperammonaemia, etc.). Diagnosis relies on the assay of urine and plasma amino acids and organic acids. Therapy entails removal of toxic compounds by extrarenal procedures or special diets.
Group 2	These disorders arise partly from a defect in utilization or production of energy due to a metabolic defect in the liver, muscle, myocardium or brain, for example glycogenosis types I and III, congenital lactic acidaemia, fatty acid oxidation defects and mitochondrial respiratory chain defects. Symptoms include hypoglycaemia, hyperlactacidaemia, severe hypotonia, myopathy, cardiomyopathy, cardiac failure and sudden infant death syndrome. These disorders may arise antenatally.
Group 3	These disorders disturb the synthesis or catabolism of complex molecules. Symptoms are permanent, progressive and not related to food intake, e.g. lysosomal disorders, peroxisomal disorders, α_1-anti-trypsin deficiency and carbohydrate-deficient glycoprotein (CDG) syndrome. As therapies are not available for most of these conditions, ascertaining the correct diagnosis is important.
Presentation of IMD in the neonatal period	For simplicity, three presentations may be described: neurological, hepatodigestive and cardiac.

1. Neurological presentations. These may present primarily as hypotonia, seizures or neurological dysfunction. |

(a) Neurological dysfunction

In group 1 (toxicity) disorders, there is often a normal pregnancy and delivery, an initial normal and symptom-free postnatal period, followed by unprovoked progressive deterioration unresponsive to symptomatic therapy. Typically the affected infant feeds poorly and then progresses into a coma with apnoeas, bradycardias, hiccups and involuntary movements (tremors, myoclonic jerks), axial hypotonia and limb hypertonia.

In group 2 (energy deficiency) disorders, there is no intervening symptom-free postnatal period. Commonly there is generalized hypotonia, rapidly progressive neurological deterioration, hypertrophic cardiomyopathy, occasional malformations and dysmorphic features.

(b) Seizures

Seizures occur as early signs of IMD in pyridoxine dependency, sulphite oxidase deficiency, non-ketotic hyperglycinaemia (NKH) and peroxisomal disorders. Of note, seizures rarely occur in organic acidurias or urea cycle defects unless the affected infant is comatose, hypoglycaemic or in a pre-existing stupor.

(c) Hypotonia

Predominant or isolated hypotonia is only seen in a few IMDs (e.g. peroxisomal disorders, NKH, respiratory chain disorders, sulphite oxidase deficiency and urea cycle defects).

2. Hepatodigestive presentations. Hepatomegaly with hypoglycaemia and seizures suggest glycogenosis types I and III, fructose diphosphatase deficiency or hyper-insulinism.

Liver failure syndrome (jaundice, haemorrhagic disease, hepatocellular necrosis with raised transaminases, ascites and hypoglycaemia) suggests galactosaemia, fructosaemia, tyrosinosis type I (after 2–3 weeks), neonatal haemochromatosis and respiratory chain disorders.

Primarily cholestatic jaundice with failure to thrive is observed in α_1-anti-trypsin deficiency, bile acid metabolic defects, peroxisomal disorders, Niemann–Pick type C disease, CDG syndrome, and Byler's disease. Hepatic presentations of fatty acid oxidation defects or urea cycle defects consist of fatty degeneration or Reye-like syndrome with slightly prolonged prothrombin time, raised transaminases, normal bilirubin levels but not true liver failure.

3. Cardiac presentations. Cardiac failure with cardiomyopathy (dilated hypertrophic), hypotonia, muscle weakness and failure to thrive suggests Pompe's disease, respiratory chain disorders, fatty acid oxidation defects or CDG syndrome. Long-chain fatty acid oxidation defects may present with conduction defects (A–V block, bundle branch blocks, ventricular tachycardia).

Investigations

Investigations must proceed alongside supportive therapy. Certain findings may be especially significant in suspected IMD, namely metabolic acidosis with large anion gap (organic acidurias), acetonuria (always abnormal in newborn), and raised lactate concentration with ketosis (especially in the absence of hypoxic insult, infection or circulatory collapse). Hyperammonaemia often suggests a urea cycle defect (with associated respiratory alkalosis), organic acidaemia (with ketoacidosis) or transient hyperammonaemia in preterm infants. Leucopenia, thrombocytopenia and even sepsis may also be present, especially in organic acidurias. Obtain adequate amounts of plasma, urine and CSF for immediate analysis and storage. Expert metabolic advice is essential.

1. Urine
- Note smell and colour.
- Reducing substances (Clinitest, Ames).
- pH (pH stix, Merck).
- Acetone (Acetest, Ames).
- Keto acids (dinitrophenylhydrazine (DNPH)).
- Sulphitest (Merck).
- Uric acid.
- Electrolytes.
- Organic acid chromatography.

Each fresh urine sample should be collected separately and either frozen ($-20°C$) for storage or kept in the fridge if not being assayed immediately.

2. Blood
- FBC.
- Blood gases.
- Blood glucose.
- Ammonia.
- Liver function tests (including transaminases).
- Coagulation screen.
- Amino acid chromatography.
- Electrolytes (check anion gap), calcium.
- Lactate and pyruvate.
- Uric acid.
- Free fatty acids.
- Acetoacetate, 3-hydroxybutyrate.

For storage, obtain 5 ml of heparinized plasma and freeze ($-20°C$), and freeze whole blood (10 ml in EDTA tube) for DNA studies. In addition, obtain blood on filter paper (Guthrie test cards). For white and red cells, spin the blood sample, separate the plasma and store frozen ($-20\,°C$), keeping the infranatant (red and white cells) at $+4\,°C$ (for up to 2 days).

3. *Other investigations*
- Lumbar puncture (CSF biochemistry, store some CSF at $-20\,°C$).
- Skin biopsy (fibroblast culture) – place in culture medium or normal saline and store at $+4\,°C$.
- Liver and muscle biopsies (before or after death). Freeze the liver biopsy tissue immediately on dry ice or in liquid nitrogen.
- Cerebral ultrasound and EEG.
- Echocardiography and ECG.
- Chest X-ray.
- Post-mortem.

Management

1. *General.* The primary goal is to correct the biochemical derangement(s) while ensuring adequate nutrition. The production of toxic metabolites should be suppressed while encouraging their elimination by extrarenal and alternate pathways.

Supportive care is required and this includes mechanical ventilation, circulatory support, maintenance of good hydration and diuresis with correction of electrolytes, correction of severe acidosis (pH <7.15) and treatment of sepsis.

2. *Specific therapies.* Peritoneal dialysis, haemodialysis and exchange transfusion (with fresh blood) may be useful in some IMDs where the accumulation of toxic metabolites is detrimental (organic acidurias, urea cycle defects). Adequate nutrition suppresses endogenous tissue breakdown. At the earliest opportunity, enteral or total parenteral nutrition should be commenced using appropriate glucose, lipid and amino acids, and mixtures built up to provide the recommended dietary allowance (RDA).

- Insulin infusion (0.2–0.3 units/kg/hour) may suppress catabolism.
- Sodium benzoate (250–500 mg/kg/day) and sodium phenylbutyrate (250–650 mg/kg/day) may be useful in urea cycle defects by enhancing nitrogen excretion as hippurate and phenylacetylglutamine, respectively.
- Arginine becomes an essential amino acid in urea cycle defects and therefore requires supplementation (at doses of 100–150 mg/kg/day) to maintain plasma concentrations of 50–200 μmol/l. Alternatively, substitute citrulline (up to 700 mg/kg/day) for arginine.
- L-carnitine (100 mg/kg/day), orally or intravenously, is useful in organic acidaemias (propionic, isovaleric and methylmalonic acidaemias, and 3-methylcrotonyl glycinuria) as it enhances specific acylcarnitine excretion.

- Dichloroacetate (DCA), a potent inhibitor of pyruvate dehydrogenase kinase, is useful in congenital lactic acidosis unresponsive to other therapies. All severe hyperlactacidaemias (primary or secondary) are DCA responsive (50 mg/kg/day).

Long-term outcome

Despite several advances in the diagnostic techniques for these disorders, the long-term outlook remains largely poor. Most patients with urea cycle defects and hyperammonaemia have a very poor outcome, with most survivors being handicapped. Those known to be affected prenatally may initially do better if treated expectantly, but a favourable long-term outlook may only be secured by liver transplantation. The organic acidaemias generally have a poor outcome and affected infants may only benefit significantly from liver transplantation or futuristic gene therapy. Isovaleric acidaemia has a better outlook than the other acidaemias, with neurodevelopmental outcome depending on early diagnosis and compliance with treatment. With early diagnosis and meticulous therapy, infants with maple syrup urine disease (MSUD) can be expected to survive long-term with at times satisfactory neurodevelopmental outcomes. The excellence of long-term metabolic control and the length of time after birth for which the plasma leucine levels are above 1 mmol/l directly influence intellectual outcome.

Further reading

Chaves-Caballo E. Detection of inherited neurometabolic disorders: a practical clinical approach. *Pediatric Clinics of North America*, 1992; **39**: 801.

Greene CL, Goodman SI. Inborn errors of metabolism. In: Hay WW, Groothuis JR, Hayward AR *et al* (eds). *Current Pediatric Diagnosis and Treatment*, 13th edn. Stamford: Appleton & Lange, 1997; 864.

Ogier de Baulny H, Saudubray JM. Emergency treatments. In: Fernandes J, Saudubray JM, Van den Berghe G (eds). *Inborn Metabolic Disease: Diagnosis and Treatment*, 2nd edn. New York: Springer-Verlag, 1995; 47–55.

Saudubray JM, Narcy C, Lyonnet L *et al*. Clinical approach to inherited metabolic disorders in neonates. *Biology of the Neonate,* 1990; **58**: 44.

Werlin SL. *E. coli* sepsis as a presenting sign in neonatal propionic acidemia. *American Journal of Medical Genetics*, 1993; **46**: 455.

Related topics of interest

INHERITED METABOLIC DISEASE – RECOGNIZABLE PATTERNS

Several clinical signs and laboratory findings are especially valuable in diagnosing metabolic IMDs. The following patterns may be recognized.

Altered neurological status

1. *Toxic type with hypertonia and abnormal movements*
   (a) Principal investigations
       Urine and plasma amino acid chromatography.
   (b) Findings
       Urine DNPH strongly positive, no acidosis and minor or no acetonuria. Normal lactate, glucose and calcium. Ammonia normal or raised.
   (c) Usual diagnosis
       MSUD (characteristic smell).

2. *Toxic type with dehydration*
   (a) Principal investigations
       Urine and plasma organic acid chromomatography, plasma and urine carnitine esters and plasma carnitine.
   (b) Findings
       Moderate acetonuria and acidosis. Urine DNPH slightly positive or negative. Ammonia raised. Lactate normal or raised, glucose and calcium normal or raised. Leucopenia and thrombocytopenia.
   (c) Usual diagnoses
       Ketolytic defects, organic acidurias (isovaleric acidaemia, propionic acidaemia, methylmalonic acidaemia).

3. *Energy deficiency type with liver or cardiac symptoms*
   (a) Principal investigations
       Plasma and urine organic acids, plasma carnitine, loading or fasting test, fatty acid oxidation studies on lymphocytes or fibroblasts.
   (b) Findings
       Acidosis without acetonuria and urine DNPH negative. Lactate and ammonia raised with low/normal calcium or glucose and normal blood count.
   (c) Usual diagnoses
       Fatty acid oxidation and ketogenesis defects.

4. *Energy deficiency type, hypotonia, tachypnoea*
   (a) Principal investigations
       Lactate/pyruvate ratios, hydroxybutyrate/acetoacetate ratio, urine organic acids, enzyme assays (muscle, fibroblast or lymphocytes).

(b) Findings

Marked acidosis, acetonuria and lactacidaemia. Ammonia normal or raised. Normal calcium and glucose.

(c) Usual diagnoses

Multiple carboxylase deficiency, congenital lactic acidosis (pyruvate carboxylase, pyruvate dehydrogenase, Krebs cycle, respiratory chain).

5. *Toxic type, hypotonia, seizures, coma and moderate hepatocellular disturbances*

(a) Principal investigations

Plasma and urine amino acids, urine organic acids, liver or intestinal enzyme studies (e.g. ornithine carbamyl transferase and carbamyl phosphate synthetase).

(b) Findings

Alkalosis without acetonuria and DNPH negative. Ammonia raised, lactate normal or raised with normal blood glucose, calcium and blood count.

(c) Usual diagnoses

Urea cycle defects, fatty acid oxidation defects (glutaric aciduria type II, carnitine palmitoyltransferase II (long-chain acyl-CoA dehydrogenase, 3-hydroxy long-chain acyl-CoA dehydrogenase).

6. *Severe hypotonia, myoclonic jerks, seizures*

(a) Principal investigations

Amino acid chromatography, CSF amino acids, plasma phytanic acid and plasma very long-chain fatty acids.

(b) Findings

No acidosis, acetonuria and DNPH negative. Ammonia, lactate, glucose, blood count all normal.

(c) Usual diagnoses

NKH, sulphite oxidase, xanthine oxidase, peroxisomal disorders, pyridoxine dependency, trifunctional enzyme.

Hepatomegaly with deranged liver function

1. *Hepatomegaly and hypoglycaemia*

(a) Principal investigations

Fasting and loading tests. Liver, fibroblast and lymphocyte enzyme studies.

(b) Findings

Acetonuria with acidosis. Ammonia normal, lactate raised, moderate hypoglycaemia and normal blood count.

(c) Typical diagnoses

Fructose diphosphatase deficiency, glycogenosis type I (acetest negative), glycogenosis type III (moderate acetonuria).

2. *Hepatomegaly, jaundice, liver failure and hepato-cellular necrosis*
(a) Principal investigations
Enzyme studies to exclude galactosaemia, fructosaemia and tyrosinaemia. Urinary organic acids.
(b) Findings
Slight acidosis and acetonuria. Ammonia normal or raised, lactate significantly raised and glucose normal or decreased.
(c) Typical diagnoses
Galactosaemia, fructosaemia, tyrosinosis type I, neonatal haemochromatosis, respiratory chain disorders.

3. *Hepatomegaly, cholestatic jaundice, chronic diarrhoea and failure to thrive*
(a) Principal investigations
Plasma and urine organic acids, protein electrophoresis, phytanic acid, very long-chain fatty acids, pipecolic acid and phytanic acid.
(b) Findings
Acidosis and ketosis are absent with normal glucose, lactate and ammonia.
(c) Typical diagnoses
α_1-anti-trypsin deficiency, peroxisomal disorders, inborn errors of bile acid metabolism.

4. *Hepatosplenomegaly, storage signs, chronic diarrhoea and failure to thrive*
(a) Principal investigations
Enzyme studies, mucopolysaccharides, sialic acid and oligosaccharides.
(b) Findings
Acidosis and ketosis are absent. Ammonia and glucose normal with normal or raised lactate.
(c) Typical diagnoses
Storage disorders, GM_1 gangliosidosis, infantile sialic acid storage disease (sialidosis II), I-cell disease, mucopolysaccharidosis type VII.

Further reading

Chaves-Caballo E. Detection of inherited neurometabolic disorders: a practical clinical approach. *Pediatric Clinics of North America*, 1992; **39**: 801.

Lyon G, Adams RD, Kolodny EH. *Neurology of Hereditary Metabolic Diseases of Children*, 2nd edn. New York: McGraw-Hill, 1996.

Saudubray JM, Ogier H, Charpentier C. Clinical approach to inherited metabolic diseases. In: Fernandes J, Saudubray J-M, Van den Berghe G (eds). *Inborn Metabolic Disease: Diagnosis and Treatment*, 2nd edn. New York: Springer-Verlag, 1995; 3–39.

Schaub J, Van Hoof F, Vis HL (eds). *Inborn Errors of Metabolism (Nestlé Nutrition Workshop Series*, Vol. 24). New York: Raven Press, 1991.

Scriver CR, Beaudet AL, Sly WS, Vale D (eds). *The Metabolic and Molecular Basis of Inherited Disease*, 7th edn. New York: McGraw-Hill, 1995.

Related topics of interest

INTRAUTERINE GROWTH RESTRICTION

The provision of adequate nutrition for the growing fetus is essential for its normal development and has implications for future health and wellbeing during childhood and adulthood. IUGR is largely a consequence of fetal malnutrition. It is well known that the lighter a newborn infant is at birth the more likely it is to become ill or die. Recently, convincing evidence has accumulated linking fetal malnutrition with an increased morbidity and mortality from cardiovascular disease in adulthood.

Pathophysiology

Most fetuses, including those in multiple gestations, follow similar growth curves during the first 20 weeks of pregnancy with any slowing of growth usually only occurring in the second half of pregnancy. Where the cause is physiological (e.g. multiple pregnancy or inherited genetic factors), slow growth is confined to the third trimester. The more severe the pathology, the earlier fetal growth restriction becomes evident. The earliest slowing of growth (during the second trimester) occurs when the fetus is inherently abnormal (e.g. congenital or chromosomal anomaly) or has sustained significant first trimester insult (e.g. from intrauterine infection or drug exposure).

Recent studies have given considerable insight into the pathophysiology of IUGR. At the start of gestation, growth appears to be controlled by nutritional input and growth factors acting locally by autocrine and paracrine mechanisms. Among these, insulin-like growth factors (IGFs, especially IGF-1) and their binding proteins (IGFBPs) appear to have a central regulatory role. Fetuses showing IUGR have low IGF-1 and IGFBP-3 levels but elevated growth hormone (GH) levels. Following birth and renutrition, a rapid increase in IGF-1 and a decrease in GH levels is observed. Thus GH, though playing a role in fetal and infantile growth, appears not to be the key hormone for fetal growth. On the other hand, insulin appears to play a major role in the regulation of fetal growth and it may exert this by increasing IGF-1 production.

Definition

Newborn infants may be described according to their birthweight for gestation as appropriate for gestational age (AGA), small for gestational age (SGA) or large for gestational age (LGA). The definition of SGA varies from a birthweight below the 10th centile to one of less than the 3rd centile. In the UK, just over 2% of all babies may be SGA, whereas in some developing nations, up to one in three newborns may be SGA and every other infant may be of low birthweight (LBW) (weighing <2.5 kg). Although the terms IUGR and SGA are often used interchangeably, IUGR is not strictly synonymous with SGA. Whereas SGA indicates an atypical growth pattern, IUGR implies either inhibition or restriction of a normal growth potential. Thus healthy SGA infants whose smallness is genetically predetermined are not IUGR.

Causes of IUGR and SGA

1. Physiological

(a) Fetal

- Multiple pregnancy.
- Inherited genetic factors.

(b) Maternal

- Small stature.
- Young or elderly mothers.

2. Pathological

(a) Fetal

- Chromosomal anomalies (2% of SGA infants).
- Congenital malformation (up to 15% of SGA infants).
- Intrauterine infection.

(b) Maternal

- Uteroplacental vascular insufficiency.
- Pregnancy-induced hypertension, pre-eclampsia, diabetes mellitus, collagen disorders, renal disease.
- Under-nutrition.
- Smoking.
- Drugs – therapeutic and addictive (e.g. cocaine.)
- Socioeconomic status.
- Irradiation.

SGA infants may be symmetrically or asymmetrically growth-restricted. Symmetrical growth restriction suggests early onset of IUGR (e.g. chromosomal anomaly, intrauterine infection or constitutionally small babies), producing equal reduction in brain and body size. Asymmetrically growth-restricted infants (majority of SGA infants) have relative sparing of head size and length but marked reduction in weight with onset of growth restriction in the last few weeks of pregnancy (e.g. placental insufficiency, pre-eclampsia, maternal smoking). Symmetrical IUGR is associated with a less favourable prognosis than asymmetrical IUGR, affecting only the weight.

Clinical correlates of SGA infants

1. Hypoglycaemia. Reduced glycogen liver stores, impaired gluconeogenesis, relative hyperinsulinaemia and deficient catecholamine secretion predispose to hypoglycaemia (symptomatic and asymptomatic).

2. Hypothermia. SGA infants have relatively large surface area to weight ratios and less subcutaneous fat, making them more vulnerable to cold stress.

3. Birth asphyxia. Fetal distress is twice as common due to the inability to maintain anaerobic metabolism. There may be a greater risk of meconium aspiration.

4. Polycythaemia. Risk is increased due to the relatively hypoxic intrauterine environment of SGA infants. A haematocrit of ≥ 0.65 may be found in 50% of SGA infants. Treatment is by partial exchange transfusion with plasma albumin.

5. Respiratory problems. Recurrent apnoeas, pulmonary haemorrhage and PPHN may be more common. RDS is less common, however.

6. Infection. Immunity is impaired with defective cell-mediated (decreased T lymphocytes) and humoral responses (deficient IgG). Furthermore, polymorphs have reduced chemotactic mobility and bactericidal capacity.

7. Neurobehavioural problems. SGA infants are less active and responsive with poor muscle tone and are jittery with variable feeding and sleeping patterns.

Detection of IUGR

Up to 90% of SGA infants may be detected by serial ultrasound measurements of the biparietal diameter, abdominal circumference (AC) and femoral lengths (FL) and comparing ratio of biparietal diameter to AC or FL to AC.

Management of IUGR

1. Prenatal
- Advise cessation of smoking.
- Treat hypertension and pre-eclampsia.
- Obtain fetal blood samples for karyotype and acid–base status in severe IUGR.
- Serial umbilical artery Doppler wave forms discriminate between fetuses at high or low risk of intrauterine/perinatal death. Absent end-diastolic flow (EDF) is associated with hypoxaemia, acidosis and an unfavourable outcome. Reversed EDF is a more ominous sign.

2. Postnatal
- Start feeds early and screen for asymptomatic hypoglycaemia (check 4-hourly capillary glucose).
- Avoid hypothermia, monitor temperature and provide a heated mattress if necessary.
- Treat polycythaemia with partial exchange transfusion.
- Avoid rapid increments of feeds and use breast milk in preference (high risk of NEC).
- If oral feeds are not tolerated, provide parenteral nutrition and gradually re-introduce enteral feeds.
- Thrombocytopenia and leucocytopenia are common. Treat suspected infection early.

Long-term outcome

The postnatal growth of infants born with IUGR is characterized by a rate of growth superior to that seen in the normal infant ('catch-up growth'). This affects first the weight then the length, and by the end of the second year the majority have attained a normal size. The severity and duration of antenatal growth restriction affects later growth potential. Infants who experience prolonged antenatal growth restriction will remain small, whereas infants who experience short periods of fetal growth restriction show catch-up growth. However, approximately 8% of IUGR infants whose birthweight or length are below the 3rd percentile will have a final adult height below the 3rd percentile. Of all the possible causes of small stature at the end of adolescence, 20% are due to IUGR. Recent therapeutic trials with GH have, however, been encouraging, suggesting that a satisfactory final adult height might be achieved with GH therapy.

Severely growth-restricted infants also have an excess of serious neuromotor impairments and deficits of cognitive function (e.g. cerebral palsy) compared to AGA infants. For the less severely affected infants, long-term outcomes in terms of physical growth, neurodevelopmental outcome or school performance may not differ significantly from matched peer groups; morbidity being largely determined by gestation. However, some recent UK epidemiological studies have suggested an increased risk of death from cardiovascular disease in adult life and an adverse effect on adult cognitive performance. These studies have shown that low birthweight is a risk factor for syndrome X, also known as insulin resistance syndrome, which includes glucose intolerance (non-insulin-dependent diabetes mellitus), hypertension and dyslipidaemia, all being risk factors for cardiovascular and cerebrovascular diseases. Although the mechanisms of these illnesses are not known, they illustrate the complex effects of fetal malnutrition on the 'programming' of illnesses in later life.

Further reading

Barker DJP. *Mothers, Babies and Health in Later Life*, 2nd edn. London: BMJ Publishing, 1998.

Barker DJP, Gluckman PD, Godfrey KM *et al.* Fetal nutrition and cardiovascular disease in adult life. *Lancet*, 1993; **341**: 938–41.

Cowett RM, Stern L. The intrauterine growth retarded infant: etiology, prenatal diagnosis, neonatal management and long-term follow-up. In: Lifshetz F (ed). *Pediatric Endocrinology*. New York: Marcel Dekker, 1990; 93–110.

Czernichow P. Pathophysiology and consequences of intrauterine growth retardation. In: Kelnar CJH (ed). *Baillière's Clinical Paediatrics, Vol. 4. No. 2, Paediatric Endocrinology*. London: Baillière Tindall, 1996; 245–57.

Eyal FG. The small-for-gestational-age preterm infant. In: Witter FR, Keith LG (eds). *Textbook of Prematurity: Antecedents, Treatment, and Outcome*. Boston: Little, Brown and Company, 1993; 361–9.

Hackett GA, Campbell S, Gamsu H, Cohen-Overbeek T, Pearce JMF. Doppler studies in the growth-retarded fetus and prediction of neonatal necrotising enterocolitis, haemorrhage, and neonatal morbidity. *British Medical Journal*, 1987; **294**: 13–16.

Setiauseil-Zipff U, Hamm W, Stenzel B, Bolte A, Gladtke E. Severe intrauterine growth retardation: obstetrical management and follow-up studies in children born between 1970 and 1985. *European Journal of Obstetrics and Gynaecology and Reproductive Biology*, 1989; 30: 1–9.

Sinclair JC, Bracken MB (eds). *Effective Care of the Newborn Infant*. Oxford: Oxford University Press, 1992.

Sorensen HT, Sabroe T, Olsen J *et al*. Birthweight and cognitive function in young adult life: historical cohort study. *British Medical Journal*, 1997; **315**: 401–3.

Stewart AL. Fetal growth: mortality and morbidity. In: Sharp F, Fraser RB, Milner RDG (eds). *Fetal Growth*. London: Royal College of Obstetricians and Gynaecologists, 1989; 403–12.

Related topics of interest

INTUBATION

Infants are most frequently intubated in the perinatal period, the primary indication being respiratory failure secondary to prematurity. Other infants requiring intubation have either failed to respond to the other means of resuscitation, including bag and mask ventilation, or are electively intubated for other reasons. Thus the procedure is done either electively or as an immediate and urgent response to the clinical condition of the infant. It is desirable for the procedure to be done calmly, which is aided by the assurance of assistance being readily available from a senior colleague if required. Practitioners who are new to the discipline should be supervised by senior colleagues until they have acquired sufficient skills and confidence to undertake the procedure independently.

Indications
- Prematurity ($\leq$28 weeks gestation).
- Failure to respond to bag and mask or T-piece ventilation.
- Respiratory distress with abnormal blood gases and an oxygen requirement ($FiO_2 \geq 0.60$).
- Poor respiratory drive with recurrent apnoeas (and bradycardias) and/or respiratory arrest.
- Planned elective intubation, e.g. for surgery.

Premedication

For non-urgent intubations such as elective intubation for surgery, it is appropriate and desirable to provide analgesia (e.g. morphine 100 μg/kg) and/or muscle relaxation (e.g. suxamethonium 2 mg/kg i.v. with atropine 15 μg/kg i.m./i.v.) just prior to intubation. This reduces the infant's stress response to the procedure and may make the procedure easier as the infant will not be struggling. It is not necessary to paralyse the infant first; this is risky if intubation fails.

Procedure

Use a laryngoscope with a short blade especially for the small preterm infant. Suction the oropharynx to clear the view. Partially extend the neck. Introduce the laryngoscope from the right side of the mouth and gradually tilt and lift the blade anteriorly but *without* resting the blade on the lower gum (traumatizes the lower gum). Gently withdraw the laryngoscope till the epiglottis flips into view. The vocal cords then immediately come into view just below the epiglottis, which may be aided by light cricoid pressure. Introduce the endotracheal (ET) tube through the open cords (without forcing) then adjust the position of the tube (depth of insertion down the trachea) by checking that air entry is equal on both sides. Secure the ET tube if artificial ventilation is to be maintained.

Common problems

1. Infant not responsive to artificial ventilation
- ET tube may have been misplaced or dislodged.
- Lung inflation pressure may be too low – increase by 5–10 cm H_2O.
- Gas flow (or oxygen) is turned off!

- A tension pneumothorax may be present (unilateral or bilateral). Transilluminate and if necessary needle the chest.

2. *Partial improvement followed by rapid deterioration*
- ET tube blocked (e.g. by meconium, blood, thick secretions) – replace ET tube.
- Acute pneumothorax – transilluminate and aspirate affected side.
- ET tube dislodged.

Failed intubation

Do not persist unnecessarily long if the initial intubation is unsuccessful! Discontinue the attempt if still unsuccessful after 2 min. Re-oxygenate the infant by bag and mask or T-piece ventilation. If still unsuccessful after two further attempts, let someone else try (do not be too proud to ask for help). Note, however, that infants can be effectively ventilated by bag and mask (or T-piece) for prolonged periods of time until assistance arrives. Infants may, on the other hand, be traumatized and subjected to repeated hypoxic insults by repeated failed intubation attempts.

Common causes of failed intubation

- Inexperience.
- Neck over-extension.
- ET tube inappropriately large.
- Inadequate visualization of airway – notwithstanding your experience, most 'blind' intubations fail!
- Rarely – unusual anatomy or congenital malformations.

Complications

- Pharyngeal tears from laryngoscope.
- Trauma to alveolar margin by laryngoscope (resting and rotating laryngoscope on gum).
- Vocal cord trauma (forcing ET tube plus introducer through closed cords or using inappropriately large ET tube).
- Tracheal, laryngeal and mediastinal perforating injuries.
- Penetrating injuries of the brain from attempted nasal intubation.
- Pneumothorax, especially right-sided (selective intubation of right main bronchus).
- Pulmonary haemorrhage.
- Marked abdominal distension from excessive mask bagging and/or oesophageal intubation.

Further reading

Angelos GM, Smith DR, Jorgenson R, Sweeny F. Oral complications associated with neonatal oral tracheal intubation: a critical review. *Paediatric Dentistry*, 1989; **11**: 133–40.

Black AE, Hatch DE, Nauth-Misir N. Complications of nasotracheal intubation in neonates, infants and children: a review of 4 years' experience in a children's hospital. *British Journal of Anaesthesia*, 1990; **65**: 461–7.

Cameron D, Lupton BA. Inadvertent brain penetration during neonatal nasotracheal intubation. *Archives of Disease in Childhood*, 1993; **69**: 79–80.

Fletcher MA, MacDonald MG (eds). *Atlas of Procedures in Neonatology*. Philadelphia: JB Lippincott Company, 1993.

Rawlings DJ, Lawrence S, Goldstein JD. Acquired tracheoesophageal fistula in a premature infant. *American Journal of Perinatology*, 1993; **10**: 164–7.

Shukla HK, Hendricks-Munoz KD, Atakent Y, Rapaport S. Rapid estimation of insertional length of endotracheal intubation in newborn infants. *Journal of Pediatrics*, 1997; **131**: 561–4.

Sutherland PD, Quinn M. Nellcor Stat Cap differentiates oesophageal from tracheal intubation. *Archives of Disease in Childhood, Fetal and Neonatal Edition*, 1995; **73**: F184–6.

Ziegler JW, Todres ID. Intubation of newborns. *American Journal of Diseases in Childhood*, 1992; **146**: 147–9.

Related topics of interest

Acute collapse (p. 6)
Complications of mechanical ventilation (p. 54)
Mechanical ventilation (p. 185)
Respiratory distress (p. 275)
Resuscitation (p. 282)

JAUNDICE

Term infants

All neonates have a transient rise in bilirubin, and some 30–50% become visibly jaundiced. Jaundice in neonates is considered as either physiological or pathological. *Physiological* jaundice is the consequence of immature liver enzymes, a high red cell mass, the short half-life of neonatal erythrocytes and increased intestinal reabsorption of bilirubin – the enterohepatic circulation. These combine to overload the pathway to conjugation and excretion of bilirubin, and there is a transient unconjugated hyperbilirubinaemia peaking around the third day, fading rapidly over the next 3 days and cleared by day 10. Prematurity, bruising, polycythaemia, breast-feeding and other factors can increase physiological jaundice (sometimes to the point of needing treatment). Jaundice is *pathological* and important if:

- It is in the first 24 hours of life – haemolysis until proven otherwise.
- It is associated with another illness.
- The bilirubin concentration is above the normal range.
- It has become prolonged (>10 days at term, >14 days in preterm infants).

The 97th centile for bilirubin concentration in the first few days of life in the well, breast-fed term baby is approximately 250 μmol/l, and 210 μmol/l in the formula-fed baby. These thresholds of concentration and time may therefore be taken as levels above which jaundice should be investigated for potentially pathological causes. They are not thresholds for initiating treatment, nor are they thresholds below which pathological causes for jaundice are absent. Vigilance is always needed.

1. Investigations. A bilirubin concentration, blood group and Coombs' test are the initial investigations in a well term baby who clinically looks jaundiced enough to need treatment. Further tests are not indicated unless the need for treatment is confirmed by a high bilirubin concentration without evidence of haemolytic disease. Tests on treated infants should include urine culture, urine reducing sugars (to exclude galactosuria, which tests positive on Clinitest, but negative on Clinistix), and further estimates of total bilirubin concentration. Liver function tests and conjugated/unconjugated bilirubin assays may be needed to exclude hepatitis and conjugated hyperbilirubinaemia, respectively, and certainly if the jaundice is prolonged. Some specific hepatic causes of jaundice are discussed in the topic 'Liver disorders'. Worldwide, G6PD deficiency is the most important cause of jaundice, especially in south-east Asia and African countries. In the UK, it is justifiable to screen jaundiced male infants who are of an ethnic origin that has a high prevalence of G6PD deficiency.

2. Management. Generally, if the baby is well and feeding well and if the concentration of bilirubin is below the treatment level, no further action should be taken unless the jaundice deepens or becomes prolonged. If the bilirubin concentration is above the treatment threshold and likely to rise to a point where kernicterus is a risk, phototherapy is needed (see *Table 1*). Kernicterus is a pathological term meaning 'yellow nuclei', referring to the appearance of the basal ganglia when the brain is examined at post-mortem: the ganglia are stained because the fat-soluble unconjugated bilirubin has entered the brain cells. Long-term neurological sequelae of this include deafness and athetoid cerebral palsy. Untreated severe hyperbilirubinaemia can cause fits, opisthotonus and death in the neonate.

There is continuing debate about the threshold above which kernicterus is likely to occur. Recent work suggests that in well term infants without haemolytic disease (including G6PD deficiency) it is higher than originally thought. The term 'vigintiphobia' (fear of the figure twenty) was coined to reflect paediatricians' fear of the total bilirubin concentration rising above 20 mg/dl (342 µmol/l) lest kernicterus ensued. Now, a gentler approach to jaundice is used, and kernicterus is considered to be a significant risk only above a bilirubin concentration of 450 µmol/l in this group of infants. The setting of this value also sets the level (450 µmol/l) at which exchange transfusion to prevent kernicterus is mandatory. In turn, phototherapy is started when the bilirubin concentration is 100 µmol/l below this exchange line. In well term infants, therefore, phototherapy is started at bilirubin concentrations as low as 80 µmol/l on day 1, rising to 350 µmol/l on day 3 and later.

In summary, the approach to jaundice in a well term baby is cascaded; starting with an examination to confirm the baby is well. If the baby looks significantly jaundiced, a single set of blood tests is performed. If treatment is indicated, phototherapy is started. This can be regarded as a treatment to avoid exchange transfusion. This in turn is the definitive treatment to prevent kernicterus. Neither phototherapy nor exchange transfusions are harmless, and should be initiated only if necessary. There is, however, a greater risk of kernicterus at lower concentrations of bilirubin if the baby is preterm, has haemolytic disease, G6PD deficiency, hypoalbuminaemia, acidosis or is receiving any drugs that may displace bilirubin from the albumin binding sites. The thresholds for action have therefore to be reduced accordingly.

Preterm infants

There are insufficient coherent data on jaundice in preterm infants below 35 weeks gestation to develop scientific evidence-based guidelines about phototherapy. *Table 1* contains some published recommendations and some extrapolations from them.

Prolonged jaundice

Jaundice is prolonged if it lasts >10 days in the term infant, and >14 days in the preterm. The most common cause for this is breast milk jaundice in a well and thriving baby who has an unconjugated hyperbilirubinaemia secondary to an increased enterohepatic circulation. Unfortunately there is no specific 'test' for this, and it is always a diagnosis of exclusion after other more sinister diagnoses, including biliary atresia, are ruled out. Investigation starts with the question: is the hyper-bilirubinaemia unconjugated or conjugated? If *unconjugated*, first check:

- Liver function.
- Thyroid function.
- Urine culture.
- Haemoglobin and red cell morphology.

If these are negative and the baby is a well, thriving and breast-fed, it is safe to watch for a further 2–3 weeks during which time the jaundice should fade and the baby remain well. If this does not happen, then more extensive investigations into causes of haemolysis, repeat liver function tests and specific conditions such as Gilbert's and Crigler–Najjar syndromes should be performed.

If *conjugated*, it is pathological: there is a need for prompt diagnosis and referral to a specialist centre at the outset is often the best way to achieve this. Among the important diagnoses to be considered and excluded are:

- Biliary atresia.
- Neonatal hepatitis.
- α_1-anti-trypsin deficiency.
- Inspissated bile syndrome.
- Dubin–Johnson and Rotor syndromes.
- Choledocal cyst.
- CF.

Table 1. Guidelines for jaundice therapy

Gestation	Postnatal age and bilirubin level (μmol/l) for phototherapy			
	<1 day	1–2 days	2–3 days	>3 days
≤27 weeks or <1000 g	85	100	100–150	150–175
28–32 weeks	85–120	100–150	125–175	175
32–35 weeks	100–150	150–200	220	220
≥37 weeks	85–170	170–260	260–350	>350

Further reading

Dodd K. Neonatal jaundice – a lighter touch. *Archives of Disease in Childhood*, 1993; **68**: 529–32.

Maisels MJ. Neonatal jaundice. In: Sinclair JC, Bracken MB (eds). *Effective Care of the Newborn Infant*. Oxford: Oxford University Press, 1992; 507–58.

Maisels MJ, Newman TB. Jaundice in full-term and near-term infants who leave the hospital within 36 hours: the pediatrician's nemesis. *Clinics in Perinatology*, 1998; **25**: 295–302.

Modi N. Jaundice. In: Harvey D, Cooke RWI, Levitt GA (eds). *The Baby Under 1000 g*. London: Butterworth, 1989; 120–33.

Newman TB, Maisels MJ. Evaluation and treatment of jaundice in the term newborn: a kinder, gentler approach. *Pediatrics*, 1992; **89**: 809–18.

Seidman DS, Gale R, Stevenson DK. What should we do about jaundice? In: Hansen TN, McIntosh N (eds). *Current Topics in Neonatology, No. 2*. London: W.B. Saunders, 1997; 125–41.

Volpe JJ. Bilirubin and brain injury. In: *Neurology of the Newborn*, 3rd edn. Philadelphia: W.B. Saunders, 1995; 490–513.

Watchko JF, Oski FA. Bilirubin = 20 mg/dl = vigintiphobia. *Pediatrics*, 1983; **71**: 660–3.

Related topics of interest

JITTERINESS

Jitteriness is a fine rhythmic 5–6 Hz tremor of the arms and legs. It is the most common involuntary movement in newborn babies. In the majority of jittery babies there is no associated pathology.

Aetiology
- Idiopathic.
- Hypoglycaemia.
- Hypocalcaemia.
- Drug withdrawal.
- Prematurity.
- Intrauterine growth restriction.
- Infants of diabetic mothers.

Differential diagnosis The challenge is to distinguish 'jitters' from fits. The main feature is that jitteriness stops when the limb is held or gently restrained, whereas fits continue. Also there are no abnormal eye movements, and jitters can be provoked by stretching and then releasing a limb in contrast to the spontaneous onset of fits.

Management Hypoglycaemia and hypocalcaemia must be excluded or treated if necessary. While hypocalcaemia is benign, jitteriness of hypoglycaemia may be a heralding sign of a more profound hypoglycaemia with more severe symptoms. Jitteriness as part of a drug withdrawal syndrome in a neonate occurs after marijuana, caffeine and opiate drug withdrawal, and has also been reported in infants of mothers on selective serotonin re-uptake inhibitors. In these situations, the overall state of the baby determines therapy, rather than any one sign. Jitteriness in other babies is thought to be due to an immaturity of the nervous system, probably a lack of myelination. Up to 44% of well term babies were observed to be jittery in one series. For these babies, no treatment is needed. Jitteriness can continue into infancy, and again is benign.

Further reading

Parker S, Zuckerman B, Bauchner H *et al.* Jitteriness in full-term neonates: prevalence and correlates. *Pediatrics*, 1990; **85**: 17–23.
Rennie JM (ed). *Textbook of Neonatology*, 3rd edn. Edinburgh: Churchill Livingstone, 1998.
Taeusch HW, Ballard RA (eds). *Avery's Diseases of the Newborn*, 7th edn. Philadelphia: W.B. Saunders, 1998.

Related topics of interest

LIVER DISORDERS

Liver disorders commonly present with jaundice, abnormal liver function tests, or hepatomegaly and, less commonly, present as part of a metabolic disorder or are discovered in the context of other investigations. While the individual disorders may be quite rare, as a group these disorders are fairly common. However, the complete evaluation of some of these disorders can be technically difficult, and early referral to a specialist paediatric hepatology centre is desirable when the diagnosis remains uncertain after a detailed history and examination complemented by the appropriate laboratory investigations.

Biliary atresia

This is a congenital condition occurring in 1 in 14 000 babies in the UK. Bile cannot reach the intestine as the extra-hepatic ducts are blocked. Left untreated, 95% of babies die by 2 years of age. Treatment is by the Kasai operation – a porto-enterostomy – in which the lower surface of the liver, stripped of its capsule, is applied to an open segment of bowel to allow drainage of the bile. The earlier the operation is done, the better. Success rates of >75% are achieved with surgery before 2 months in specialized units; after that it is only 25%. Liver transplantation after failed Kasai surgery is the final option.

Early and prompt diagnosis is needed: biliary atresia is always the first diagnosis to exclude in prolonged neonatal jaundice, even if it is mild. It is a conjugated hyperbilirubinaemia that can be confirmed by appropriate blood tests and the detection of bilirubin in the urine, which is yellow, whereas the stools are pale. Differential diagnoses include intrahepatic biliary atresias, neonatal hepatitis, α_1-anti-trypsin (A_1AT) deficiency, choledocal cysts, CF, inspissated bile syndrome, and other rare metabolic or anatomical abnormalities. The complicated and urgent nature of this condition means that babies with a persistent conjugated hyperbilirubinaemia should be assessed at a specialist unit. Usually, once other disorders have been excluded, the differential diagnosis lies between a neonatal hepatitis and biliary atresia. A technetium (^{99m}Tc) di-isopropyl iminodiacetic acid (DISIDA) scan is performed to outline the biliary tree and detect bile excretion. The definitive diagnosis may be made only by open liver biopsy during an explorative laparotomy.

Neonatal hepatitis

Many use this as an umbrella term, but it is best to think of:

1. Infective hepatitis.
2. Cholestasis secondary to a metabolic disease or other cause.

1. Infective hepatitis. To make this diagnosis the baby must have symptoms consistent with infection and aminotransferase levels of >2.5 times the upper limit of normal in the absence of other liver disease. Hepatitis viruses A, B, C, and D have all been implicated. Other non-hepatitis viruses can also cause neonatal hepatitis, (e.g. rubella, CMV).

(a) Hepatitis A

Fetal transmission has not been demonstrated. Maternal peripartum hepatitis A is a threat to the baby as the virus spreads by contact with maternal blood and the faecal–oral route. Infants of mothers who develop hepatitis A within 2 weeks of delivery should receive 0.5 ml of immunoglobulin.

(b) Hepatitis B

Transmission to the baby is primarily from exposure to maternal blood at delivery, though maternal–fetal transmission is reported from Taiwan.

Babies at high risk of transmission are those whose mothers:

- Have had hepatitis B in the last trimester.
- Are from south-east Asia or from Afro-Caribbean countries.
- Are HBeAg positive.

As transmission occurs at birth, prevention is possible, and *all* babies of HbsAg-positive mothers should be vaccinated. Low-risk babies should receive a course of vaccine starting within 48 hours of birth. High-risk babies should receive vaccine and HBIG. In order to achieve this, screening of maternal hepatitis status during pregnancy is needed. This is not yet universal in the UK. Spread by the faecal–oral route is also possible and appropriate precautions should be taken. Health workers should be vaccinated and shown to be immune. Infected babies can go on to have a transient disturbance of liver enzymes, acute hepatitis that, in its worst form, can be fulminant and fatal, or a chronic hepatitis leading to cirrhosis. See 'Hepatitis B'.

2. *Cholestasis.* Cholestasis ('hepatitis') secondary to a metabolic disease or other cause including:

(a) Metabolic
- A_1AT deficiency.
- CF.
- Tyrosinaemia.
- Galactosaemia.
- Fructose intolerance.
- Lipid storage disorders.
- Peroxisomal disorders.
- Haemochromatosis.
- Hypothyroidism.
- Hypopituitarism.

(b) Other
- Down's syndrome.
- Parenteral nutrition.
- Familial cholestatic syndromes.

Of these, galactosaemia is immediately life-threatening and presents with a sepsis-like picture several days after starting to ingest milk (lactose). Bedside testing of the urine for a reducing sugar that is not glucose (positive Clinitest, negative Clinistix (Ames Laboratories, UK)) in such a jaundiced baby is mandatory. All feeds are stopped and i.v. glucose started if galactosaemia is suspected. The hepatitis resolves with a lactose-free intake – initially the i.v. glucose, then a special diet for life. The diagnosis is confirmed by assaying red cell galactose-1-phosphate uridyl transferase.

There are many genetic variations of A_1AT deficiency. Its principal function is the inhibition of neutrophil elastase, and when deficient, neutrophil-mediated inflammation can progress in the liver and lungs. When it is suspected, phenotype testing is undertaken: measurement of A_1AT itself can be misleading in the presence of hepatitis. The normal phenotype is the so-called PiMM (Pi – protease inhibitor), and the one most commonly associated with neonatal liver disease is PiZZ. There is geographical variation in the frequency of the genes: in the UK, southern Europe and the USA, about 1 in 3000 babies is born with PiZZ. Ten per cent of such infants develop cholestasis in infancy, though 50% may have abnormal liver function tests by the end of the first year. A_1AT deficiency must be excluded in cases of late haemorrhagic disease of the newborn. Most with cholestasis progress relentlessly to cirrhosis and liver failure. Treatment is supportive until transplantation is necessary.

Specific disorders of bile metabolism

Two steps in the conversion of unconjugated bilirubin to a conjugated water-soluble form involve uridine diphosphate glucuronyl transferase (UDPGT) which converts bilirubin to bilirubin monoglucuronide and is also capable of converting that to the diglucuronide. Bilirubin monoglucuronide dismutase catalyses the conversion to the diglucuronide.

1. Syndromes with UDPGT deficiency
(a) Crigler–Najjar syndrome (type 1)
- Autosomal recessive.
- Complete absence of hepatic glucuronyl transferase.
- Persistent unconjugated hyperbilirubinaemia, usually >340 μmol/l.
- Kernicterus in infancy.
- Death in infancy, some surviving to adulthood then developing kernicterus.

- Treatment – phototherapy.
- Transplantation – prior to neurological complications.
- Phenobarbitone has no effect.

(b) Crigler–Najjar syndrome (type 2)
- Autosomal recessive/dominant (variable penetrance).
- Less severe persistent unconjugated hyperbilirubinaemia.
- Treatment with enzyme-inducing phenobarbitone and phototherapy reduces bilirubin levels.
- Neurological problems unusual.

(c) Gilbert's syndrome
- Autosomal dominant.
- Affects 5% of the population.
- Benign, mild, chronic unconjugated hyperbilirubinaemia.
- Bilirubin clearance about one-third of normal.
- Impaired UDPGT activity and impaired hepatic uptake.
- 50% of cases have reduced red-cell survival.
- Bilirubin rises with fasting, exercise, intercurrent illnesses.
- Rarely recognized before puberty.
- Phenobarbitone reduces jaundice.

(d) Dubin–Johnson syndrome
- Autosomal recessive.
- Chronic conjugated hyperbilirubinaemia.
- Jaundice may be seen after birth, but may not appear until fourth decade.
- Diagnosis by exclusion of other causes of conjugated hyperbilirubinaemia and by typical liver biopsy appearance of deposition of melanin-like pigment.
- No treatment necessary.

(e) Rotor's syndrome
- Autosomal recessive.
- Predominantly conjugated hyperbilirubinaemia.
- Benign.

Further reading

Altschuler SM, Liacouras CA. *Pediatric Gastroenterology and Liver Disease*. Edinburgh: Churchill Livingstone, 1998.
Mowat AP. *Liver Disorders in Childhood*, 3rd edn. Oxford: Butterworth Heinemann, 1994.

Related topics of interest

Inherited metabolic disease – investigation and management (p. 156)
Jaundice (p. 173)

MATERNAL DRUG ABUSE

Drug addiction during pregnancy has deleterious effects on the mother, her fetus, the immediate family and the rest of society. A high proportion of drug-abusing women are in relationships with men who also abuse drugs with up to two-thirds having been subjected to physical and sexual abuse. Mental health problems are frequent among drug-abusing individuals. Self-care and diet therefore tend to be neglected with consequential fetal compromise.

Drug abuse is on the increase particularly in the developed nations though prevalence rates vary widely, being highest (up to 15%) in inner-city areas. It is not only confined to women of low socioeconomic status but occurs in all social groups regardless of income level or ethnic/racial identity. Mood-altering drugs are often used along with alcohol with a tendency for the younger age group (under 30s) to use two or more drugs. Of the infants diagnosed as having AIDS in the UK in 1996, outside London, approximately three-quarters of the mothers or their partners contracted HIV infection through i.v. drug abuse.

Indicators of possible drug abuse in pregnancy

1. Medical
- Self admission of use.
- Sporadic or no prenatal care before delivery.
- Preterm labour and delivery or abruptio placenta.
- Stillbirth or birth of infant with anomalies.

2. Social
- Frequent changes of residence or employment.
- Past drug or alcohol abuse.
- Imprisonment.
- Family violence.
- Removal of other children from the home.
- A disruptive or dysfunctional lifestyle.

Commonly abused drugs
- Alcohol (fetal alcohol syndrome).
- Cocaine (microcephaly, cardiac malformations).
- Amphetamines.
- Marijuana.
- Cannabis.
- Heroin.
- Codeine.
- Barbiturates.

Management during pregnancy

Encourage the mother to enter an alcohol and drug treatment programme, often in conjunction with a psychiatrist specializing in drug and substance abuse. Mothers addicted to narcotics may be switched to methadone (decreased risk of infection) which can be gradually weaned. Methadone, however, has more prolonged and severe withdrawal effects.

Mothers should be screened for possible hepatitis B and HIV infection following appropriate counselling. Social services should be involved with the appointment of a key worker with arrangements for long-term follow-up.

Neonatal presentation of maternal drug abuse

Most infants will present with symptoms of drug withdrawal. These are not drug-specific but the timing of withdrawal symptoms is characteristic with some drugs. Opiate withdrawal (e.g. heroin) has a rapid onset (maximum intensity on day 2–4 and fading by 10–14 days) whereas methadone withdrawal persists over weeks or months. Withdrawal symptoms may resolve within a few days or persist for several weeks, while the growth impairment and neuro-behavioural effects may last for several months.

Symptoms of withdrawal syndrome

1. Central nervous system
- Restlessness.
- Irritability.
- Tremulousness.
- Hyperactivity (with rub marks).
- High-pitched cry.
- Hyperacusis.
- Hypertonus.
- Yawning.
- Photophobia.
- Seizures.

2. Respiratory system
- Tachypnoea.
- Stuffy nose.
- Rhinorrhoea.
- Sneezing.
- Hiccups.
- Apnoeas.
- Respiratory distress.

3. Gastrointestinal system
- Salivation.
- Vomiting.
- Diarrhoea.
- Poor feeding.
- Poor weight gain.

Management of the infant

1. Acute
- Aim to promote normal sleep patterns.
- Nurse in quiet environment.
- Monitor blood glucose especially in low birthweight infants with feeding difficulties.
- Firm wrapping reduces irritability and hyperactivity.
- For severe irritability with feeding difficulties, give chlopromazine (1–3 mg/kg/day at 3–6-hourly intervals) or opiates titrating against symptoms. Prophylactic therapy is not appropriate – only treat if symptomatic.
- The use of 'score charts', comprising a record of withdrawal signs and symptoms against time, provides an

objective assessment of the infant's clinical status and can guide treatment.

- Treat seizures with phenobarbitone, phenytoin, clonazepam or paraldehyde.
- Taper drug therapy gradually (over weeks to months).
- Breast-feeding is contraindicated.

2. Long-term. Assess social circumstances with social services to decide whether the child can be allowed home and decide on long-term follow-up. Infants with fetal alcohol syndrome require appropriate neurodevelopmental follow-up. Neurodevelopmental outcome may be suboptimal, particularly in infants born to mothers abusing alcohol and cocaine and those brought up in families with disruptive or dysfunctional lifestyles.

Further reading

Chasnoff IJ (ed). Chemical dependency and pregnancy. *Clinics in Perinatology*, 1991; **18**: 1–191.

Chasnoff IJ, Scholl SH. Consequences of cocaine and other drug use in pregnancy. In: Washton A, Gold MS (eds). *Cocaine: A Clinicians Handbook*. New York: Guildford Press, 1987; 241.

Durand DJ, Espinoza AM, Nickerson BG. Association between prenatal cocaine exposure and sudden infant death syndrome. *Journal of Pediatrics*, 1990; **117**: 909.

Fetters L, Tronick EZ. Neuromotor development of cocaine-exposed and control infants from birth through 15 months: poor and poorer performance. *Pediatrics,* 1996; **98**: 938–43.

Finnegan LP. Perinatal substance abuse: comments and perspectives. *Seminars in Perinatology*, 1991; **15**: 331.

Harrison M. Drug addiction in pregnancy: the interface of science, emotion and social policy. *Journal of Substance Abuse and Treatment*, 1991; **8**: 261.

Nicoll A, McGarrigle C, Brady T *et al*. Epidemiology and detection of HIV-1 among pregnant women in the United Kingdom: results from national surveillance 1988–1996. *British Medical Journal*, 1998; **316**: 253–8.

Niebyl JR. *Drug Use in Pregnancy*, 2nd edn. Philadelphia: Lea & Febiger, 1988.

Shaw NJ, McIvor L. Neonatal abstinence syndrome after maternal methadone treatment. *Archives of Disease in Childhood*, 1994; **71**: F203–5.

Related topics of interest

MECHANICAL VENTILATION

Mechanical ventilation using positive airway pressure is indicated for babies with respiratory failure secondary to lung or cardiac disease, for some with recurrent apnoeas or fits, and during deep sedation or anaesthesia. The ventilators used are traditionally time-cycled, pressure-limited ventilators, i.e. the time of the inspiratory and expiratory phases are set, and the ventilator delivers certain preset pressures. Such ventilators have been adapted for trigger ventilation. HFOV, volume-controlled ventilation and liquid ventilation are also used. In severe respiratory failure with ventilation–perfusion mismatch, NO may be introduced into the inspiratory gases to dilate the pulmonary vasculature and ECMO may be used in near-term infants with severe respiratory failure.

Continuous positive airway pressure (CPAP)

CPAP is an attempt to mimic the positive-end expiratory pressure a baby generates by grunting during expiration against a closed glottis. The generated positive pressure reduces atelectasis. CPAP can be administered by face mask, endotracheal tube or nasal prongs. Increasingly it is applied by short, soft nasal prongs on the end of a CPAP driver circuit. These devices sense airway pressure changes secondary to the baby's spontaneous respiratory effort and alter gas flows to maintain a near constant airway pressure. This may reduce the work of breathing. A comparison of neonatal outcomes in American units showed that the unit using early CPAP and tolerating slightly higher $PaCO_2$ had the lowest incidence of chronic lung disease. At the same time, reports from Scandinavia using similar techniques suggested benefits of early CPAP, and this modality of treatment is currently being re-explored.

Preterm babies extubated during recovery from respiratory distress onto nasal CPAP are less likely to need reintubation than those extubated into a headbox. CPAP is also an important treatment of obstructive and mixed apnoeas, in which the soft structures of the upper airway may collapse inwards during the baby's negative pressure inspirations. CPAP 'splints' open the airway.

Intermittent positive pressure ventilation (IPPV)

In IPPV, the inspiratory and expiratory pressures, inspired oxygen fraction (FiO_2), inspiratory time (Ti), expiratory time (Te) and hence the rate (bpm) and the Ti/Te ratio can all be controlled.

1. Target ranges for blood gases
- pH – arterial pH should preferably be ≥ 7.25 (≥ 7.3 in the first week of life).
- PaO_2 – the recommended range is 6–10 kPa.
- $PaCO_2$ – this should be ≥ 5 kPa. If the pH is >7.25, there may be an advantage in letting the $PaCO_2$ rise towards 7.5 kPa in the hope of avoiding baro- and volutrauma. There is

increasing evidence linking early hypocapnia with an increased incidence of BPD and PVL.
- SaO_2 – a range of 90–95% is best, but arterial gases are needed to confirm adequate oxygenation and pH.

2. *Arterial oxygenation (PaO_2).* This can be controlled by:

- Changing the FiO_2.
- Changing the mean airway pressure by:
    Changing the peak inspiratory pressure (PIP).
    Changing the PEEP.
    Changing the Ti/Te ratio.
    Lengthening the inspiratory plateau (increasing inspiratory gas flows).

As PaO_2 varies directly with mean airway pressure (MAP) between 5 and $15\,cmH_2O$, increasing MAP will improve oxygenation.

3. *Arterial carbon dioxide tension ($PaCO_2$).* This varies inversely with minute volume, the product of rate and stroke (tidal) volume, which is 5–8 ml/kg in conventionally ventilated babies. Thus $PaCO_2$ can be controlled by:

- Changing the rate.
- Changing the tidal volume by:
    Changing the PIP.
    Changing the PEEP (likely to have the greater effect for the same degree of change).

Remember that CO_2 retention can be caused by inadvertent PEEP (PEEP higher than set) during high-rate ventilation with short expiratory times. Acute unexpected rises in $PaCO_2$ often indicate an endotracheal tube blockage or pneumothorax.

Synchrony between the baby and the ventilator

In IPPV, the ventilator and the baby may breathe independently of one another, causing inefficient ventilation, variable tidal volumes and high intrapulmonary pressures that result in an increased incidence of pneumothoraces. The ventilator–baby interaction should be studied to ensure that the baby is breathing synchronously. This is achieved by the following:

1. *Capturing the baby's respiration.* This is done by increasing the ventilator rate to just above the baby's spontaneous rate (often 80 bpm or more in babies <1250 g), at which point the baby tends to synchronize with the ventilator.

2. *Sedation.* The baby should be sedated to the point where the baby's own respiratory drive is depressed but not abolished.

3. *Paralysis.* This guarantees 'synchrony', but has several disadvantages, including the loss of the baby's own considerable respiratory effort.

4. Trigger ventilation. This is where the baby's own breath initiates a ventilator breath. The most efficient systems detect early inspiratory gas flow with an anemometer or early inspiratory pressure changes with a pneumotachygraph in the circuit. To achieve synchrony, there must be minimal delay between the baby starting the breath and the ventilator's response; Ti must be set between 0.25 and 0.3 s as a baby's spontaneous Ti is of that order.

The ventilator can be triggered either with every breath, or intermittently with a certain number of breaths per minute. A back-up rate is set so that the ventilator takes over in an 'IPPV' mode if the baby becomes apnoeic. Babies probably benefit from being on caffeine to stimulate their respiration during trigger ventilation and to aid early weaning. With minor variations, control of PaO_2 and $PaCO_2$ is as above. Despite its theoretical appeal, there are few controlled trials on trigger ventilation, and its benefits over well-performed IPPV have yet to be established. The (UK) collaborative randomized controlled trial of trigger versus conventional ventilation in over 900 preterm infants (<32 weeks gestation) with RDS showed no significant difference in outcomes.

High frequency oscillatory ventilation (HFOV)

In HFOV, the inspiratory gases are oscillated around a mean airway pressure by a piston or diaphragm cycling at ~10 Hz (600 bpm). Tidal breaths such as those seen in spontaneous breathing, IPPV or trigger ventilation are not generated. Gas dispersion occurs primarily through diffusion and convection, but also by pendelluft, asymmetric velocity profiles and turbulence in the small airways and tidal ventilation of very short path alveoli. Pendelluft is the generation of local oscillating currents between neighbouring respiratory units of different physical properties and time constants.

Recruitment of alveoli is important: the MAP is increased until the baby is in an FiO_2 of 0.3–0.4 and/or nine posterior ribs are seen above the diaphragm on the chest X-ray. Babies with the most severe lung disease will still be in a high FiO_2 even with the lungs radiologically expanded, but many will have diminished their oxygen demand as additional alveoli were recruited. Oxygenation is controlled by changes in FiO_2 and MAP. CO_2 elimination varies with the amplitude of the oscillation. It is remains uncertain whether HFOV alters long-term outcomes such as death or chronic lung disease. Also unclear is whether babies should be ventilated on HFOV throughout their respiratory illness, or be transferred to it when pressures during IPPV reach a yet to be determined threshold.

Volume controlled ventilation (VCV)

VCV might reduce chronic lung disease if that is caused by (or partly by) volutrauma as opposed to barotrauma. In time-cycled, pressure-limited ventilation, the tidal volume varies from breath to breath and over-distension with some breaths may be traumatic. The constant tidal volumes of VCV may induce less damage, even if occasional high airway pressures have to be used. Limited experience with babies >1200 g has been reported, and it is also uncertain whether the technique can be applied to the more difficult population of babies <750 g.

Further reading

Avery ME, Tooley WH, Keller JB *et al.* Is chronic lung disease in low birthweight infants preventable? A survey of eight centers. *Pediatrics,* 1987; **79**: 26–35.

Bancalari E, Sinclair JC. Mechanical ventilation. In: Sinclair JC, Bracken MB (eds). *Effective Care of the Newborn Infant.* Oxford: Oxford University Press, 1992; 200.

Goldsmith JP, Karotkin EH (eds). *Assisted Ventilation of the Neonate,* 3rd edn. Philadelphia: W.B. Saunders, 1996; 215–28.

Goldsmith JP, Spitzer AR (eds). Controversies in neonatal pulmonary care. *Clinics in Perinatology,* 1998; **25** (1).

Related topics of interest

MECONIUM ASPIRATION SYNDROME

This life-threatening condition occurs with increasing frequency as gestation advances. The incident of MAS varies in different parts of the world ranging from 1 to 5 per 1000 births. Higher rates are reported from North America and the Middle East compared to Europe. Though up to 15% of all deliveries may be complicated by meconium staining of amniotic fluid, only 5–10% of babies born through meconium-stained liquor develop pulmonary disease. *In utero* passage of meconium is uncommon because of the good anal sphincter tone, lack of strong intestinal peristalsis and the meconium normally plugging the rectum. Acidosis, asphyxia and compression of the fetal head all stimulate relaxation of the anal sphincter and intestinal peristalsis. Fetal hypercarbia and hypoxia stimulate gasping which can lead to meconium aspiration. Passage of meconium before 34 weeks is rare but consider listeriosis (causes liquefaction of meconium) if it occurs.

Pathogenesis	Aspirated meconium reaches the peripheral airways, causing partial or complete obstruction. Partial obstruction causes gas trapping and lung over-distension (a 'ball-valve' effect). Complete obstruction leads to atelectasis and ventilation–perfusion mismatch. Meconium inhibits surfactant action, the normal bacteriostatic qualities of amniotic fluid, and also produces a chemical pneumonitis. Furthermore, hypoxia, acidosis and hypercarbia produce pulmonary vasoconstriction leading to pulmonary hypertension, right-to-left shunting and worsening gas exchange.
Clinical features	<ul><li>Fetal distress during labour.</li><li>Post-term and/or IUGR.</li><li>Meconium staining of the skin, nails, umbilical cord.</li><li>Hypoglycaemia.</li><li>Metabolic acidosis.</li><li>Cyanosis and hypoxaemia.</li><li>Tachypnoea or gasping respiration.</li><li>Pneumothorax (30% with severe MAS).</li><li>Post-asphyxial signs (CNS, renal or cardiovascular).</li><li>PPHN.</li></ul>
Diagnosis	This is based on the presence of meconium-stained liquor, meconium below the cords or chest radiological appearances (lung over-inflation, widespread coarse, fluffy opacities, pneumothorax and pneumomediastinum).
Management	Admit all infants with meconium below the cords for observation. Symptomatic infants should have pulse oximetry, supplemental oxygen (as required), blood gas analysis and a chest X-ray. Commence broad-spectrum antibiotics after cultures. Respiratory failure and severe hypoxaemia requires intubation and mechanical ventilation. Surfactant administration, fast rates and low PEEP, high-frequency ventilation may improve

gas exchange. Inhaled NO (a selective pulmonary vasodilator) may further improve oxygenation when used in conjunction with conventional or high-frequency ventilation. Refractory hypoxaemia unresponsive to the above measures is an indication for ECMO. Asphyxiated infants with MAS may have multisystem involvement (e.g. renal failure, seizures, hypotension) which need specific therapy.

Prevention

Identify fetuses at risk of asphyxia (IUGR, post-term, oligohydramniotic) and monitor carefully during labour.

A skilled neonatal resuscitator should attend deliveries complicated by meconium staining of liquor. Clear mouth and pharynx when head is delivered, and following delivery view the larynx. If meconium is present aspirate carefully. If thick meconium is present or meconium is seen below the cords, aspirate the trachea using a large-bore suction catheter or carefully intubate then repeatedly aspirate the trachea.

Endotracheal tube adapters or other mechanical aspirators should be used to prevent the resuscitator from being contaminated with any infectious agents (e.g. HIV) present in the amniotic and vaginal fluids.

Although up to half of all meconium-stained infants may have meconium in their trachea, and 1 in 10 may have meconium below the cords despite it being absent from the mouth or pharynx, intubation of all meconium-stained infants is associated with a greater morbidity.

Prognosis

Mild disease not requiring mechanical ventilation has an excellent prognosis with recovery within a few days. Recently, mortality from severe MAS has declined from almost 50% to 4–18%. Most deaths are due to air leaks, PPHN, respiratory failure or associated perinatal asphyxia. There is an increased risk of asthma and exercise-induced bronchial reactivity in survivors. The use of hyperventilation-induced hypocapnia ($PaCO_2$ <25 mmHg or <3.5 kPa) in treating PPHN is associated with adverse neurodevelopmental outcome (e.g. sensorineural hearing loss and low psychomotor developmental test scores). Perinatal asphyxia is associated with a mortality and neurodevelopmental morbidity related to the severity of the asphyxial insult.

Further reading

Cunningham AS, Lawson EE, Martin RJ *et al.* Tracheal suction and meconium: a proposed standard of care. *Journal of Pediatrics*, 1990; **138**: 153.

Halahakoon CN, Halliday HL. Other acute lung disorders. In: Yu VYH (ed). *Baillière's Clinical Paediatrics, Vol. 3. No. 1, Pulmonary Problems in the Perinatal Period and their Sequelae.* London: Baillière Tindall, 1995; 87–114.

Halliday HL. Other acute lung disorders. In: Sinclair JC, Bracken MB (eds). *Effective Care of the Newborn Infant*. Oxford: Oxford University Press, 1992; 359–84.

Spitzer AR (ed). *Intensive Care of the Fetus and Neonate*. St. Louis: C.V. Mosby, 1996.

Wiswell TE, Tuggle JM, Turner BS. Meconium aspiration syndrome: have we made a difference? *Pediatrics*, 1990; **85**: 715–21.

Related topics of interest

MULTIPLE PREGNANCY

Multiple pregnancy rates vary worldwide. For instance, the prevalence of twin births varies from 6.7 per 1000 deliveries in Japan to 40 per 1000 deliveries in Nigeria. This is due largely to variations in dizygotic twinning, as the prevalence of monozygotic twinning is relatively constant worldwide at 3.5 per 1000 births. Dizygotic twins arise when two ova are released and fertilized in one menstrual cycle; monozygotic twins arise when one ovum is fertilized and the resulting zygote divides into two.

Over the last two decades, the incidence of twins and higher order births has been rising, partly due to the more widespread use of assisted reproductive techniques. However, multiple pregnancy is associated with greater risks for both mothers and fetuses compared with a singleton pregnancy. This is because every complication of pregnancy occurs more commonly. The most important complication of multiple pregnancy is preterm delivery, with its concomitant increased perinatal morbidity and mortality. Thus twins account for only 2% of births, but 9% of all perinatal deaths due to their prematurity and low birthweight. The perinatal mortality rate among higher order births is directly related to the number of fetuses. The average length of a twin pregnancy is 20 days shorter than a singleton one. The mean duration of pregnancy decreases as the number of fetuses *in utero* increases. Approximately 25% of twins are born preterm. The mean gestational age at delivery for triplets is 33 weeks (with 85–90% delivering before 37 weeks and 20–30% before 32 weeks). Almost all quadruplets experience preterm delivery (half before 32 weeks gestation).

Maternal risks associated with multiple pregnancy

- Increased symptoms of early pregnancy (e.g. nausea and vomiting).
- Increased risk of miscarriage.
- The vanishing twin syndrome.
- Preterm labour and delivery.
- Hypertension (pre-eclampsia and eclampsia).
- Antepartum haemorrhage.
- Hydramnios (in up to 12% of multiple pregnancies).
- Possible need for prenatal hospitalization for prolonged periods.
- Antepartum fetal death (risk of DIC in up to 25%).
- Risk of operative delivery (increased risk of trauma and infection).
- Increased likelihood of Caesarean delivery.
- Post-partum haemorrhage.
- Postnatal problems (e.g. increased risk of depression).

Fetal risks associated with multiple pregnancy

- Stillbirth or neonatal death (perinatal mortality rate of twins is up to 10 times that of singletons).
- Preterm labour and delivery (rates of 30–50%).
- IUGR (25–33% have birthweight <10th centile).
- Congenital abnormalities (twice as common compared with singletons).
- Twin to twin transfusion.
- The 'stuck' twin phenomenon (occurs in 8% of twin pregnancies but mortality is >80% for both twins).

- Hydramnios (malpresentation).
- Cord accidents (carry a perinatal mortality of up to 50%).
- Risk of asphyxia (mortality risk from asphyxia for twins is four to five times that of a singleton).
- Operative vaginal delivery.
- Death of a co-twin.
- Twin entrapment (rare, typically occurs in monoamniotic twins, incidence of 1 in 800, high risk of fetal death).

Specific problems associated with multiple pregnancy

1. Determining zygosity. This is of importance as monozygotic pregnancies have increased morbidity and mortality. Twins of different sex are obviously dizygotic. Monozygosity can be proven on the basis of a monochorionic placenta. However, monozygotic twins with dichorionic placentas may only be distinguished reliably from like-sex dizygotic twins by blood grouping, red cell and tissue enzymes, serum proteins or minisatellite DNA probe tests.

2. Fetal nutrition and growth. Multiple fetuses of necessity compete for nutrition. Fetal growth in twins is usually similar to that of singletons until approximately 24 weeks' gestation. Thereafter, bodyweight falls disproportionately more than head growth. The average birthweight of a newborn twin is 500 g less than a singleton. Dichorionic twins are heavier than monochorionic twins.

3. Twin–twin transfusion syndrome. Placental arterio-venous vascular anastomoses can result in the twin–twin transfusion syndrome, usually in monozygotic monochorionic twins. A cord blood haemoglobin difference of at least 5 g/dl is noted between the twins. An incidence of 5–15% of all twin pregnancies has been reported, and the acute severe twin–twin transfusion syndrome occurs in 1% of monochorionic gestations. The donor twin becomes anaemic, hypovolaemic, oligohydramniotic and growth-restricted. The recipient twin becomes polycythaemic, hypervolaemic, polyhydramniotic and may develop cardiac failure, ascites, and pleural and pericardial effusions. Hydrops fetalis may develop in both. Antenatal treatment includes laser ablation of anastomoses, repeated amniocentesis, transfusion of donor and exsanguination of recipient. Mortality may be high (80–100%) for twins presenting acutely at 18–26 weeks gestation.

4. 'Stuck' twin phenomenon. One fetus in a diamniotic pregnancy lies in a severely oligohydramniotic sac while the co-twin lies in a severely polyhydramniotic sac. Mortality is high (>80%). Most result from twin–twin transfusion syndrome.

5. Congenital anomalies. Major anomalies are twice as common in multiple pregnancies compared with singletons.

Cardiac anomalies, bowel atresia, neural tube defects and chromosomal abnormalities are more common in multiple pregnancies. Certain malformations uniquely occur in monozygotic twins (namely conjoined twins) (1 in 50 000 pregnancies), the commonest form being thoracopagus and acardia (1 in 30 000–35 000 deliveries).

6. *Death of a co-twin.* Fetal demise of one twin occurs in 0.5–6.8% of twin pregnancies after the first trimester. The emboli and debris from the dead fetus may enter the circulation of the surviving (monochorionic) twin, producing multiple brain, gastrointestinal and renal lesions. In contrast, surviving dichorionic twins have a good prognosis. Regardless of zygosity, males fare less well than females and male–male pairs have the highest perinatal mortality rates. In male–female pairs, female infants fare better. The second-born twin may be at greater risk of death and morbidity.

Further reading

Fowler MG, Kleinman JC, Kiely JL, Kessel SS. Double jeopardy: twin infant mortality in the United States, 1983 and 1984. *American Journal of Obstetrics and Gynecology*, 1991; **165**: 15–22.

Fusi L, McParland P, Fisk N, Nicolini U, Wigglesworth J. Acute twin–twin transfusion: a possible mechanism for brain-damaged survivors after intrauterine death of a monochorionic twin. *Obstetrics and Gynecology*, 1991; **78**: 517–20.

Hawrylyshyn PA, Barkin M, Bernstein A, Papsin FR. Twin pregnancies – a continuing perinatal challenge. *Obstetrics and Gynecology*, 1982; **59**: 463–6.

Keith LG, Papiernik E, Keith DM, Luke B (eds). *Multiple Pregnancy. Epidemiology, Gestation and Perinatal Outcome*. London: Pathernon Publishing Group, 1995.

Little J, Bryan E. Congenital anomalies. In: MacGillivary I, Campbell DM, Thompson B (eds). *Twinning and Twins*. Chichester: John Wiley, 1988; 207–40.

Related topics of interest

Congenital malformations and birth defects (p. 70)
Intrauterine growth restriction (p. 165)
Pregnancy complications and fetal health (p. 247)
Prenatal diagnosis (p. 253)

NECROTIZING ENTEROCOLITIS

The first reported cases of NEC were made over 150 years ago, although the term NEC was first used in the 1950s. NEC is a maladaptive response of the immature gastrointestinal tract to perinatal/postnatal injury. Damage to the intestinal mucosa in the presence of intraluminal feeds and microbial infection are important aetiological factors. Intestinal ischaemia, from any cause, rapid oral feeds, non-human milk formula and bacterial infection are thought to be particularly important. Abnormal prenatal umbilical wave forms (absent and reversed end-diastolic flow) and marked IUGR are particularly associated with NEC. Approximately 90% of cases occur in premature infants, with the incidence varying with gestational age from 0.1 per 1000 live births in term infants to almost 8% in the very low birthweight infants. It is most frequently seen within the first 2 weeks of life although it may occur in infants who are several weeks old. Approximately 300 cases occur annually in the UK with 70–100 deaths.

Although the caecum, ascending colon and terminal ileum are the most commonly affected sites, any part of the gastrointestinal tract may be involved. The affected segment of gut may only show small perforations or be severely affected and necrotic.

Clinical features

These are varied, from the non-specific signs of hypotonia, lethargy, and apnoeas with temperature instability, to the signs of septic shock with hypotension, bradycardia, pallor with abdominal distension, bloody stools, bilious aspirates and DIC. A silent tender abdomen with a red and indurated abdominal wall suggests a perforation.

Investigations

1. Radiology. Plain abdominal X-ray shows thickened dilated loops of bowel (which may be fixed) occasionally with fluid levels. In the acute phase of the disease, daily radiographs should be performed. A lateral abdominal film (right side up for better air–liver contrast) is important in the acute stage of the disease, as perforations may be difficult to detect other-wise. Typical radiographs show intramural gas (pneumatosis intestinalis) and in later stages, air may also be seen in the liver, along with ascites. Intra-abdominal abscesses and ascites may be more readily recognized with ultrasound.

2. Haematology
- FBC.
- Coagulation screen.

3. Biochemistry
- U&E.
- Blood gases.

4. Microbiology. Perform a full septic screen (omit LP if diagnosis is clear).

Management

Stop oral feeds to rest the gut and commence parenteral nutrition for at least 10 days. Deflate the abdomen with a naso-gastric tube on free drainage. Administer FFP in the acute phase of the disease at 10–20 ml/kg depending on the clinical state (wide core–peripheral temperature gap, poor capillary refill, hypotension). Transfuse with packed red cells if anaemic. Support the blood pressure (keep mean arterial blood pressure ≥35 mmHg) with colloids and inotropes (dopamine 10–20 µg/kg/min or dobutamine 10–30 µg/kg/min). Monitor arterial blood gases, correct acidosis and commence ventilation if hypoxic and retaining carbon dioxide in the presence of apnoeas. Carefully monitor electrolytes and hydration with 6–12-hourly electrolytes in the acute phase of the disease, then less frequently later when more stable. Control infection with i.v. broad-spectrum antibiotics including metronidazole. Correct DIC and transfuse platelets if marked thrombocytopenia is present (platelet count <20 × 10^3/mm^3). Provide adequate analgesia by infusing opiates (e.g. 10–40 µg morphine/kg/hour). Treat intercurrent problems such as electrolyte imbalance and hypoglycaemia promptly.

Surgery is required when a perforation has occurred or when there is continuing deterioration (with persistent acidosis) despite adequate medical treatment. In the unstable sick very low birthweight infant, simple drainage of the peritoneal cavity under local anaesthetic may be a useful interim measure until the infant is fit for surgery.

Enteral feeds (preferably expressed breast milk or a simplified formula, e.g. Prejestimil™, Mead Johnson) may be recommenced slowly in the well infant after 10–14 days (or longer if surgery was required). Relapses may occur in up to 10% of cases following re-introduction of enteral feeds. Complications include stricture formation with intestinal obstruction and short bowel syndrome following bowel resection.

Further reading

Bauer CR. Necrotizing enterocolitis. In: Sinclair JC, Bracken MB (eds). *Effective Care of the Newborn Infant.* Oxford: Oxford University Press, 1992; 602–16.

Stoll BJ, Kliegman RM (eds). Necrotizing enterocolitis. *Clinics in Perinatology*, 1994; **21** (2).

Related topics of interest

NEONATAL SCREENING FOR INHERITED DISEASE

Mass screening of newborns for metabolic disorders was introduced by Bob Guthrie (Guthrie test for phenylketonuria (PKU)) some three decades ago. Conditions which merit screening occur frequently, have gradual onset (allowing time for detection before the onset of symptoms) and can be detected by inexpensive and accurate assays. Early treatment should produce a good outcome. This is ideal for PKU.

Phenylketonuria

PKU has an incidence of 1 in 12 000 births and in the classic form is due to phenylalanine hydroxylase deficiency. However, tetrahydrobiopterin co-factor defects may also produce PKU. The PKU screening test identifies all infants with elevated serum phenylalanine. An amino acid chromatogram is performed on a heel prick spot of blood collected onto filter paper. Other disorders can also now be detected from this same blood sample including tyrosinaemia, MSUD as well as some genetic disorders (from DNA analysis).

Infants with serum phenylalanine values persistently above 1.0 mmol/l (18 mg/dl) need treatment. Infants with phenylalanine levels of 0.2–0.6 mmol/l (4–10 mg/dl) on the first test should have a repeat test. Levels of ≥0.6 mmol/l (10 mg/dl) need further assessment and may need treatment. Infants should be tested when on full feeds (commonly days 4–6) and off i.v. fluids.

Treatment should be carried out by those expert in this area. In essence, most of the amino acid requirements are provided in synthetic form and natural proteins only used in sufficient amounts to supply the phenylalanine requirements for growth, leaving no excess to be broken down to tyrosine.

Hypothyroidism

Hypothyroidism has an incidence of 1 in 3500 births. Most screening programmes use a single blood sample taken at day 5–10 (when relative stability has returned to the thyroid axis after the abrupt changes at birth). A heel prick spot of blood is collected onto filter paper at the same time and onto the same paper as the PKU test. Thyroxine screening alone is inadequate because of the overlap between normal and hypothyroid values. Thyroid-stimulating hormone (TSH) assay is the primary test performed (though this may miss the rarer cases of secondary hypothyroidism (pituitary or hypothalamic hypothyroidism with an incidence of 1 in 60 000–100 000 births).

Normal TSH levels are <25 mU/l. Levels of 25–80 mU/l are equivocal and the infant should be retested. Levels of >80 mU/l are abnormal and the infant should be recalled urgently for full thyroid function tests. Treatment should be started as soon as possible (without waiting for results) with thyroxine 8–10 µg/kg/day (once-daily dose).

The commonest cause of congenital primary hypothyroidism is thyroid dysgenesis (dysplasia). It is associated with trisomy 21, with females affected twice as often as males and with an incidence of 1 in 3500. The second commonest cause is thyroid dyshormonogenesis (autosomal recessive biochemical defects of iodothyronine synthesis), which has a frequency of 1 in 30 000–50 000, equal sex incidence and accounts for 10–15% of infants detected by screening.

Galactosaemia

Galactosaemia has a prevalence of 1 in 60 000 births and screening detects 60–70% while they are still asymptomatic. The effect of screening at 4–6 days upon final outcome is still uncertain. Routine screening is not practised in the UK.

Hereditary tyrosinaemia

Screening for this uncommon disorder is only routine in certain parts of the world, such as Norway, Sweden and Quebec in Canada. There is a defect in fumaryl aceto-acetate and excretion of succinylacetone in urine is diagnostic. Treatment is with low tyrosine and phenylalanine milk. If undetected, there is progressive liver dysfunction, hypoglycaemia, renal tubular defects and eventually cirrhosis. However, a transient tyrosinaemia is common in preterm infants (responds to 50 mg vitamin C daily for 1 week).

Cystic fibrosis

DNA analysis now affords a useful screening tool for CF, especially where there is a strong family history of the disorder or one parent is known to be affected. Routinely the commonest mutations are screened for, namely ΔF508, 621+1G>T, G542X, G551D and R553X. Absence of these mutations gives an 80% certainty of excluding CF as a diagnosis in the indigenous UK population. An optimal screening programme should screen for the most common mutations in a given population as these vary in different ethnic groups and geographic locations. Meconium ileus in the neonatal period is associated with CF. Fifteen per cent of infants with CF present with bowel obstruction caused by meconium ileus, but only 75% of infants with meconium ileus have CF. Blood immunoreactive trypsin (IRT) level should be assayed. Elevated IRT (normal values <70 µg/l) suggests CF. Similarly, low tryptic activity (normal faecal chymotrypsin 120 µg/g) in the stool suggests CF.

Haemoglobinopathies

The two most important haemoglobinopathies, numerically and clinically, are sickle cell disease (SCD) and thalassaemia major (homozygous β-thalassaemia). Both are β-globin chain defects and therefore rarely cause problems before 3–6 months of age, when the β-chain of adult haemoglobin (HbA;

$\alpha_2\beta_2$) normally becomes predominant as fetal haemoglobin (HbF; $\alpha_2\gamma_2$) disappears. The thalassaemia syndromes are the commonest inherited single gene defects in the world. The main 'at-risk' groups are individuals from the Mediterranean region, the Middle East, Asians, Afro-Caribbeans and orientals.

Sickle haemoglobin can be identified by alkaline cellulose acetate electrophoresis backed by acid citrate-agarose electrophoresis of a haemolysate of packed red cells.

Thalassaemia can be diagnosed by analysis of globin chain synthesis and gene mapping. α-thalassaemia (homozygous $\alpha°$-thalassaemia) presents as hydrops fetalis and is incompatible with survival.

Further reading

Bickel H, Guthrie R, Hammersen G (eds). *Neonatal Screening for Inborn Errors of Metabolism*. Berlin: Springer-Verlag, 1980.

Gaston M. Why we should screen newborns for sickle cell disease. *Contemporary Pediatrics*, 1989; **1**: 175.

Griffiths P, Mann JR, Darbyshire PJ, Green A. Evaluation of eight and a half years of neonatal screening for haemoglobinopathies in Birmingham. *British Medical Journal*, 1988; **296**: 1583–5.

Hall DMB, Michel JM. Screening in infancy. *Archives of Disease in Childhood*, 1995; **72**: 93–6.

Phelan PD. Neonatal screening for cystic fibrosis. *Thorax*, 1995; **50**: 705–6.

Scriver CR, Beaudet AL, Sly WS, Valle D (eds). *The Metabolic and Molecular Basis of Inherited Disease*, 7th edn. New York: McGraw-Hill, 1995.

Wonke B, Modell B. Impact and future of screening for haemoglobin disorders. *Current Paediatrics*, 1998; **8**: 55–61.

Related topics of interest

NEONATAL SURGERY

Several medical conditions presenting in the neonatal period require surgical intervention. Such surgery is best performed in a dedicated surgical unit where anaesthetists experienced in neonatal anaesthesia are available along with designated paediatric surgeons. The need for surgery may arise unexpectedly or have been previously anticipated and therefore planned.

Pre-operative preparations

- Obtain parental consent in good time.
- Cross-match an appropriate amount of blood if peri-operative blood loss is likely. A maternal blood sample is required for this in the newborn period.
- Obtain a baseline FBC and electrolytes, especially if the infant is several days old.
- Secure adequate venous and arterial access for the pre-operative administration of colloid and crystalloid and continuous peri-operative monitoring of blood pressure and blood gases for infants who are ready for surgery.
- In the immediate pre-operative period it may be necessary to intubate and ventilate infants requiring general anaesthesia for their surgical procedures. Check endotracheal tube placement radiographically and adjust ventilation if necessary, following some baseline blood gases.

Intra-operative medical management

During surgery, several parameters should be monitored to maintain the infant in an optimal physical and metabolic status.

- Monitor temperature and provide additional heating to prevent excessive cooling.
- Monitor blood pressure (invasively where possible).
- Monitor blood gases and blood glucose during prolonged surgical procedures.
- Maintain an i.v. infusion of a dextrose solution (newborns) or dextrose/electrolyte solution (older infants) administering colloid (e.g. blood or 4.5% human albumin) should blood losses become significant (falling BP, rising pulse).
- Where necessary, administer antibiotics with induction of anaesthesia.

Post-operative management

This is determined partly by the surgical procedure previously performed, especially whether major or minor, and the general condition of the infant (i.e. whether well or critically ill). Following minor surgery (e.g. uncomplicated hernia repair), the infant may be otherwise well and only require minimal analgesia which may be administered orally. Oral or i.v. feeds may be commenced soon after the infant has recovered from anaesthesia. Following major surgery, however, intensive care monitoring is usually necessary with particular reference to the following:

- Monitor urine output aiming to maintain a urine flow rate of ≥1 ml/kg/hour; patients with renal failure should be closely monitored to avoid hyperkalaemia, fluid overload, acid–base disturbance and drug toxicity (e.g. from amino-glycosides).
- Monitor BP and support if necessary with colloid (blood, 4.5% albumin or FFP) and inotropes (dopamine/dobutamine 10–30 µg/kg/min).
- Monitor adequacy of peripheral circulation/perfusion by monitoring core–peripheral temperature gap (maintain <2°C) and/or capillary refill time (normal <3 s); administer colloid if above parameters are unsatisfactory.
- Continue infusion(s) of analgesia in appropriate amounts (e.g. morphine 40 µg/kg/hour or fentanyl 1–2 µg/kg/hour) following an appropriate loading dose, and if necessary an i.v. sedative (e.g. midazolam 0.05–0.1 mg/kg).
- Restrict crystalloids after major surgery because of inap-propriate ADH secretion as fluid overload may otherwise develop.
- Monitor U&E, FBC, blood glucose and, if still ventilated, arterial blood gases.
- Commence total parenteral nutrition (via central venous line if possible) if full enteral nutrition is likely to be delayed (e.g. after repair of abdominal wall defects).
- Ongoing losses (e.g. secondary to nasogastric suctioning, drainage through stoma fistula, dressing) should be replaced 2–4-hourly with normal saline to avoid dehydration.
- Monitor wound healing and if wound appears infected, swab and commence antibiotics empirically. Review choice of antibiotics with culture results.

The place for surgery

In most neonatal centres, surgery is performed in the operating theatre not in the intensive care unit, on the assumption that the neonatal intensive care unit (NICU) does not provide a suffi-ciently clean area, and so predisposes the infant to a higher risk of infection. However, when the patient undergoing surgery is an unstable extremely low-birthweight infant, the need for transportation (at times to an off-site centre), the extra handling and change of ventilator equipment all increase the risk of dis-rupting vascular lines or chest tubes, accidentally dislodging the endotracheal tube and hypothermia which may all further compromise the ill pre-operative infant. With good planning and organization, an area of the NICU can easily be set aside for the surgery of critically ill preterm or more mature infants who would be too unwell to transfer to a dedicated operating theatre. The surgical team, anaesthetists, operating theatre staff and the NICU staff can work quite harmoniously on the NICU, allowing continuity of care for the infant (and the continued use of 'neonatal' technologies such as high-frequency ventilation), while avoiding transportation of the infant and its associated complications. With good organization, both minor operations and some major procedures may be performed on the unit without placing the infant at disadvantage.

Further reading

Gavilanes AWD, Heineman E, Herpers MJHM, Blanco CE. Use of neonatal intensive care unit as a safe place for neonatal surgery. *Archives of Disease in Childhood, Fetal and Neonatal Edition*, 1997; **76**: F51–3.

Puri P (ed). *Newborn Surgery*. London: Butterworth-Heinemann, 1995.

Reyes HM, Vidyasagar D (eds). Neonatal surgery. *Clinics in Perinatology*, 1989; **16 (1)**.

Rowe MI, Lloyd D. Pre-operative and post-operative management. In: Spitz L, Nixon HH (eds). *Rob and Smith's Operative Surgery, 4th edn. Paediatric Surgery*. London: Butterworths, 1988; 4–10.

Spitz L, Steiner GM, Zachary RB. *A Colour Atlas of Paediatric Surgical Diagnosis*. London: Wolfe Medical Publications, 1981.

Stringer MD, Oldham KT, Mouriquand PDE, Howard ER (eds). *Pediatric Surgery and Urology: Long-term Outcomes*. Philadelphia: W.B. Saunders, 1998.

Wetzel RC. Pediatric anesthesia. *Pediatric Clinics of North America*, 1994; **41 (1)**.

Related topics of interest

Abdominal distension (p. 1)
Anaesthesia and post-operative analgesia (p. 13)
Congenital malformations and birth defects (p. 70)
Hirschsprung's disease (p. 110)
Necrotizing enterocolitis (p. 195)
Surgical emergencies (p. 312)

NEURAL TUBE DEFECTS

In the human embryo, the developing CNS becomes recognizable by day 19 as the neural plate. This differentiates into the neural tube, the forerunner of all the major structures of the brain and the spinal cord. Defects in the early organogenesis of the neural tube lead to the host of developmental defects manifest as brain and spinal cord malformations, often accompanied by unfavourable neurodevelopmental outcome.

In recent years there has been a consistent steady decline in the incidence of congenital CNS malformations. Neural tube defects (NTDs) occur less frequently in the higher social classes. Maternal serum alpha-fetoprotein (AFP) is raised in pregnancies with open NTDs. Folic acid (4 mg daily) appears effective in preventing the first occurrence as well as the risk of recurrent NTDs if administered periconceptually. Detailed antenatal ultrasound examination will detect most fetuses with severe NTDs.

Anencephaly

The posterior skull fails to develop exposing a rudimentary brain with absent cerebral hemispheres, associated with poly-hydramnios and spina bifida. It is incompatible with life. There is an increased risk of NTDs in future pregnancies.

Spina bifida occulta

This may affect approximately 1 in every 20 individuals. It has an excellent prognosis. Defects are often only detected by chance on spinal X-rays but few have outward signs (hairy path, dimple, naevus). There is no increased risk of NTDs in future pregnancies.

Meningocele

Meningocele is a relatively benign condition where the spinous process is absent and a CSF-containing sac protrudes through the gap. It may be sited anywhere from the cervical spine to the sacral region. Hydrocephalus may develop (10%) but is less severe and may resolve spontaneously. Operative closure is advised and prognosis is excellent. Antenatally, AFP is not raised and unless detailed spinal ultrasound views are obtained, the diagnosis may be missed antenatally.

Myelomeningocele

This is usually thoracolumbar (worst prognosis) but may be lumbar, sacral or lumbosacral. Defects often span several segments of the spinal cord with various vertebral anomalies (wedge-shaped or hemivertebrae, fusion or absence of some ribs, splayed out spinal laminae) and spinal scoliosis. Occasionally, defects of the skull membranous bones are present (craniolacunia) with characteristic radiological appearance. The site and size of exposed abnormal neural elements (the 'neural plaque') partly determine the outcome.

1. Common clinical findings
- Flaccid paralysis and analgesia: affects lower limbs. Cervical/upper thoracic lesions may affect upper limbs similarly.

- Lower limb deformities: due to imbalanced paralysis of muscle groups (commonly with flexed and abducted hips, hyperextension of knees, talipes, calcaneovalgus – lesion below L3).
- Paralysed sphincters and urinary tract anomalies: dribbling incontinence, paralysed rectal sphincters and patulous anus and associated retention of urine, bladder trabeculation, hydronephrosis and/or ureteric reflux. Other renal defects (pelvic kidney, duplex collecting system, horseshoe kidney) are also more common.
- Hydrocephalus: present at birth in 90% (head shape and size may be normal).

2. Investigations
- Spinal X-rays (to determine extent of skeletal anomalies).
- Cranial ultrasound scan (to assess severity of hydrocephalus).
- Renal ultrasound scan.
- Micturating cystourethrogram (bladder anomalies, ureteric reflux).
- Electrolytes (excessive sodium loss with CSF leak).

3. Management. Treatment is now selective. Infants with serious defects and a projected poor outcome receive palliative care (with parents' agreement). Determine the neurological deficits – assess sensory and motor levels of the lesions. Orthopaedic assessment is required (fixed anomalies of spine and limbs and hip anomalies).

4. Indications for palliative care
- Gross hydrocephalus.
- Paralysis below L3.
- Marked kyphosis and scoliosis.
- Associated major congenital malformations.
- Thoracolumbar or thoracolumbosacral lesion.

If the outcome is favourable, active treatment may be undertaken ideally in a specialized unit, beginning with closure of the lesion. Mild to moderate hydrocephalus may be treated medically and then surgically if this fails (see 'Hydrocephalus').

Cranial meningocele

The skull bone is deficient and a cystic swelling (containing CSF only) projects through the defect (usually occipital). It has a good outcome.

Encephalocele

Abnormal brain tissue is in a sac protruding from the occipital, parietal or frontal areas or into the upper nasal cavity. Microcephaly and hydrocephaly are common. Associated anomalies include myelomeningocele, Klippel–Feil syndrome. Small encephaloceles may be treated surgically but large lesions have a poor prognosis (cortical blindness or partial sight, spastic quadriplegia, epilepsy and death). The worst prognosis is associated with large lesions and microcephaly.

Agenesis of the corpus callosum
Whole or part of the corpus callosum is missing so the third ventricle extends between hemispheres to the skull. This is associated with hypertelorism and megalencephaly. Cranial ultrasound or CT scan will reveal absent corpus callosum.

Holoprosencephaly
Holoprosencephaly is a rare condition with absent olfactory bulbs and tracts and failure of cleavage of forebrain. A large single dilated ventricle is present and the corpus callosum may also be absent. It is associated with other major malformations including chromosomal defects (e.g. trisomy 13), and has a high mortality as no treatment is available. Genetic counselling is needed as recurrence is common.

Megalencephaly
This is usually a benign familial tract with a large head without the signs of hydrocephalus, and growth at the normal rate. Measure siblings' and parents' head circumference, which should also be large.

Hydranencephaly
Hydranencephaly is a rare condition in which the cerebral hemispheres have been destroyed or have failed to develop. The infant's head freely transilluminates (distinguish from extreme hydrocephalus) and prognosis is poor with high mortality despite surgical treatment (shunt insertion).

Microcephaly
Microcephaly is very common. It has multiple aetiologies ranging from infection (e.g. CMV, rubella, toxoplasmosis), part syndromic (e.g. fetal alcohol, Roberts' and Seckel syndromes) and chromosomal defects (e.g. autosomal recessive familial type). Head circumference is below the 2nd centile related to birthweight with sloping forehead. Prognosis is poor with neurodevelopmental delay, spasticity and seizures.

Further reading

Chervenak FA, Isaacson G, Lorber J. *Anomalies of the Fetal Head, Neck and Spine: Ultrasound Diagnosis and Management.* Philadelphia: W.B. Saunders, 1988.
Czeizel AE, Dudas I. Prevention of the first occurrence of neural-tube defects by periconceptional vitamin supplementation. *New England Journal of Medicine*, 1992; **317**: 1832–5.
Levene MI, Liford RJ, Bennett MJ, Punt J (eds). *Fetal and Neonatal Neurology and Neurosurgery*, 2nd edn. Edinburgh: Churchill Livingstone, 1995.
MRC Vitamin Study Research Group. Prevention of neural tube defects. Results of the Medical Research Council Vitamin Study. *Lancet*, 1991; **338**: 131–7.
Volpe JJ. *Neurology of the Newborn*, 3rd edn. Philadelphia: W.B. Saunders, 1995.

Related topics of interest

NEUROLOGICAL EVALUATION

History

Often overlooked, the history is an important part of neonatal assessment. It includes:

- Family history.
- Outcome of previous pregnancies.
- Current pregnancy, and mode of delivery.
- Evidence of fetal distress, Apgar scores, cord blood pH.
- Behaviour prior to examination, especially fits, jitteriness, feeding difficulties.

Clinical examination

This assesses four main areas:

- Tone.
- 'Automatic' or 'primitive' responses.
- Conventional signs as elicited in older children.
- Behaviour.

1. Tone. This is the resistance of muscles to stretch. It is generally lower when the baby is asleep. Passive tone is reflected in the posture of a baby. Active tone is elicited by manoeuvres such as pulling to sit from a supine position (head-lag), and in the resistance to stretching of a flexed limb. Healthy full-term neonates lie in a flexed posture, with the hips flexed and adducted, and the knees flexed so that the legs are drawn up under the body. The shoulders are adducted, the elbows flexed. This posture persists for a week or so after birth before flexor tone diminishes. Preterm babies have lower tone, so the tight flexion is not seen: the very preterm baby lies with arms and legs abducted and extended.

The normal active tone of an alert term baby will enable him/her to briefly hold his/her head in line with the body during 'pull to sit' and ventral suspension manoeuvres. The degree of recoil when a limb is extended is also a useful sign of tone. As tone varies with gestational age, it is used in gestational age assessment. Conversely, it is important to know the gestation of a baby in order to assess the appropriateness of a baby's tone when neurological compromise is suspected.

2. Primitive reflexes. These are complex responses present in newborns, but then diminishing and disappearing. Persistence beyond the normal age suggests that higher cortical centres are not gaining control of tone and movement as expected, and can, for example, be an early sign of cerebral palsy.

- The *Moro* (startle) reflex is elicited by gently dropping the head of a baby from one hand into the palm of the other some 5 cm below. The full reflex shows abduction and extension of the arms with hand opening followed by adduction and flexion of the arms over the chest with hand closure. It wanes rapidly after 1–2 months and is abnormal if it persists at all beyond 6 months. The Moro reflex is often absent in preterm babies.

- Primitive *walking* is elicited by holding an alert baby vertically with the feet firmly in contact with a flat surface and leaning him/her slightly forwards. It has usually disappeared by 4–6 weeks. It can also be started through a 'placing reaction', in which the dorsum of a baby's foot is brought up against the underside of a tabletop. The baby then raises the foot and places it on the table, and may then begin primitive walking.

- The *asymmetric tonic neck reflex* is most marked at 2–4 months and may not be easily elicited in the newborn. The head is turned to one side to elicit extension of the arm on that side with some extension of the ipsilateral leg. It has usually disappeared by 6–7 months.

- The *palmar grasp* disappears by 8 weeks to be replaced by voluntary grasp 6–8 weeks later as cortical control develops.

- *Rooting* persists until 3–4 months, after which visual cues predominate in the normal baby, who will recognize the breast or the bottle and move towards them, but no longer root and suck on a finger placed at the corner of the mouth.

3. *Conventional signs.* These include:

- Maximum head circumference and examination of the head shape, sutures and fontanelles.

- Eye examination that must include eliciting a 'red reflex'. The light of an ophthalmoscope reflected from the red retina is absent in congenital cataracts and retinoblastomas. This examination may also pick up colobomata of the iris. Corneal haziness can be caused by oedema in congenital glaucoma (buphthalmos), which needs immediate referral to an ophthalmologist. In the very preterm baby, the lens remains vascularized up to 32 weeks and this may initially prevent the red reflex. Such a baby should be seen anyway by an ophthalmologist for retinopathy screening. Given time, sophisticated assessment of a baby's eyes and visual behaviour can be achieved, but at routine neonatal examination the one thing that *must* be checked is red reflex. Missed cataracts can lead to permanent reductions of visual acuity if they are removed too late.

- Gross movements of the limb should be noted during examination. Knee and biceps jerks are easily elicited, the others less so. Isolated sustained clonus at the ankles can occur in jittery babies. Plantar reflexes are variable.

Responses should be symmetrical. Asymmetry may indicate a unilateral peripheral nerve palsy or unilateral brain damage, though the signs of the latter can be very subtle in the newborn baby.

4. Behaviour. This is important, and not just during examination. These responses have been quantified by a number of workers including Brazelton, who produced a Neonatal Behavioural Assessment Scale, which includes the arousal sequence described below. Use of these scales requires training, experience and patience on the part of the neonatologist. If approached when asleep, the normal term infant may progress from:

(1) being deeply asleep with eyes closed, regular breathing and no movements, to
(2) light sleep with rapid eye movements, some random movements and irregular breathing, onto
(3) a drowsy state with eyes open and small movements, to
(4) being alert, looking bright and having minimal movements, then to
(5) grosser movements with fussing, and finally onto
(6) crying.

At the correct state of arousal and with some patience on the part of the examiner, a term baby will fix and follow an interesting object such as a face or a brightly coloured ball, though following up to 8 weeks post-term does not depend on an intact visual cortex. Babies will also respond to sound. Abnormal neurological signs can be elicited in babies with HIE, PVL and with IVHs. These detailed and sometimes subtle signs again require particular expertise to elicit, and tend not to be used regularly by clinicians, particularly for PVL and IVH, which can be more readily detected by ultrasound scanning.

In addition to history and clinical examination, a number of techniques can contribute to the neurological evaluation of a newborn baby:

- Ultrasound scanning of the brain.
- CT scan.
- MRI, including diffusion-weighted and perfusion MR imaging.
- Magnetic resonance spectroscopy (^{31}P- and ^{1}H-MR spectroscopy).
- EEG.
- Auditory evoked brain stem responses.
- Visual evoked responses.

Further reading

Brazelton TB. *Neonatal Behavioural Assessment Scale*, 2nd edn. London: Spastics International Medical Publications, 1962.

Brett EM. Neurology of the newborn. In: Brett EM (ed). *Paediatric Neurology*. Edinburgh: Churchill Livingstone, 1991; 1–25.

Dubowitz LMS. *The Neurological Assessment of the Preterm and Full-term Infant*, 2nd edn. Clinics in Developmental Medicine, No. 148. Cambridge: Cambridge University Press, 1998.

Levene MI, Liford RJ, Bennett MJ, Punt J (eds). *Fetal and Neonatal Neurology and Neurosurgery*, 2nd edn. Edinburgh: Churchill Livingstone, 1995.

Paneth N, Rudelli R, Kazam E, Monte W (eds). *Brain Damage in the Preterm Infant*. Clinics in Developmental Medicine, No. 131. London: MacKeith Press, 1994.

Volpe JJ. *Neurology of the Newborn*, 3rd edn. Philadelphia: W.B. Saunders, 1995.

Related topics of interest

Childbirth complications and fetal outcome (p. 46)
Germinal matrix-intraventricular haemorrhage (p. 93)
Hypotonia (p. 126)
Hypoxic–ischaemic encephalopathy (p. 128)
Neuromuscular disorders – muscular (p. 210)
Neuromuscular disorders – neurological (p. 214)
Periventricular leucomalacia (p. 234)
Postnatal examination (p. 244)
Seizures (p. 294)

NEUROMUSCULAR DISORDERS – MUSCULAR

Congenital muscular dystrophy

Congenital muscular dystrophies (CMDs) are autosomal recessive muscle disorders which may be classified into two major groups, depending on the association with structural brain anomalies. CMDs without structural CNS anomalies (the 'classic' or 'occidental' CMDs) form a heterogeneous group of disorders. In those with associated structural CNS anomalies, eye involvement and neurological abnormalities are common. In CMDs, the muscle biopsy is abnormal though no unique identifying features exist.

Congenital muscular dystrophies without structural CNS anomalies

- These can now be sub-classified on the basis of merosin (laminin α_2-chain) staining. The merosin gene maps to chromosome 6q22.
- The merosin-negative sub-group is more severely affected clinically with peripheral nerve involvement and has associated hypomyelination of brain white matter on cranial MRI scans and relatively high serum CPKs. Most will be unable to walk, in contrast to merosin-positive patients, most of whom will walk.
- Both sub-groups can present in the neonatal period with weakness, hypotonia, raised CPK and joint contractures.
- Diagnosis is made from EMG, nerve conduction studies, elevated CPK, muscle biopsy and merosin staining and cranial CT or MRI.

Congenital muscular dystrophies with structural CNS anomalies

1. *Fukuyama muscular dystrophy*
- Most common form of CMD with brain anomalies, mainly found in Japan.
- Inheritance is autosomal recessive and the gene locus is on chromosome 9q31–33.
- At birth there is hypotonia, generalized weakness, joint contractures, depressed deep tendon reflexes, microcephaly, with neurodevelopmental delay, convulsions (50%) and raised CPK.
- Death occurs by age 10 years.

2. *Walker–Warburg syndrome*
- Predominantly inherited as an autosomal recessive trait.
- There is weakness, hypotonia, macrocephaly, hydrocephaly and eye abnormalities.
- CNS malformations include lissencephaly, cerebellar hypoplasia, Dandy–Walker malformation, hydrocephalus, absent corpus callosum and heterotopias.
- Most die in early infancy.

3. *Muscle–eye–brain disease*
- Inheritance is autosomal recessive.
- Similar to Walker–Warburg syndrome though the phenotype is milder.
- Early hypotonia, delayed development, seizures, hydrocephalus and eye involvement (optic atrophy, retinal dysplasia, progressive visual failure).
- Death occurs between 6 and 16 years.

Congenital myotonic dystrophy

This autosomal dominant, multisystem disorder is the most prevalent form (5 per 100 000) of muscular dystrophy that is inherited almost exclusively from mothers.

- Severe neonatal disease is associated with polyhydramnios, poor fetal movements and premature delivery.
- Clinical features include hypotonia, talipes, poor respiratory function, impaired sucking and swallowing, 'tented upper lip', facial weakness, ptosis, dilation of cerebral ventricles and moderate intellectual impairment.
- Mortality is high (up to 50%).
- The milder form is non-lethal and so can occur in all age groups and initial hypotonia resolves.
- Management is supportive and prolonged ventilation may be required.
- Always examine mothers for myotonia or weakness of distal muscles and neck flexors.
- Diagnosis is by DNA assay for a trinucleotide CTG repeat located in the 3′ untranslated region of a gene coding for myotonin protein kinase on chromosome 19q13.3. Disease severity is related to the length of the expansion, with normals having up to 37 repeats, mildly affected individuals or asymptomatic mutation 'carriers' 50–99 repeats, and the severely affected ('full mutation') individuals 100 to ≥2000 repeats. Disease severity increases in successive generations (the phenomenon of genetic anticipation).
- Prenatal diagnosis is possible.

Congenital myopathies

These disorders are characterized by hypotonia and weakness at birth with scoliosis, ptosis and ophthalmoplegia often developing in late infancy/early childhood. In general, congenital myopathies have distinctive muscle biopsy findings, their names reflecting their myopathological features. In contrast, the muscle biopsy findings are dystrophic and non-specific in congenital muscular dystrophies. The CPK is normal or slightly raised (moderately or markedly raised in congenital muscular dystrophies). The main disorders are as follows.

- Nemaline myopathy. Muscle biopsy is diagnostic (characteristic nemaline bodies).
- Central core disease (autosomal dominant). Chromosome 19q13.1 implicated and muscle biopsy is diagnostic (central cores evident).
- Centronuclear/myotubular myopathy. The most common type (the neonatal form) is X-linked, has severe symptoms and a very high mortality, with muscle biopsy showing

central nuclei and type 1 fibre predominance. The myotubularin gene (locus Xq28) is implicated.

Metabolic myopathies

1. Pompe's disease (infantile acid maltase deficiency or glycogen storage disease II. Acid maltase releases glucose from glycogen, oligosaccharides and maltose. Absence leads to glycogen storage. This autosomal recessive disorder presents in the first 3 months of life with rapidly progressive weakness, hypotonia and enlargement of liver, heart and tongue. CNS glycogen storage causes hypo-reflexia and diminished alertness. Feeding and respiratory difficulties are common and so is death before the age of 2 years. Diagnosis is by assaying acid maltase activity in muscle, lymphocytes or urine. Muscle biopsy shows large vacuoles full of glycogen (PAS-positive) and strongly reactive for acid phosphatase. The gene defect maps to chromosome 17q23. No therapy exists.

2. Cytochrome c oxidase deficiency. At least two forms are recognizable, benign infantile myopathy and fatal infantile myopathy. Fatal infantile myopathy presents soon after birth with severe lactic acidosis, marked weakness, hypotonia, respiratory and feeding difficulties. Most infants die before the age of 1 year. Muscle biopsy and histochemistry shows ragged-red fibres with lipid and glycogen accumulation and no cytochrome oxidase activity. The benign form is distinguished from the fatal form by immunological detection of the enzyme by enzyme-linked immunosorbent assay (ELISA) in muscle tissue (enzyme protein is absent in the fatal form).

3. Fatty acid oxidation defects. These disorders include the carnitine deficiency syndromes and fatty acid oxidation enzyme defects which generally present in infancy with generalized weakness, hypotonia, lethargy or coma. Muscle biopsy shows lipid accumulation and enzymatic deficiency in muscle tissue or cultured skin fibroblasts.

Mitochondrial myopathies

- Multisystem disorders with growth failure, muscle fatigue with exercise, myopathic facies, microcephaly, mental retardation, myoclonic seizures, ataxia and stroke-like episodes.
- Fluctuating neurological abnormalities are characteristic.
- Maternal inheritance pattern (maternal transmission of mitochondrial DNA).

Non-lysosomal glycogenoses

- *Phosphofructokinase deficiency.* Diagnosis is by muscle biopsy with immunohistochemistry (glycogen deposition, absence of phosphofructokinase) and enzyme assays (diminished muscle phosphofructokinase activity).
- *Phosphorylase deficiency.* Muscle biopsy and immunohistochemistry are diagnostic (myopathic changes, glycogen deposition, absent phosphorylase activity).

Prader–Willi syndrome

- Presents with profound hypotonia at birth, feeding difficulties necessitating tube feeding but no respiratory difficulties.
- Facies are characteristic with a high forehead, dolicephalic head, small almond-shaped eyes, open triangular mouth, fair hair and blue eyes with small hands and feet.
- The cry is weak and high-pitched.
- Hypotonia gradually improves and the infants achieve independent mobility after the age of 2 years.
- There is a tendency to gross generalized obesity after the child starts walking.
- Males have undescended testes, rudimentary scrotum and are infertile.
- There is intellectual impairment with IQs in the low normal to mildly retarded range.

Diagnosis. Although the karyotype appears normal, specific DNA probes reveal in most cases a deletion of the proximal arm of the *paternally* inherited chromosome 15 (15q11–13). Most cases are sporadic. Patients without the deletion (15–20% of cases) have two copies of the *maternal* chromosome and no paternal contribution (an example of maternal disomy or genomic imprinting). These can be isodisomic, where the child receives two copies of the same autosome, or heterodisomic, where the child receives a pair of autosomes from a single parent. Infants with Angelman's syndrome have a similar deletion (15q11–13) but involving the *maternal* contribution, and those without the deletion may be disomic for the paternal chromosome.

Further reading

Darras BT. Neuromuscular disorders in the newborn. *Clinics in Perinatology*, 1997; **24**: 827–44.

Dubowitz V. Colour Atlas of Muscle Disorders in Childhood. St Louis: Mosby, 1989.

Dubowitz V. *Muscle Disorders in Childhood*, 2nd edn. London: W.B. Saunders, 1995.

Rosenberg RN, Pruiser SB, DiMauro S *et al. The Molecular and Genetic Basis of Neurological Disease*. Stoneham, MA: Butterworth-Heinemann, 1993.

Related topics of interest

NEUROMUSCULAR DISORDERS – NEUROLOGICAL

Neuromuscular disease in the newborn period is uncommon and often presents a major diagnostic challenge. As weakness is one of the primary presentations of neuromuscular disorders, it is useful to go though the exercise of determining whether the weakness is primarily due to a 'peripheral' neuromuscular disorder or a primary central neurological disorder. Primary neuromuscular disorders are often associated with a normal level of consciousness, decreased or normal tendon reflexes, poor limb recoil and minor dysmorphic features or congenital anomalies, whereas central neurological disorders have associated decreased consciousness, seizures, cranial nerve signs, normal or brisk reflexes, strong limb recoil, a tendency for muscle tone to improve with time and major congenital anomalies. Enquiry into the family history (including consanguinity), delayed milestones, and childhood deaths are most important. Polyhydramnios, decreased fetal movements, breech presentation, abnormal labour and birth asphyxia also suggest neuromuscular disease. Enquire from the mother and examine for signs of myotonic dystrophy or myasthenia gravis.

Clinical features

- Reduced tone, power and muscle bulk.
- Myotonia, fasciculations, facial diplegia and ptosis.
- Examine the parents (e.g. for myotonia and easy muscle fatigue in the mother with myotonic dystrophy and myasthenia gravis).
- Common congenital anomalies include micrognathia, prominent forehead, high-arched palate, undescended testes, congenital dislocation of the hips, scoliosis and contractures.

Investigations

1. *Biochemical*
- Creatine phosphokinase (CPK) – elevated with skeletal and cardiac muscle damage. May need to assay CPK isoenzyme levels which will differentiate between brain, cardiac and muscle.
- Asparate aminotransferase (AST) – persistently elevated in neuromuscular disorders with liver involvement, e.g. Pompe's.
- CSF – raised CSF protein in peripheral nerve disease.
- Serum lactate – raised in mitochondrial cytopathies.

2. *Genetic.* Detection of an increasing number of recognized gene deletions by molecular genetic techniques which also enable prenatal diagnosis to be made. DNA may be extracted and stored for future genetic analysis.

3. *Imaging*
- Radiographs – thin ribs; cardiomegaly – e.g. metabolic cardiomyopathy.
- Cranial CT/MRI/ultrasound – brain malformation, e.g. cerebral dysgenesis and decreased white matter in

congenital muscular dystrophy, dilated ventricles in congenital myotonic dystrophy.
- Muscle ultrasound – assessing muscle bulk; adipose or connective tissue infiltration increase muscle echogenicity.

4. *Neurophysiology*
- Nerve conduction velocity – diminished in peripheral neuropathy.
- Electromyogram (EMG) – assess intrinsic muscle electrical activity (e.g. shows fibrillation in peripheral neuropathy and anterior horn cell disease, and fasciculations in anterior horn cell disease). Maternal electrophysiology studies may be more informative than the infant's (e.g. myotonic dystrophy and myasthenia gravis).

5. *Histopathology.* Needle and open muscle biopsy for immunohistochemistry and electron microscopy may give definitive diagnosis.

Management

Supportive care is required – supplemental oxygen, assisted ventilation, prevention of contractures by physiotherapy and nasogastric tube feeding. Prolonged assisted ventilation, prematurity and multiple congenital anomalies are associated with poor outcome.

Anterior horn cell disease

Spinal muscular atrophies (SMA)

There are three clinical variants based on rate of progression and age at onset of disease:

1. Acute SMA or SMA type I or Werdnig–Hoffman disease.
2. Intermediate SMA or SMA type II.
3. Chronic SMA or SMA type III or Kugelberg–Welander disease.

After cystic fibrosis, SMA is the second commonest lethal autosomal recessive disorder with an incidence of 1 in 6000 births.

In SMA type I there is progressive, severe degeneration of anterior horn cells in spinal cord and cranial nerve motor nuclei. The clinical features are diminished fetal movements, respiratory distress at birth, alertness, paradoxical respiratory movements, frog-leg position, with contractures being uncommon. Cranial nerve involvement results in impaired sucking and swallowing with atrophy and fasciculations of the tongue. Examination shows hypotonia, areflexia and weakness affecting the lower extremities earlier and more severely than the upper extremities, and proximal muscles more than distal ones. As the disease advances, there is paralysis of the bulbar muscles, loss of cough reflex and an inaudible cry. EMG shows spontaneous fasciculations and fibrillations. CPK is normal or mildly to moderately elevated (up to five times the upper limit of normal). There is rapid deterioration and respiratory death in the first 2 years of life.

All three types of autosomal recessive SMA have been mapped to a single locus on chromosome 5q11.2–13.3 with preferential deletion of two genes, the survival motor neurone and the neuronal apoptosis inhibitory protein gene. Prenatal and postnatal genetic diagnosis is therefore now possible. Current treatment of SMA type I is supportive only, given the poor prognosis. Most patients with SMA types II and III are normal at birth, usually sit unsupported (but never stand), with death occurring after age 2 years (SMA type II) or adulthood (SMA type III).

Peripheral nerve disease

Examples include giant axonal neuropathy, inflammatory neuropathies, metabolic neuropathies (Leigh's disease) and sensory neuropathies (e.g. congenital sensory neuropathy) characterized by hypotonia and generalized weakness, more pronounced distally with absent tendon reflexes. Cranial nerve and respiratory muscle involvement, feeding difficulties and joint contractures are common. CSF protein may be raised. CSF and plasma lactate are raised in Leigh's disease. Muscle biopsy shows denervation.

Neuromuscular junction disorders

Transient neonatal myasthenia gravis

This develops in 15% of infants of mothers with myasthenia gravis. Maternal anti-acetylcholine receptor antibodies or immunocytes cross the placenta and symptomatic infants may also synthesize acetylcholine receptor antibodies. Clinical features are severe hypotonia (69%), weak suck, dysphagia, ptosis (50%), ophthalmoplegia and respiratory failure (65%). Diagnosis is confirmed by demonstrating high serum concentration of acetylcholine receptor antibody in newborn infants and reversal of symptoms with edrophonium chloride (Tensilon test) – 0.04–0.15 mg/kg i.m. or s.c. injection (preferred route) or 0.04 mg/kg i.v. Clinical improvement is evident within minutes and lasts 10–15 min. Exchange transfusion may be helpful in severe cases. For treatment, use pyridostigmine (5–10 mg orally, 4-hourly) or neostigmine (1–5 mg orally, 4-hourly).

Congenital myasthenic syndromes

These can be classified according to the site of the defect, that is, presynaptic (familial infantile myasthenia, autosomal recessive), post-synaptic or synaptic (congenital end-plate acetylcholinesterase deficiency, autosomal recessive; classic slow channel syndrome, autosomal dominant; congenital acetylcholine receptor deficiency, autosomal recessive) or mixed. Presenting symptoms in infancy include fluctuating weakness, weak cry and suck, generalized hypotonia, respiratory distress and feeding difficulties. Tests for anti-acetylcholine receptor antibodies are negative. The Tensilon test is positive except in the classic slow channel syndrome and in congenital end-plate acetylcholinesterase deficiency. The diagnosis is based on history and examination, EMG studies, Tensilon test, response to acetylcholinesterase inhibitors and muscle biopsy. Long-term treatment with neostigmine or pyridostigmine may be used if the Tensilon test is positive.

1. Metabolic and toxic junction disorders. Hypermagnesaemia from therapy with magnesium sulphate for maternal eclampsia may produce severe weakness, apnoea, bulbar dysfunction and autonomic dysfunction. Aminoglycosides may produce a very similar picture.

2. Infantile botulism. Infants are normal at birth but develop symptoms between the ages of 10 days and 6 months. This results from intestinal absorption of ingested *Clostridium botulinum* toxin. Clinical features include marked weakness, hypotonia, absent reflexes, bulbar dysfunction, ophthalmoplegia, constipation and respiratory insufficiency. Examination reveals diffuse hypotonia and weakness, ptosis, mydriasis, reduced gag reflex and preservation of deep tendon reflexes. Diagnosis is by culturing *C. botulinum* from stools, and EMG shows increasing response to repetitive nerve stimulation. Respiratory support and anti-toxin therapy may be required. Symptoms last 2–6 weeks.

Further reading

Darras BT. Neuromuscular disorders in the newborn. *Clinics in Perinatology*, 1997; **24**: 827–44.
Dubowitz V. Colour Atlas of Muscle Disorders in Childhood. St Louis: Mosby, 1989.
Dubowitz V. *Muscle Disorders in Childhood*, 2nd edn. London: W.B. Saunders, 1995.
Rosenberg RN, Pruiser SB, DiMauro S *et al. The Molecular and Genetic Basis of Neurological Disease*. Stoneham, MA: Butterworth-Heinemann, 1993.

Related topics of interest

Feeding difficulties (p. 84)
Hypotonia (p. 126)

Neurological evaluation (p. 206)
Neuromuscular disorders – muscular (p. 210)

NITRIC OXIDE THERAPY

The discovery in 1987 of NO as an endogenous biological mediator and the elucidation of its biological roles has been one of the most significant recent developments in medicine. NO is now recognized to be involved in the physiology of almost every life form and organ system, being involved in functions as diverse as central and autonomic neurotransmission, hormonal release, bacterial cell killing, platelet inhibition and smooth muscle relaxation. Of current interest to the care of newborns is the role of NO in smooth muscle relaxation.

Nitric oxide and vascular biology

Vascular endothelial cells synthesize NO from the amino acid L-arginine and oxygen by the enzyme nitric oxide synthase (NOS). The released NO, being a lipophilic molecule, travels freely through cell membranes and can act on the neighbouring vascular smooth muscle cell immediately beneath it. Within the vascular smooth muscle, NO binds to the enzyme soluble guanylate cyclase (sGC), stimulating it to produce cyclic guanylate monophosphate (cGMP) from guanosine triphosphate. cGMP activates protein kinases and leads ultimately to the dephosphorylation of myosin light chains and muscle relaxation. Any NO released from the abluminal surface of the endothelial cell into the bloodstream is rapidly bound to haemoglobin and converted to nitrate, which is finally excreted in urine.

Nitric oxide in the perinatal period

- NO mediates the normal pulmonary vascular adaptation at birth.
- Inhibition of endogenous NO synthesis results in a failure of the postnatal pulmonary vascular adaptation and the development of PPHN.
- Hypoxia and hypertension, which characterize PPHN, inhibit release of endogenous NO.
- A lower synthetic rate of NO has been reported during the acute phase of PPHN and L-arginine, a substrate for NO synthesis, may be deficient in some infants with PPHN.
- Inhaled NO therapy, therefore, circumvents a deficiency in the two substrates for NO synthesis, oxygen and L-arginine, and supplies the vasodilator directly to the pulmonary vasculature.
- Inhaled NO is effective in reversing the hypoxaemia due to PPHN.
- Infants with CHD and pulmonary vascular disease have endothelial dysfunction and impaired endogenous NO production manifest as pulmonary hypertension. This is responsive to inhaled NO therapy.
- Inhaled NO therapy has become the therapy of choice in disorders characterized by PPHN.

Advantages of inhaled nitric oxide over intravenous vasodilators	• Selective pulmonary vasodilation without systemic hypotensive effects. • Improves ventilation–perfusion matching (may be made worse by i.v. vasodilators). • Vasodilatory effect rapidly instituted and terminated (onset of pulmonary vasodilation may be slow with i.v. agents and any systemic hypotensive effects profound and slow to reverse, especially with tolazoline).
Disadvantages of inhaled nitric oxide therapy	• Cost of administration equipment. • Equipment not readily portable – problems with transferring infants receiving treatment (e.g. to ECMO centre) if portable NO administration equipment is not available. • Dependence on NO, even in the absence of obvious beneficial effect. • Undefined NO toxicology profile in newborns, both in the short term and long term. • Considerable expertise required to administer the therapy safely. • Potential toxicity to attendant medical and nursing staff.

Respiratory conditions amenable to nitric oxide therapy	• PPHN of any cause.
	• Conditions characterised by ventilation–perfusion mismatch with or without PPHN.
	    Pneumonias.
	    Paediatric ARDS.
	    Respiratory distress syndrome.
	    Aspiration syndromes (MAS, blood, vomitus).
	    BPD (acute deteriorations, e.g. with pneumonia).

Administration of inhaled nitric oxide	The following requirements must be met: • Reliable equipment to continuously monitor the concentration of administered NO and NO_2. • The duration of contact and mixing between NO and the administered oxygen before inhalation by the patient is minimal (sufficient to allow adequate mixing of NO and O_2 but not the excessive oxidation of NO to NO_2). • NO and NO_2 are scavenged from the exhaust gases. • Full intensive care monitoring and support exists including blood methaemoglobin measurement. • Adequate environmental and safety checks are in place. • Staff administering NO therapy must be familiar with the equipment, the safe administration and monitoring of NO therapy and the potential adverse effects.
Special notes	• As NO inhibits platelet aggregation, NO therapy may be inappropriate in haemorrhagic disorders (e.g. recent severe IVH or pulmonary haemorrhage).

- NO doses of 1–40 ppm appear optimal. If there is no response to 40 ppm NO, further increments in the dose are unlikely to produce a response.
- A starting dose of 5–10 ppm is probably optimal.
- Use the lowest effective dose of NO (maintenance therapy may be possible with ~1 ppm or less).
- Monitor methaemoglobin levels at least daily (normal level <2%). Reduce the NO dose if methaemoglobin levels exceed 2% and treat methaemoglobinaemia with methylene blue.
- As NO is not yet a licensed drug, obtain parental consent for the therapy.
- Prescribing NO on a drug treatment chart encourages adherence to the treatment regimen.
- Providing a local policy and/or guidelines facilitates the safe administration of NO by all members of staff.
- Currently, inhaled NO therapy is only of *proven* benefit in term or near-term infants with PPHN. Infants with CDH have a poor response to NO therapy.
- NO therapy is more effective when administered by HFOV as compared with conventional ventilation.

Further reading

Edwards AD. The pharmacology of inhaled nitric oxide. *Archives of Disease in Childhood*, 1995; **72**: F127–30.

Mupanemunda RH. Current status of inhaled nitric oxide therapy in the perinatal period. *Early Human Development*, 1997; **47**: 247–62.

Mupanemunda RH, Edwards AD. Treatment of newborn infants with inhaled nitric oxide. *Archives of Disease in Childhood*, 1995; **72**: F131–4.

Mupanemunda RH, Edwards AD. Nitric oxide: physiology, pathophysiology, and potential clinical applications. In: David TJ (ed). *Recent Advances in Paediatrics, No. 15*. New York: Churchill Livingstone, 1997; 119–36.

Zapol WM, Bloch KD (eds). *Nitric Oxide and the Lung*. New York: Marcel Dekker, 1996.

Related topics of interest

NUTRITION

The provision of adequate oxygen, nutrition and warmth to the vulnerable small preterm infant forms the basis of modern neonatal medicine. A fetus *in utero* doubles its weight from 500 g to 1000 g between 22 and 27 weeks, and in the following 4 weeks (27–31 weeks) acquires a further 500 g of weight, a rate unmatched at any other time in the normal human lifespan. Achievement of similar growth rates for the new VLBW infant presents a formidable nutritional challenge due to the relative inability of these infants to metabolize nutrients and excrete waste products. Furthermore, as the majority of energy and nutrient stores are laid down in the third trimester, preterm delivery puts the VLBW infant at considerable disadvantage. Nutritional goals for extremely preterm infants are therefore to supply energy nutrients not only to meet basic needs but also to promote growth. The optimal diet for preterm infants is one that supports growth at intrauterine rates but without imposing stress on the infant's immature metabolic and excretory functions.

Parenteral nutritional requirements

In the immediate postnatal period, the extremely preterm infant experiences marked tissue catabolism from stress, infection and under-nutrition, reflected by a 5–15% weight loss in the first week of life. Should the energy intake be increased beyond that required for maintenance, the infant starts gaining weight by the end of the first week of life, with birthweight being regained in 10–17 days.

- Energy intakes of 110–165 kcal/kg/day are required to meet maintenance energy needs and growth (100 ml/kg/day of 10% dextrose only provides 40 kcal/kg/day).
- Under-nutrition affects pulmonary maturation, growth, immunity, long-term growth and neurodevelopment.
- Plasma concentrations of most amino acids fall precipitously within hours after birth if protein is not administered.
- Nutritional support should be commenced in the ELBW infant (or the sick, more mature infant) at the earliest opportunity.
- Delayed onset of i.v. nutrition (total parental nutrition, TPN) is accompanied by a loss of endogenous protein of 0.5–1 g/kg/day.
- Early amino acid intake in ELBW infants reverses the nitrogen loss (as little as 1.15 g amino acid/kg/day with energy intake <30 kcal/kg/day may improve nitrogen retention).
- As insulin secretion depends on the plasma concentration of certain amino acids (e.g. leucine, arginine), low plasma levels of amino acids not only limit protein metabolism but also predispose to hyperglycaemia (reduced glucose uptake secondary to reduced insulin secretion in response to low plasma concentration of amino acids responsible for stimulating insulin).

- Commence TPN in the ELBW infant as soon as is possible after birth if the infant is not receiving enteral feeds.
- The TPN content of proteins, lipids, carbohydrates, electrolytes, minerals, vitamins and trace elements can be adjusted as the total amount of TPN administered and the duration of TPN administration increases. Maximum amounts of lipid and protein are 3 g/kg/day and 4 g/kg/day, respectively.
- Lipid emulsions should be given as a 20% solution, rather than 10%, as this results in lower plasma concentrations of phospholipid, cholesterol and triglycerides.
- Certain nutrition deficiencies at this critical period in life may have a profound influence on the development of disease in later childhood and adulthood.

Administration and monitoring of parenteral nutrition

- Central venous catheters inserted percutaneously into a central position are preferable to peripheral vein infusions, which carry the risk of skin necrosis from extravasation of nutrient infused into subcutaneous tissue.
- Central venous catheters allow administration of hyperosmolar solutions (e.g. when fluid volumes must be restricted with a symptomatic PDA) for prolonged periods.
- TPN administration via central venous catheters, however, has several complications, including:

- Cardiac arrhythmias.
- Cardiac tamponade.
- Cholelithiasis.
- Cholestatic jaundice (10–14%).
- Impaired immunity.
- Pleural effusion or chylothorax.
- Intracardiac thrombi.
- Pulmonary embolism.
- Sepsis (*S. epidermidis*, *Candida*, *Malassezia*).
- Thrombosis of the major vessels in which catheter is placed.
- Perforation of the inferior vena cava with abdominal ascites (TPN found when abdomen is drained).

Regular biochemical monitoring is required (initially daily U&E and blood glucose with weekly liver function tests, then less frequently once the infant is in a steady metabolic state).

Initiation and advancement of enteral feeds

- Intraluminal nutrition is necessary for normal gastrointestinal structure and functional integrity.
- Enteral feeds have direct trophic effects and indirect effects secondary to release of intestinal hormones.
- The provision of minimal enteral feedings (trophic feedings)

primes the gastrointestinal tract prior to more substantial enteral nutrition. This results in a reduction of feeding intolerance, earlier attainment of full enteral feeding, reduced levels of serum bilirubin and a reduction in the incidence of cholestasis.

- Intermittent gavage feeds (nasogastric or orogastric) are a convenient way of safely providing enteral feedings to ELBW infants who are relatively stable.
- Gradually reduce TPN volumes as more feeds are tolerated enterally.
- Rapid advancement of enteral feeds (>20 ml/kg/day) is associated with increased risk of NEC.
- Infants may be fed with an indwelling umbilical artery catheter (UAC). This is *not* associated with an increased incidence of NEC.
- Mother's own milk is ideal food for the preterm or term infant. It is better tolerated and confers some immunological protection as well as neurodevelopmental advantages. If not available, donor breast milk may be used.

Breast versus formula feeds

- Whenever possible, breast milk should be used for feeding preterm infants, especially SGA and VLBW infants.
- The incidence of NEC may be up to six times greater in formula-fed infants.
- Observational studies suggest that breast-feeding may advantage the infant in cognitive and intellectual development compared to infants fed formula milk. This advantage was evident at 18 months and 7.5–8 years even after adjusting for social and educational differences between groups. The advantage was related to being fed milk by tube in the neonatal period and not with subsequent breast-feeding, and was dose-related to the proportion of breast milk consumed.
- Breast milk should be fortified when given to preterm infants, as this improves growth and bone mineral content.
- In the absence of breast milk, preterm formula should be used.
- Long-chain polyunsaturated fatty acids (LCP) may have important roles in brain and retinal development and are present in breast milk. Most infant formulas do not yet contain LCP, and this should perhaps be recommended.
- Additional supplements of carbohydrate (e.g. Maxijul, SHS International Ltd, UK), or carbohydrate and fat (Duocal, SHS International Ltd, UK) may be required in enterally fed infants when weight gain is poor.
- Breast-feeding is contraindicated if the mother has HIV infection or is taking certain medications (e.g. cytotoxics).

Further reading

Barker DJP. *Mothers, Babies and Health in Later Life*, 2nd edn. Edinburgh: Churchill Living-stone, 1998.

Heird WC. Parenteral feeding. In: Sinclair JC, Braken MB (eds). *Effective Care of the New-born Infant*. Oxford: Oxford University Press, 1992.

Heird WC, Kashyap S. Intravenous feeding. In: Hay WW (ed). *Neonatal Nutrition and Metab-olism*. St Louis: Mosby–Year Book, 1991; 237–59.

Steer PA, Lucas A, Sinclair JC. Feeding the low birthweight infant. In: Sinclair JC, Bracken MB (eds). *Effective Care of the Newborn Infant*. Oxford: Oxford University Press, 1992; 94–140.

Tsang RC, Lucas A, Uauy R, Zlotkin S (eds). *Nutritional Needs of the Preterm Infant: Scien-tific Basis and Practical Guidelines*. Baltimore: Williams & Wilkins, 1993.

Related topics of interest

Feeding difficulties (p. 84)
Fluid and electrolyte therapy (p. 87)
Gastro-oesophageal reflux (p. 90)
Necrotizing enterocolitis (p. 195)
Trace minerals and vitamins (p. 317)

OESOPHAGEAL ANOMALIES

Oesophageal atresia and tracheo-oesophageal fistula

Oesophageal atresia (OA) and tracheo-oesophageal fistula (TOF) are due to a failure of early embryonic differentiation of the oesophagus and trachea. At least five types are recognized, the commonest being OA with distal TOF (87%). OA without fistula is the second commonest type (8%), followed by the 'H'-type TOF (4%).

OA presents with excessive dribbling of saliva and episodes of cyanosis and respiratory distress on the first day of life. The lack of fetal swallowing during the pregnancy usually causes polyhydramnios, and this in turn may cause preterm labour and delivery. The diagnosis is confirmed by failure to pass a naso-gastric tube into the stomach. X-ray of the chest and abdomen will show the tube lodged in the blind end of the upper oesophageal pouch. At least 85% of babies with OA have a TOF. Usually this connects with the lower oesophagus, and so air enters the stomach and may cause distension. The incidence is approximately 1 in 3500. There is the infrequent familial occurrence.

Clinical features

Respiratory distress results from airway obstruction by secretions, aspiration of secretions or milk into the lungs or a distended abdomen. When OA occurs without a TOF, or with one that connects with the upper pouch, no air enters the abdomen, which is then scaphoid rather than distended. There may be associated abnormalities of the vertebrae, an imperforate anus, tracheo-oesophageal fistula, and renal abnormalities to constitute the acronymic VATER syndrome. Infants who have an 'H'-type TOF but no OA usually present after the neonatal period with frequent lower respiratory infections and/or respiratory difficulties during feeds. Cinefluoroscopy and bronchoscopy/oesophagoscopy reveal the fistula.

Management

Prior to surgery, the infant is best nursed head-up at 45°, and the oesophagus is aspirated either with a multiple end-hole suction catheter (Replogle), or by aspirating a wide bore nasogastric tube every 5 min. If possible, ventilation should be avoided as it can cause excessive gastric distension.

The operation of choice is a primary end-to-end anastomosis as soon as the baby is stable. A nasogastric silastic feeding tube is passed through the anastomosis at the time of surgery. This nasogastric tube must be very secure; another cannot be passed post-operatively for fear of damaging the anastomosis. Post-operative nutrition is initially parenteral, but as the bowel recovers, enteral feeding can be started slowly. Prior to commencing oral feeds, a barium swallow is performed to check the integrity of the anastomosis.

When primary anastomosis cannot be achieved, a gastrostomy is created for decompression, feeding and to allow intermittent insertion of a bougie to stretch the lower oesophageal pouch. The upper pouch can also be stretched intermittently. An oesophagostomy is created in the neck to allow external drainage of the saliva and allow sham feeding. In time, end-to-end anastomosis can be achieved.

Complications   Post-operative complications include stenosis of the circumferential oesophageal scar: this is treated by dilatation. A persistent brassy 'TOF-cough' may persist for years and is due to the abnormalities of the trachea. These infants may be especially difficult to feed, particularly if a long period elapses without oral feeds. GOR is common and requires medical and sometimes surgical therapy. The anastomosis may also break down with recurrence of the fistula.

Further reading

Ein SH, Shandling B. Pure esophageal atresia: a 50-year review. *Journal of Pediatric Surgery*, 1994; **29**: 1208–11.

Fanaroff AA, Martin RJ. *Neonatal–Perinatal Medicine: Diseases of the Fetus and Neonate*, 6th edn. St Louis: Mosby, 1997.

O'Neill Jr JA, Rowe MI, Grosfeld JL, Fonkelsrud EW, Coran A. *Pediatric Surgery*, 5th edn. St Louis: Mosby, 1998.

Stringer MD, Oldham KT, Mouriquand PDE, Howard ER. *Pediatric Surgery and Urology: Long-term Outcomes*. Philadelphia: W.B. Saunders, 1998.

Related topics of interest

ORTHOPAEDIC PROBLEMS

Congenital dislocation of the hips

Although its strict definition means 'a partial or complete displacement of the femoral head from the acetabulum', the term congenital dislocation of the hips is frequently used to embrace a spectrum of abnormalities embracing dislocation, sub-luxation and even dysplasias. Congenital hip instability is found in 15–20 per 1000 babies. Most of these resolve spontaneously. Unscreened and untreated, about 1 in 1000 babies go on to develop a dislocated hip. Risk factors include:

- A family history.
- Breech presentation.
- Female sex.
- Neuromuscular disease.

There has been concern that some neonatal screening programmes failed to reduce the incidence of congenital dislocation of the hips needing surgery, but a consensus view has emerged that screening will minimize but not prevent its late diagnosis. Debate continues as to the most efficacious, cost-effective and feasible way to screen all babies. At present, screening is by physical examination alone, or ultrasound scan (which may be universal or for selected high-risk babies), or both.

1. Physical examination
- Is the hip dislocated at the start of the examination?
  If so, full abduction of the thigh with forward pressure on the greater femoral trochanter from the middle finger will reveal a positive Ortolani sign (a clunk as the femoral head relocates into the acetabulum), or prove impossible, indicating an irreducible hip.
- Can the hip be dislocated, i.e. is it unstable?
  Barlow's manoeuvre attempts to lift the femoral head anteriorly from the acetabulum and then displace it latero-posteriorly. If the joint subluxates, movement may be felt with the impression of the femoral head sliding laterally. Ortolani's test will then be positive, even if it was negative when the hips were first abducted.

The management of each hip must be planned, and in centres where ultrasound scanning is only selectively available for those with a recognized risk factor or abnormal examination, a scheme similar to that below will be followed:

- Clinically normal and low risk. No action – discharge.
- Clinically normal and high-risk history. Follow-up and early scan.

- Clinically abnormal or suspicious. Follow-up and early scan.
- Dislocated or dislocatable. Refer to physiotherapist and orthopaedic surgeon for splinting and investigation.

Ultrasound scanning does not just detect dislocated hips but also shallow acetabula and dysplasia of the femoral head and acetabulum. While congenital dislocation of the hips can be treated and the outcome for that treatment (and missed cases) is clear, there is no treatment for dysplastic hips, but now that they can be detected early, their natural history will become clearer.

2. *Treatment.* The underlying principle is that the femoral head is held within the acetabulum so that the two can grow together and mould to each other. In unstable hips, this can be achieved by gently splinting the legs in abduction until the joint is stable. Splinting can be left for several weeks in an unstable hip, and then applied only to those with continuing clinical or sonographic abnormalities. If abduction can be achieved only with some force, there is a risk of avascular necrosis of the femoral head secondary to the pressure generated by the pull of the stretched adductor muscles. Therefore, some hips are splinted after an adductor tenotomy to relieve the pressure. In irreducible congenital dislocation of the hips an open surgical reduction is necessary.

Talipes

This is the inability to place the foot plantigrade on a flat surface. Risk factors include a family history, neuromuscular disease and oligohydramnios. The legs (and spine) must be carefully checked for signs of neuromuscular disease. Talipes is described by the position of the foot: plantar-flexed (equino-), dorsi-flexed (calcaneo-), hooked or twisted inwards (varus) or everted (valgus). Many feet with talipes need only massage and stretching exercises. Strapping can be used to bring an equino-varus foot into a better position. It is applied so as to pull on the foot when the knee is extended. More severe talipes may need serial plasters and surgery.

Positional talipes is an oxymoron. Whatever the posture of the foot at rest, talipes is 'positional' if the foot can be placed plantigrade on a flat surface in mid-position without force. It does not need treating.

Fractures

Fractures tend to occur in three groups of babies:

- Healthy large term babies with difficult deliveries.
- Preterm babies with osteopaenia of prematurity.
- Babies with congenital bone abnormalities.

The first group is the commonest. Neonatal fractures heal rapidly with extensive callus formation. Very little treatment is needed apart from analgesia if necessary and gentle immobilization of the fractured bone if possible.

1. Skull. Cephalhaematoma may rarely be associated with a fracture. If confirmed on X-ray, consider CT scanning.

2. Humerus. This may be fractured during a difficult extraction. This is very painful and produces a pseudo-palsy and crepitus. Use a vest to splint the arm to the chest wall. Check vascular and nerve supply to the forearm and hand. The bone should heal with no long-term problems.

3. Clavicle. May be fractured during delivery. Often not diagnosed until the callus is palpable, although the baby may be irritable initially. Difficult to diagnose on X-ray prior to callus formation because of the curvature of the clavicle. No specific treatment is necessary.

4. Ribs. Fractures may occur spontaneously or during physiotherapy in babies with osteopaenia of prematurity. Diagnosis is usually retrospective when callus seen on chest X-ray.

5. Femur. Fractures may occur during breech extraction, or postnatally in infants with neuromuscular disorders. This is very painful with accompanying crepitus. Bleeding into the thigh may cause shock. Healing and remodelling will occur without Gallows traction. Support limb gently during handling and nappy changes.

Further reading

Jones DA. *Hip Screening in the Newborn*. London: Butterworth-Heinemann, 1998.
Lennox IAC, McLauchlan J, Murali R. Failures of screening and management of congenital dislocation of the hip. *Journal of Bone and Joint Surgery*, 1993; **75**: 72–5.

Related topics of interest

PATENT DUCTUS ARTERIOSUS

The natural history of a patent ductus arteriosus (PDA) in healthy term and preterm infants (regardless of gestational age) is of spontaneous closure by the fourth day of life. Infants with RDS have delayed closure of the duct which causes clinical problems with increasing frequency as birthweight and gestational age decreases. The incidence of clinically significant PDA in preterm infants with RDS has been reported to vary from 7% (birthweight >1500 g, or ≥33 weeks gestation) to 51% (birthweight <1000 g or <28 weeks gestation). The incidence of PDA also varies with the severity of RDS and is influenced by acute perinatal stress, hypoxia, acidosis, fluid therapy, surfactant therapy and prenatal medication.

Pathophysiology

Normal postnatal ductal closure is mediated by a complex mechanism involving oxygen and other mediators. Hypoxia relaxes the ductus, whereas hyperoxia constricts it. There are developmental changes in the sensitivity of the ductus to oxygen, increasing sensitivity being seen with increasing gestational age. Prostaglandins (PG), particularly PGE_2, also relax the ductus, the ductus of the immature infant being more sensitive to PG than that of the more mature infant. Furthermore, the ductus remains reactive to PG even after initial constriction, accounting for the observed PDA recurrence observed in preterm infants. Steroids decrease the sensitivity of the ductus to PGE, hence prenatal administration of steroids decreases the incidence of PDA. During the acute stage of RDS, PGE levels are elevated and this may influence ductal patency. With resolution of RDS, there is a reduction in pulmonary vascular resistance and a rise in pulmonary blood flow and a congestive circulatory state. This may increase ventilatory requirements and increase the risk of developing chronic lung disease, NEC and IVH.

Prevention

- Antenatal dexamethasone reduces the severity of RDS *and* the incidence of symptomatic PDA (sPDA).
- Fluid restriction (<140 ml/kg/day) during the first week of life reduces the incidence of sPDA.
- Inappropriate use of plasma expanders for hypotension may predispose to the development of an sPDA.
- Prophylactic administration of indomethacin decreases the incidence of sPDA without convincingly reducing morbidity and mortality and is therefore not generally recommended.
- Prophylactic ductal ligation in infants of birthweight <1000 g does not reduce mortality or morbidity (apart from decreasing the incidence of NEC) and would result in surgery being performed in many infants who did not require it.

Clinical features

The PDA in preterm infants may be subclinical (no murmur) or clinical (murmur present), while clinical PDA may be non-significant (no cardiopulmonary dysfunction) or significant (with cardiopulmonary dysfunction). In the absence of a ductus murmur, a PDA can only be diagnosed non-invasively by Doppler echocardiography. A non-significant clinical PDA presents with only a heart murmur (at the left sternal border, second intercostal space) which is largely systolic although it may continue into the diastolic phase.

Significant clinical PDA
- Precordial murmur (commonly purely systolic) in the pulmonary area.
- Hyperactive precordium.
- Bounding pulses.
- Resting tachycardia.
- Cardiomegaly on chest X-ray.
- Carbon dioxide retention.
- Frequent apnoeas.
- Failure to wean off the ventilator at the expected time or unexplained deterioration of respiratory status.

Diagnosis
- Pulmonary plethora or congestion with cardiomegaly on chest radiograph.
- Direct visualization of PDA on two-dimensional Doppler colour-flow echocardiography.
- Left atrial enlargement with increase in LA/AO ratio (>1.3) on echocardiogram (normal values 0.66–1.06).
- High left ventricular function index (shown by left ventricular shortening fraction) (normal value $34 \pm 3\%$).

Management
- Optimize oxygenation.
- Restrict fluids to 80–120 ml/kg/day.
- Correct anaemia (maintain haematocrit >40%).
- Diuretics, for fluid overload or congestive heart failure. Use frusemide 0.5–1 mg/kg/dose once or twice daily (1–3 mg/kg i.v. for congestive heart failure). For maintenance therapy use chlorothiazide 20 mg/kg/dose once or twice daily with amiloride 0.2 mg/kg, as frusemide will cause significant electrolyte imbalance. Do monitor electrolytes. Note that frusemide also promotes ductal patency by stimulating renal PGE_2 production.
- Spontaneous closure may occur in 22–28% of patients with the above measures.

Pharmacological closure of the ductus should be employed if the above measures are not sufficient. Indomethacin, a PG synthetase (cyclo-oxygenase type 1) inhibitor has been the primary agent used for many years. A dose of 0.2 mg/kg i.v. over 30 min 8–12-hourly for a total of three doses (or 0.3 mg/kg i.v. 12-hourly $\times$ 3 for infants over 4 weeks of age), or the prolonged low-dose regimen of 0.1 mg/kg/dose daily for 6 days are generally used. However, indomethacin decreases platelet aggregation (increasing the risk of haemorrhage), cerebral blood flow (but with no long-term neurological deficits), gastrointestinal perfusion (increasing the risk of NEC, gastrointestinal haemorrhage or perforation) and renal blood flow (causing transient renal dysfunction with reduced glomerular filtration rate (GFR) and urine output and a dilutional hyponatraemia, necessitating a 20% reduction in administered fluids during treatment). Prolonged low-dose administration causes less renal dysfunction, has a lower recurrence rate (~50% less) and is equally effective. The renal side-effects of indomethacin may also be prevented by the simultaneous administration of frusemide (1 mg/kg) without reducing its efficacy. The overall efficacy of indomethacin in effecting ductal closure during the first 14 days of life (in infants of <1750 g) is ~70%. After 14–21 days, efficacy is reduced and it is ineffective in infants aged >6 weeks. Efficacy is also reduced in both the very small preterm infant (<800 g birthweight) and infants of high post-conceptional age. In view of the above side-effects of indomethacin, ibuprofen, another non-steroidal anti-inflammatory drug, is now also being used, at a dose of 10 mg/kg i.v. followed by 5 mg/kg 24 and 48 hours later. Ibuprofen appears as effective as indomethacin but with fewer cerebral, gastrointestinal and renal side-effects. Second courses may be given to infants who do not respond to the first course or with recurrent PDA, although the response is often poor. Non-response to a single course in infants of <1000 g birthweight is an indication for surgery.

Relative contraindications for pharmacological therapy

- Shock.
- NEC.
- Haemorrhagic disease.
- Thrombocytopenia (platelets <50 000/mm^3).
- Recent (<48 hours) IVH.
- Renal impairment (blood urea >14 mmol/l, creatinine >140 μmol/l, or persistent oliguria of <1 ml/kg/hour).

Surgical closure of PDA

Prior to surgery, detailed echocardiography should be performed to exclude associated CHD with duct-dependent lesions. Indications for surgery are a strong contraindication or side-effect to indomethacin or ibuprofen therapy, failure to respond to indomethacin or ibuprofen therapy (once in infants of birthweight <1000 g or twice in infants >1000 g), or the presence of a large sPDA (echocardiographically) in an infant of birthweight <1000 g. Ductal ligation may be performed on the neonatal unit in small preterm infants, obviating the need to transport such infants to operating theatres on or off site with the attendant complications of hypothermia, interruption of vascular access and accidental extubation. Surgery has a more predictable outcome and may be preferable in very small preterm infants, but complications include pneumothorax, pleural effusion (serous or chylous), excessive intra-operative blood loss, phrenic and recurrent laryngeal nerve injuries.

Further reading

Burch M, Archer N. *Pediatric Cardiology*. London: Chapman & Hall, 1998.

Evans N. Diagnosis of patent ductus arteriosus in the preterm newborn. *Archives of Disease in Childhood*, 1993; **68**: 58–61.

Gavilanes AWD, Heineman E, Herpers MJHM, Blanco CE. Use of neonatal intensive care unit as a safe place for neonatal surgery. *Archives of Disease in Childhood, Fetal and Neonatal Edition*, 1997; **76**: F51–3.

Nehgme RA, O'Connor TZ, Lister G, Bracken MB. Patent ductus arteriosus. In: Sinclair JC, Bracken MB (eds). *Effective Care of the Newborn Infant*. Oxford: Oxford University Press, 1992; 281–324.

Reller MD, Rice MJ, McDonald RW. Review of studies evaluating ductal patency in the premature infant. *Journal of Pediatrics*, 1993; **122**: S59–62.

Rennie JM, Cooke RWI. Prolonged low-dose indomethacin for the persistent ductus arteriosus of prematurity. *Archives of Disease in Childhood*, 1991; **66**: 55–8.

Yeh JF, Lin YJ, Wu JM. Patent ductus arteriosus. In: Yu VYH (ed). *Baillières Clinical Paediatrics, Vol. 3, No. 1. Pulmonary Problems in the Perinatal Period and their Sequelae*. London: Baillière Tindall, 1995; 131–46.

Related topics of interest

Congenital heart disease – congestive heart failure (p. 61)
Congenital heart disease – cyanotic defects (p. 65)
Fluid and electrolyte therapy (p. 87)
Necrotizing enterocolitis (p. 195)
Neonatal surgery (p. 200)
Respiratory distress syndrome (p. 278)

PERIVENTRICULAR LEUCOMALACIA

Periventricular leucomalacia (PVL) refers to necrosis of white matter dorsal and lateral to the external angles of the lateral ventricles, involving particularly the centrum semiovale (frontal horn and body), the optic (trigone and occipital horn) and acoustic (temporal horn) radiations. The incidence of PVL at autopsy shows great variation, and during life one recent report gave a peak incidence of 15.7% at 28 weeks gestation falling to 4.3% at 32 weeks gestation (overall 9.2%) when PVL was determined by cranial ultrasonography. PVL is most often seen in preterm infants, infants with cardiorespiratory disturbance and infants with a postnatal survival of more than a few days (commonly 1–3 weeks). Recently, an association has also been recognized between ventilation-induced hypocapnia and PVL, particularly in the preterm infant.

Neuropathology

PVL has distinctive pathological features consisting of both focal periventricular necrosis and more diffuse cerebral white matter injury. The focal necrotic lesions occur primarily in the distribution of the end zones of the long penetrating arteries. The two commonest sites for PVL focal necrosis are in the white matter near the trigone of the lateral ventricles and around the foramen of Monro. These sites are the arterial end and border zones (i.e. watershed areas) between the terminal branches of the long penetrating branches of the middle cerebral artery and the posterior cerebral artery (peritrigonal white matter) or the anterior cerebral artery (frontal white matter).

The more diffuse regions of cerebral white matter injury are characterized by diffuse loss of oligodendrocytes and a corresponding increase in hypertrophic astrocytes. These diffuse lesions are less likely to undergo major cystic changes, and therefore more commonly go undetected by cranial ultrasonography during life. Diminished cerebral white matter volume and an increase in ventricular size are more readily noted.

Pathogenesis

Three major interacting factors have important roles in the pathogenesis of PVL:

1. The intrinsic vulnerability of the cerebral white matter in the preterm newborn.
2. A pressure-passive cerebral circulation.
3. The unique periventricular vascular anatomy in preterm newborns.

Infection and inflammatory cytokines may also have minor roles. The periventricular vascular supply in preterm infants is derived from deep penetrating basal cerebral arteries which have few side branches and anastomoses, making these areas most susceptible to falls in perfusion pressure and cerebral blood flow. With increasing gestational age there is an increase in anastomoses of the periventricular vasculature, making these deep periventricular regions less susceptible to ischaemia. An additional factor in the pathogenesis of PVL is the presence of a pressure-passive cerebral circulation where cerebral blood flow falls with a decrease in blood pressure. This cerebrovascular autoregulatory defect predisposes the periventricular arterial border zones and end zones in cerebral white matter to ischaemia. A third important parameter is the inherent vulnerability of cerebral white matter to injury, due to the marked sensitivity of the early differentiating oligodendro-cytes to free-radical attack. Large amounts of free radicals are generated under conditions of ischaemia-reperfusion which is central to the pathogenesis of PVL.

Diagnosis

The principal diagnostic tool is cranial ultrasonography. The acute lesions appear as bilateral echodensities or 'flares' distributed diffusely in the periventricular white matter or localized to the main sites of predilection for PVL, namely around the foramen of Monro or near the trigone of the lateral ventricles. The localized echodensities may resolve over the next 1–3 weeks and be replaced by multiple small echolucent cysts giving rise to a 'Swiss cheese appearance'. After 1–3 months, well delineated cysts disappear with gliosis and collapse of cyst walls, leaving enlarged ventricles and decreased cerebral myelin. Ultrasonography, however, is relatively insensitive and may miss up to 70% of PVL detected by histopathology, especially small focal areas of necrosis and more diffuse white matter injury. However, once detected, periventricular cysts are the most sensitive and specific neurosonographic predictors of cerebral palsy in preterm infants. The parasagittal measurements of the anteroposterior dimensions of cystic PVL best predict which infants will have quadriplegia (more common with cystic PVL ≥ 20 mm) and the more severe cognitive and sensory impairments.

Prognosis

Developmental sequelae, including the type of cerebral palsy, degree of functional motor deficits, and associated disabilities, are closely linked with the location and extent of the cystic PVL. Cysts that are limited to the frontal or anterior periventricular region have not usually been associated with cerebral palsy. Bilateral multiple cysts involving the middle (centrum semiovale) or posterior periventricular regions have been associated with cerebral palsy and other disabilities. The periventricular locus of PVL is such that it affects the descending fibres from the motor cortex, primarily those subserving the function of the lower limbs (giving rise to spastic diplegia), with severer lesions progressively involving motor fibres of the upper limbs and finally intellectual functions as well, with corresponding marked intellectual deficits. PVL may also impair subsequent cortical neuronal organization and cognitive function. In surviving infants with cystic PVL, the prevalence of all types of cerebral palsy has ranged from 38–93%, spastic cerebral palsy being present in all (but 21–69% being diplegia, 27–71% quadriplegia, and 0–33% hemiplegia). In general, once cystic PVL and ventricular dilatation (indicative of white matter atrophy) have developed, 60–90% of such infants will develop spastic diplegia and other neurological deficits.

Prevention

As PVL is primarily due to cerebral ischaemia, avoidance of systemic hypotension and hypocarbia is important. Infants with a pressure-passive cerebral circulation are especially susceptible to PVL. Near-infrared spectroscopy (still largely a research tool) is currently the main technique for detecting this circulatory abnormality.

Further reading

Fazzi E, Orcesi S, Caffi L *et al*. Neurodevelopmental outcome at 5–7 years in preterm infants with periventricular leucomalacia. *Neuropediatrics*, 1994; **25**: 134.

Gannon CM, Wiswell TE, Spitzer AR. Volutrauma, PaCO$_2$ levels and neurodevelopmental sequelae following assisted ventilation. *Clinics in Perinatology*, 1998; **25**: 159–75.

Perlman JM, Risser R, Broyles RS. Bilateral cystic periventricular leucomalacia in the premature infant: associated risk factors. *Pediatrics*, 1996; **97**: 822–7.

Rogers B, Msall M, Owens T, Guernsey K, Brody A. Cystic periventricular leucomalacia and type of cerebral palsy in preterm infants. *Journal of Pediatrics*, 1994; **125**: S1–8.

Volpe JJ. Brain injury in the premature infants – neuropathology, clinical aspects, pathogenesis and prevention. *Clinics in Perinatology*, 1997; **24**: 567–87.

Zupan V, Gonzalez P, Tacaze-Masmonteil T *et al*. Periventricular leucomalacia: risk factors revisited. *Developmental Medicine and Child Neurology*, 1996; **38**: 1061–7.

Related topics of interest

PERSISTENT PULMONARY HYPERTENSION OF THE NEWBORN

Since the original description by Gersony and colleagues of the 'PFC' syndrome in the late 1960s, there have been considerable advances in our understanding of the developmental biology and pathophysiology of persistent fetal circulation, now known as persistent pulmonary hypertension of the newborn (PPHN). However, the clinical management of this disorder is not uncommonly frustrating, not least because the diagnostic criteria are inadequately standardized and the optimal therapy is often disputed. Adding to the confusion is that PPHN is not a single disease entity but a complex of diverse causes, all with a similar clinical picture. It is unlikely, therefore, that a single therapeutic intervention will cure all infants with PPHN.

In PPHN, the high fetal pulmonary vascular resistance and pulmonary arterial pressure do not fall after birth or subsequently rise. As pulmonary arterial pressure exceeds the systemic arterial pressure, right-to-left shunting occurs across the patent foramen ovale (PFO) (right atrium to left atrium) or through the PDA (pulmonary artery to aorta), leading to systemic hypoxaemia.

The disorder occurs in term and preterm infants. The incidence varies worldwide from approximately 1 in 500 live births to 1 in 1500. It is more common in the USA, where it may count for 3.4% of all neonatal admissions (~10 000 newborns annually) and is the most common cause of death in infants of birthweight >1000 g.

Pathophysiology

There are physiological (or functional) factors and anatomical (or structural) factors which contribute to the development of PPHN.

1. Physiological factors. These produce pulmonary vasoconstriction via local vasoactive mediators, e.g. prostaglandins, thromboxanes, leucotrienes, bradykinin, endothelin-1, NO and platelet activating factor. There are a normal number of arteries and normal muscularization.

- Hypothermia.
- Hypoglycaemia.
- Perinatal asphyxia.
- Bacterial pneumonia.
- Severe hypoxia or acidosis.
- MAS.
- RDS.
- Polycythaemia-hyperviscosity syndrome.

2. Anatomical factors
(a) Decreased number of arteries with decreased cross-sectional area of pulmonary vascular bed
- CDH.
- Primary pulmonary hypoplasia.
- Peripheral pulmonary artery stenosis.
- Congenital alveolar capillary dysplasia.
(b) Normal number of arteries but with increased muscularization of arteries

- Post-maturity.
- Placental insufficiency.
- Chronic fetal hypoxia.

Clinical features

- Lability of oxygenation.
- Prominent right ventricular impulse with narrowly split and loud second heart sound.
- Tricuspid, mitral or pulmonary incompetence murmur.
- Hepatomegaly, signs of heart failure.
- Lung fields commonly clear or oligaemic on chest x-ray.
- Blood gas: severe hypoxaemia with mild acidosis, slightly elevated or normal carbon dioxide.
- ECG – right ventricular dominance, right axis deviation, and right atrial enlargement.

Diagnosis

There is no specific ideal test for PPHN. When hypoxaemia is out of proportion to the degree of parenychmal lung disease and there is no evidence of cyanotic CHD, consider PPHN as a diagnosis. The following signs are helpful:

- Lability of oxygenation, unprovoked wide swings in PaO_2.
- Preductal and post-ductal PaO_2 differences. Simultaneous preductal and post-ductal monitoring of oxygen saturation or PaO_2 shows a difference of 5–10% or >2.5 kPa, respectively.
- Hyperoxia–hyperventilation test. A brief (~10 min) period of hyperventilation induces alkalosis and pulmonary vasodilation with a consequent rise in PaO_2. This manoeuvre is associated with increased risk of pneumothorax and further lung damage, particularly as hyperventilation tends to be continued should oxygenation improve.
- Two-dimensional Doppler echocardiography is the most useful and accurate diagnostic technique. Right-to-left shunting of blood through the PDA and PFO can be visualized and the magnitude of pulmonary hypertension estimated from the flow velocity of the regurgitant jet at the pulmonary or tricuspid valve. CHD (especially anomalous venous drainage) can also be excluded at the same time.

Management – general

1. Stabilize the patient to prevent swings in oxygenation and other vital parameters
- Identify and correct any physiological abnormalities likely to increase pulmonary vascular resistance (e.g. hypoglycaemia, acidosis).
- Sedate (opiates, benzodiazepines) – paralyse to facilitate synchrony with ventilator.
- Avoid excessive handling.

2. *Maintain systemic arterial pressure*
- Correct hypotension with volume expanders (albumin, FFP, blood) and/or commence inotropes (dopamine, dobutamine).

3. *Reduce pulmonary arterial pressure*
- Choice of i.v. and inhaled agents.

4. *Assess severity of the impairment of gas exchange.* This helps predict the outcome and gauge response to therapy. Use OI for this purpose.

$$OI = \frac{\text{Mean airway pressure (cmH}_2\text{O)} \times \text{FiO}_2 \times 100\%}{\text{PaO}_2\,\text{(mmHg)}}$$

Management of ventilation

- Administer surfactant (whether patient has pneumonia, MAS, or idiopathic PPHN). MAS requires several doses of surfactant.
- Hyperventilation is now obsolete as it is associated with increased pulmonary morbidity from chronic lung disease and adverse neurodevelopmental outcome (especially sensorineural hearing impairment and impaired psychomotor development). Hypocapnia decreases CBF.
- Induced metabolic alkalosis has theoretical advantages of hyperventilation-induced alkalosis. No studies have evaluated the efficacy of this therapy. Hypernatraemia may ensue from sodium bicarbonate administration.
- 'Conservative' ventilation may be equally effective or superior to hyperventilation. This is deliberate hypoventilation allowing high PaCO$_2$ in order to diminish lung injury. The target pH is ≥7.25 as compared to ≥7.5 with hyperventilation.
- High frequency ventilation, particularly HFOV, may be superior to conventional ventilation in improving outcome, as HFOV improves lung recruitment. HFJV may be as effective as HFOV.
- Vasodilator therapy has a definite role in improving oxygenation in PPHN.

Intravenous vasodilators

Intravenous vasodilators may be less effective than inhaled vasodilators as the former produce concomitant hypotension. The most commonly used i.v. vasodilators are as follows:

- Nitroprusside 0.2–6 μg/kg/min.
- Prostacyclin 1–40 ng/kg/min.
- PGD$_2$ 1–25 μg/kg/min.
- Nitroglycerine 0.5–12 μg/kg/min.
- Tolazoline 1–2 mg/kg bolus, followed by 1–2 mg/kg/hour.
- Magnesium sulphate 200 mg/kg over 20–30 min followed by 20–150 mg/kg/hour to maintain serum magnesium concentration of 3.5–5.5 mmol/l.

Inhaled vasodilators	Inhaled vasodilator therapy is dominated by NO, the recently discovered potent endogenous vasodilator. Nebulized prostacyclin has also been used, as a selective pulmonary vasodilator with good effect. To date, five randomized trials with over 700 term or near-term infants have been completed in North America. ECMO use was decreased in the NO-treated groups (one fewer ECMO patient for every six patients treated with NO). However, up to 40% of infants failed to respond to NO.
	ECMO is indicated when medical therapy fails and/or when the OI >35 (or perhaps lower) with an 84% survival (86% of survivors being neurodevelopmentally normal). ECMO-treated infants do not have increased morbidity compared with infants treated with conventional ventilator therapy.
Prognosis	Deaths from PPHN have decreased in recent years, perhaps due to earlier diagnosis and treatment, with an overall survival rate of 77%.

Further reading

Kinsella JP, Abman SH. Recent developments in the pathophysiology and treatment of persistent pulmonary hypertension of the newborn. *Journal of Pediatrics*, 1995; **126:** 853–64.

Morin FC, Davis JM. Persistent pulmonary hypertension. In: Spitzer AR (ed). *Intensive Care of the Fetus and Neonate*. St Louis: CV Mosby, 1996; 506.

Truog WE. Inhaled nitric oxide: a tenth anniversary observation. *Pediatrics,* 1998; **101:** 696–7.

Walsh-Suskys MC. Persistent pulmonary hypertension of the newborn. The black box revisited. *Clinics in Perinatology*, 1993; **20:** 127–43.

Yu VYH, Fox WW. Persistent pulmonary hypertension. In: Yu VYH (ed). *Pulmonary Problems in the Perinatal Period and their Sequelae*. Bailliere's Clinical Paediatrics, Vol. 3, No. 1. London: Baillière Tindall, 1995; 115–30.

Related topics of interest

POLYCYTHAEMIA

Marked polycythaemia gives rise to the hyperviscosity syndrome, which is associated with a significant morbidity. Blood viscosity is determined by haematocrit, red cell deformability and plasma viscosity, the haematocrit being most important. Polycythaemia is present when the central venous haematocrit is $\geq 65\%$. Peripheral venous haematocrits are significantly higher than central ones. The haematocrit rises in the first 24 hours as plasma volume decreases. Prevalence rates of 2–4% have been reported. It is more common in babies born at high altitude. It is the hyperviscosity secondary to polycythaemia which causes most of the clinical problems.

Aetiology

Polycythaemia may be passive (fetus receives a transfusion of red cells) or active (fetus produces excessive red cells in response to intrauterine stimuli).

1. *Passive*
- Twin–twin transfusion.
- Maternal–fetal transfusion.
- Delayed clamping of cord.

2. *Active*
- Intrauterine hypoxia (hence elevated levels of erythropoietin), especially placental insufficiency/pre-eclampsia, small-for-gestation infants, post-term infants, and maternal smoking.
- Chromosomal abnormalities, especially trisomy 13, 18 and 21.
- Severe maternal heart disease.
- Beckwith's syndrome.
- Neonatal thyrotoxicosis.
- Congenital adrenal hyperplasia.
- Maternal diabetes.

Pathophysiology

It is unclear whether these symptoms are due primarily to the sluggish circulation and poor oxygen delivery or the accompanying hypoglycaemia. Hypoglycaemia is due in part to the high red cell mass and low plasma volume with a low intra-erythrocytic glucose level which reduces the overall glucose content of blood. In severe polycythaemia, sludging of the red cells and platelets in a sluggish peripheral circulation may occur, resulting in tissue hypoxia and thrombosis. This is most serious in the brain where it may cause convulsions and infarcts.

Clinical features

Signs commonly appear when the normal physiological reduction in plasma volume occurs (first 24 hours).

- Hypotonia and lethargy.
- Difficulty in arousal.

- Irritability.
- Easily startles.
- Tremulousness.
- Poor feeding.
- Vomiting.

Complications

1. *Early*
- Hyperbilirubinaemia (kernicterus).
- Cardiac and renal failure.
- Hypoglycaemia and hypocalcaemia.
- Respiratory distress.
- Thrombocytopenia.
- Seizures.
- Priapism and testicular infarction.
- Renal vein thrombosis.
- NEC.
- Distal bowel obstruction.

2. *Late*
- Speech and fine motor abnormalities.
- Spastic diplegia.
- Neurodevelopmental delay.
- Low IQ.

Investigations
- FBC.
- Determine haematocrit by centrifugation (calculated values from automatic electronic counters are inaccurate and lower than values obtained by centrifugation).
- Coagulation screen (in the presence of thrombocytopenia).
- Serum bilirubin.
- Blood glucose.
- Serum calcium.
- Abdominal X-ray (suspected NEC or obstruction).
- U&E (in presence of poor renal function).
- Head ultrasound scan (in presence of seizures).

Management

A partial exchange transfusion replaces infant's whole blood with FFP or 4.5% human albumin (when FFP is not readily available), aiming for a haematocrit of 55%. However, crystalloids (e.g. Ringer's solution) may be used effectively, especially if there is hypervolaemia secondary to twin–twin transfusion. Blood volume to be exchanged is approximately 20 ml/kg. Alternatively, use the formula: exchange volume = total infant's blood volume (85 ml × birthweight) × (observed haematocrit minus desired haematocrit) ÷ observed haematocrit. Perform the partial exchange in small volumes (5–10 ml aliquots) using peripheral veins (using umbilical vessels increases the risk of NEC).

For significant symptoms, perform a partial exchange transfusion promptly. For mild or minor symptoms, keep the infant well hydrated and warm. Screen high-risk infants by performing capillary haematocrit and if this is ≥65–70% perform venous haematocrit. Screen for and treat hypoglycaemia. If symptoms do not develop within 48 hours and the baby is feeding well, complications are unlikely.

Further reading

Black VD. Neonatal hyperviscosity syndromes. *Current Problems in Paediatrics*, 1987; **17:** 73–130.

Delaney-Black V, Camp BW, Lubchenco LO *et al*. Neonatal hyperviscosity association with lower achievement and IQ scores at school age. *Pediatrics*, 1989; **83:** 662.

Hann IM, Gibson BES, Letsky EA (eds). *Fetal and Neonatal Haematology*. London: Baillière Tindall, 1991.

Oski FA, Naiman JL. *Hematologic Problems in the Newborn*, 3rd edn. Philadelphia: W.B. Saunders, 1982.

Ramamurthy RS. Postnatal alteration in haematocrit and viscosity in normal infants and in those with polycythemia. *Journal of Pediatrics*, 1989; **114:** 169–70.

Related topics of interest

Anaemia (p. 9)
Intrauterine growth restriction (p. 165)
Jaundice (p. 173)
Transfusion of blood and blood products (p. 323)

POSTNATAL EXAMINATION

All infants, including those allowed home within a few hours of birth, should have a full examination within the first day of life. Ideally the mother should be present to enable her to ask any questions she may have. In addition, any problems noted can then be discussed immediately.

History

As always, the examination must be complemented by a history. Quickly note the maternal past obstetric and medical histories (e.g. hepatitis B infection). Note also significant social problems (e.g. drug abuse, child protection issues) and the family history (e.g. tuberculosis). Finally, run through the pregnancy details and note any complications (e.g. polyhydramnios, abnormal fetal scans), labour (e.g. intrapartum pyrexia) and delivery including details of the resuscitation, Apgar scores and birthweight. Progress since birth (feeding, passage of stools or urine and any other problems noted) should also be quickly reviewed.

Initial examination

Note age at time of examination. Check weight, length and head circumference and plot on centile chart if necessary. Undress the infant completely and check whether the appearance of the infant and posture are normal. Note the colour (e.g. pale, cyanosed, jaundiced, plethoric), skin condition (e.g. dry, peeling) and any blemishes. Examine each region in turn starting from the head down.

1. Head and neck. Note shape of skull and check sutures, fontanelle and the rest of the scalp (cephalhaematoma?), facies (any asymmetry, anomalies), eyes (shape, size, epicanthic folds), iris (colobomata), cornea (diameter >11 mm and hazy in congenital glaucoma), cataracts (absent red retinal reflex), ears (shape, size, low-set?), nasal airway (check patency), mouth (check hard and soft palate intact), neck (any soft tissue swellings, clavicles intact?).

2. Chest. Shape and breathing pattern and effort. Check heart sounds (murmurs?).

3. Abdomen and genitalia. Note liver, spleen and kidney size, and number of cord vessels. Feel femoral pulses. Check anus is patent and genitalia are normal with descended testes. If genitalia are ambiguous say so and do not assign a sex!

4. Spine and limbs. Check spine is straight with no dimples and hairy patches. Check upper and lower limbs are of normal shape, have full range of movements and are symmetrical with normal palmar creases. Check hips have full range of movements and do not dislocate.

5. *Activity and behaviour.* Note muscle tone and activity (symmetrical movements) with appropriate reflexes (grasp, suck, Moro, step) and normal cry. Asymmetrical movements may suggest birth injury-related palsies (e.g. Erb's palsy) or a fracture.

6. *Special notes.* Infants should pass meconium within 48 hours. Failure to do so suggests bowel obstruction (vomiting, abdominal distension) or anorectal anomalies (e.g. imperforate anus). Passing a small finger per rectum may encourage passage of a meconium plug followed by meconium. Consider the possibility of Hirschsprung's disease or CF in infants with a meconium plug and delayed passage of meconium (>48 hours). Serum immunoreactive trypsin level, stool tryptic activity or a sweat test may be required in the follow-up period. Urine should also be passed within 48 hours of birth or look for evidence of urinary obstructions (enlarged bladder, urethral valves) or reduced urine production (e.g. renal agenesis, renal vein thrombosis, acute tubular necrosis).

Ascertain that the infant has received vitamin K prophylaxis. BCG vaccination should be given where appropriate (e.g. family history of tuberculosis) and infants born to hepatitis B-positive mothers should receive hepatitis B vaccine (0.5 ml i.m. at birth and repeated at age 1 and 6 months). Infants whose mothers are e-antigen positive and e-antibody negative should also receive human anti-hepatitis B immunoglobulin (200 IU by deep i.m. injection) within 48 hours of birth to confer immediate protection until the vaccine is effective. This should be followed by a full course of vaccinations and a review at 1 year to assess the serological evidence of immunity.

Discharge examination

This is similar to the initial examination with some additional points being noted.

- Feeding (breast or bottle) should be established.
- Any parental concerns should be addressed and any questions answered.
- Marked jaundice should be investigated and discharge allowed only if the serum bilirubin is falling or stable.
- Pending investigations should be discussed fully and details of follow-up arrangements finalized.
- Complete and sign (legibly) the discharge record with copies being forwarded to all appropriate personnel in the community.

Further reading

Johnson PB. *The Newborn Child*, 8th edn. Edinburgh: Churchill Livingstone, 1998.
Jones DA. *Hip Screening in the Newborn*. London: Butterworth-Heinemann, 1998.
O'Doherty N. *Atlas of the Newborn*, 2nd edn. Lancaster: M.T.P. Press, 1985.
Roberton NRC. *A Manual of Normal Neonatal Care*, 2nd edn. London: Edward Arnold, 1996.
Thomas R, Harvey D. *Neonatology: Colour Guide*, 2nd edn. Edinburgh: Churchill Livingstone, 1997.

Related topics of interest

Assessment of gestational age (p. 19)
Birth injuries (p. 21)
Congenital malformations and birth defects (p. 70)
Hepatitis B (p. 105)
Immunization (p. 132)
Jaundice (p. 173)
Prenatal diagnosis (p. 253)

PREGNANCY COMPLICATIONS AND FETAL HEALTH

As maternal health is intricately linked with that of the fetus, serious complications of pregnancy invariably also affect the fetus. A selection of some of the common complications of pregnancy and their attendant effects on the fetus are presented.

Antepartum haemorrhage (APH) This constitutes bleeding from the genital tract from 28 weeks gestation up to delivery of the fetus. APH can have serious consequences for both the mother and fetus. It is associated with a marked increase in perinatal mortality and is also a significant cause of maternal mortality. The two main causes are placenta praevia and placental abruption. The latter is more serious and is associated with a twofold increase in mortality.

1. *Placental abruption.* This is due to placental separation with attendant maternal and fetal blood loss (often concealed) and fetal compromise.

(a) Maternal clinical features
- Painful bleeding from the genital tract.
- Blood loss out of proportion to mother's condition, progressing to shock.
- Uterus tense, tender, irritable and at times hard.
- Fetal parts and heart rate difficult to ascertain.

(b) Fetal risks
- Fetal blood loss and asphyxia.
- Preterm delivery (RDS).
- Intrauterine death.

(c) Management
- Immediate maternal resuscitation with fresh blood transfusion.
- Coagulation defects rectified.
- Fetal viability ascertained ultrasonically.
- If fetus is dead, labour induced (after resuscitating mother), aiming for vaginal delivery.

2. *Placenta praevia.* The placenta encroaches upon the lower uterine segment and may partially or completely cover the cervix.

(a) Maternal clinical features
- Recurrent painless bleeding from the genital tract.
- Maternal condition is proportional to blood lost.

(b) Fetal risks
- Preterm delivery (RDS).

(c) Management
- Position of placenta ascertained ultrasonically.
- Emergency delivery by Caesarian section for severe bleeding.
- Expectant management aiming to prolong pregnancy to 37–38 weeks for minor haemorrhages.
- Elective Caesarian section at 37–38 weeks for all but minor degrees of placenta praevia.

Pre-eclampsia

Also called pregnancy-induced hypertension, pre-eclampsia (PE) is characterized by hypertension and proteinuria during pregnancy (mostly third trimester) and immediate puerperium. Severe PE consists of hypertension and proteinuria (>0.25 g/l) and mild PE, hypertension without proteinuria. With an incidence of up to 1 in 10 pregnancies, PE and related hypertensive disorders are still a significant cause of maternal morbidity and death. PE may rapidly progress through the pre-eclampsia state to eclampsia which is characterized by seizures. PE may also develop into a serious hypertensive disorder with elevated liver enzymes, epigastric pain and low platelets (HELLP syndrome).

1. *Maternal clinical features*
- Hypertension (blood pressure (BP) $\geq$140/90) – mild PE.
- Hypertension with proteinuria – severe PE.
- Agitation, confusion, visual disturbance, epigastric pain, nausea and vomiting with brisk reflexes – PE state.
- Seizures (with above) – eclampsia state.

2. *Fetal risks*
- Acute or chronic placental insufficiency with IUGR.
- Placental abruption and fetal asphyxia and intrauterine death.
- Preterm delivery.

3. *Management*
- Bed rest in hospital.
- Prevention of disease progression to the most severe spectrum.
- Antihypertensive therapy (methyldopa, hydralazine, β-blockers).
- Anticonvulsant therapy (diazepam, chlormethiazole, magnesium sulphate).
- For severe disease, prompt delivery by Caesarean section is often necessary.

Preterm rupture of membranes (PROM)

Before 34 weeks, management of PROM is conservative. Tocolytics (betamimetics) may be used temporarily, affording the opportunity to induce pulmonary maturity by corticosteroids.

1. *Fetal risks*
- Preterm delivery.
- Pulmonary hypoplasia with prolonged and early PROM.
- Limb contractures.
- Idiopathic RDS.
- Amnionitis and fetal infection.

2. *Management.* Maternal intrapartum antibiotics following high vaginal and cervical swabs.

Preterm labour and birth

This constitutes labour and birth before 37 weeks gestation. Prematurity is the single largest contributor to the early neonatal mortality rate.

1. *Aetiology and risk factors*
- Preterm rupture of membranes.
- Antepartum haemorrhage.
- Incompetent cervix.
- PE and related disorders.
- Poor socioeconomic background.
- Multiple pregnancy.
- Polyhydramnios.
- Maternal infection (e.g. urinary tract infection (UTI)).

2. *Management*
- Maternal ultrasound scan to assess fetal maturity, growth, presentation and exclude obvious anomalies.
- Tocolysis if labour not advanced (cervix <4 cm) and gestation <34 weeks.
- Corticosteroids to reduce incidence of RDS (and also IVH and NEC). Betamethasone 4 mg i.m. 8-hourly for 48 hours or dexamethasone 12 mg i.m. 12-hourly for 48 hours (repeated weekly should pregnancy continue beyond 7 days).

Prolonged pregnancy

Prolonged pregnancy (beyond 42 weeks gestation) carries risks for both mother and fetus.

1. *Fetal risks*
- Difficult and prolonged labour.
- Chronic fetal malnutrition.
- Fetal distress and meconium aspiration.
- Birth asphyxia.
- Unexpected intrauterine death.
- Perinatal mortality after 42 weeks gestation is twice that at 38–42 weeks gestation.

2. *Management*
- Regular and careful assessment of fetal wellbeing.
- Induction of labour.

Polyhydramnios

In polyhydramnios, the amniotic fluid volume exceeds 2000 ml. The majority of mild polyhydramnios has no obvious cause, whereas most severe polyhydramnios (amniotic fluid index >24 cm or deepest pool ≥15 cm) has an identifiable cause. Polyhydramnios may be secondary to maternal factors (especially diabetes) or fetal factors (e.g. oesophageal atresia, multiple pregnancy, anencephaly, high intestinal obstruction, hydrops fetalis, Down's syndrome, diaphragmatic hernia, neuromuscular disorders or Beckwith–Weidemann syndrome). Major malformations may be found in up to 40% of the infants, with 5% having chromosomal anomalies.

1. Maternal clinical features
- Maternal discomfort.
- Uterine size appears large for dates.

2. Fetal risks
- Preterm rupture of membranes.
- Preterm labour.
- Abruption (following amnioreduction).
- Twin–twin transfusion (in twin pregnancy).

3. Management
- Mothers should have a glucose tolerance test and detailed fetal scan.
- In severe polyhydramnios, fetal karyotyping may be required.
- Amnioreduction to relieve maternal discomfort (large volume taps may precipitate an abruption).
- Maternal indomethacin (75–200 mg/day) which reduces fetal urine production may be beneficial.
- Look for possible anomalies in the infant following birth.

Oligohydramnios

Mid-trimester oligohydramnios is associated with increased mortality from premature rupture of membranes (pulmonary hypoplasia), urinary tract malformations (e.g. renal agenesis) and IUGR. Amnioinfusion of a warmed physiological solution permits better imaging of the fetus and confirms premature rupture of membranes. Abnormal karyotypes are present in 5–10%.

1. Fetal risks
- Fetal death.
- Pulmonary hypoplasia.
- Limb contractures.

2. Management
- Obtain detailed fetal scans.
- Obtain fetal karyotype where indicated.
- Perform an ultrasound examination of newborn infant's renal tract.

Gestational diabetes

This is defined as impaired glucose tolerance during pregnancy which reverts to normal after the puerperium. It is associated with an increased incidence of fetal malformations and perinatal complications.

1. Maternal clinical features
- Polyhydramnios.
- Hyperglycaemia and glycosuria.
- Delivery complications.

2. Fetal risks
- Diabetic embryopathy (e.g. caudal regression, anencephaly, meningocele, vertebral dysplasia, congenital heart disease, small left colon).
- Hypertrophic cardiomyopathy.
- Polycythaemia.
- Sudden fetal demise.

3. Perinatal risks
- Birth injury and asphyxia (large size).
- RDS (relative surfactant deficiency).
- Hypoglycaemia.
- Hypocalcaemia.
- Feeding difficulties (immature sucking and swallowing).
- Jaundice.
- Renal vein thrombosis.

4. Management of the fetus/infant
- Induction of labour at 38 weeks gestation.
- Operative delivery if fetus is large.
- Early feeding (orally or intravenously with 10–15% dextrose).
- Blood glucose monitoring after birth for 24–48 hours till blood sugars consistently ≥4 mmol/l.
- Respiratory distress, jaundice and polycythaemia should be managed expectantly.
- Commence antibiotics (following cultures) if respiratory distress persists.
- Where appropriate, exclude other malformations (e.g. vertebral or cardiac) by appropriate radiographs and echocardiography.

Further reading

Chalmers I, Enkin M, Keirse MJC (eds). *Effective Care in Pregnancy and Childbirth, Volume 1 – Pregnancy*. Oxford: Oxford University Press, 1992.
Creasy R, Resnik R (eds). *Maternal–Fetal Medicine: Principles and Practice*, 3rd edn. Philadelphia: W.B. Saunders, 1994.

Fanaroff AA, Martin RJ (eds). *Neonatal–Perinatal Medicine: Diseases of the Fetus and Neonate*, 6th edn. St. Louis: Mosby, 1997.

Whitfield CR (ed). *Dewhurst's Textbook of Obstetrics and Gynaecology for Postgraduates*, 5th edn. Oxford: Blackwell Science, 1995.

Related topics of interest

Childbirth complications and fetal outcome (p. 46)
Congenital malformations and birth defects (p. 70)
Intrauterine growth restriction (p. 165)
Multiple pregnancy (p. 192)

PRENATAL DIAGNOSIS

The last decade has witnessed many significant advances in prenatal diagnosis. Improvements in ultrasound imaging techniques, the application of biochemical and DNA analysis and karyotyping to samples of fetal tissue obtained by chorion villus sampling (CVS), amniocentesis and fetal blood sampling have all greatly extended the scope of prenatal diagnosis to a host of structural malformations, chromosomal abnormalities, specific gene defects and several metabolic disorders.

Structural malformations In the UK, routine scans are performed at 18–19 weeks gestation to screen for congenital malformations. Screening detects 55% of the major and 35% of minor malformations. The most commonly detected malformations are listed below on a systems basis:

1. CNS
- Anencephaly.
- Open spina bifida.
- Hydrocephalus.
- Hydranencephaly.
- Holoprosencephaly.
- Encephalocele.
- Dandy–Walker malformation.
- Intracranial cysts.
- Haemorrhage.
- Agenesis of the corpus callosum.

2. Respiratory system
- Congenital diaphragmatic hernia.
- Congenital cystic adenomatoid malformation of the lung.
- Lung sequestration.
- Mediastinal tumours.

3. Gastrointestinal system
- Duodenal atresia (with 'double bubble', suggests trisomy 21).
- Bowel perforations with ascites and gut hyperechogenicity.
- Omphalocele (high incidence of cardiac and chromosomal abnormalities).
- Gastroschisis.

4. Genitourinary system. The commonest congenital anomalies detected on ultrasound (20–30% of all). Lesions vary from renal agenesis, hydronephrotic kidneys, multicystic kidneys and other features of an obstructive uropathy (e.g. thick walled bladder and dilated upper urethra in posterior urethral valves).

5. Musculoskeletal system. Over 100 skeletal dysplasias are now diagnosable prenatally from the detection of abnormal skeletal shape (e.g. camptomelic and thanatophoric dysplasia) or bone mineralization (e.g. hypophosphatasia and achondrogenesis) while fractures and callus formation may be seen in osteogenesis imperfecta (types II–IV). Akinesia and severe contractures may be seen in neuromuscular disorders such as arthrogryposis multiplex congenita.

6. Miscellaneous anomalies. Cleft lip (and palate) may be readily detected along with other soft tissue anomalies, e.g. hydrops and cystic hygromas.

Invasive diagnostic techniques

1. Amniocentesis. Usually performed in the second trimester (at 15–16 weeks) under ultrasound guidance. The procedure has a 1% risk of spontaneous abortion. Up to 20 ml of amniotic fluid is aspirated and cells from this are cultured (2–4 weeks) then subjected to cytogenetic, DNA or enzymatic analysis. The main disadvantage is the slow turnaround time, necessitating terminations at 20 weeks. Amniocentesis may also be used for amnioinfusion (oligohydramnios) and amniotic fluid drainage (polyhydramnios). This procedure is associated with pulmonary hypoplasia.

2. Chorionic villus sampling. This has been in use over the last 12 years with great success. This is performed earlier (8–12 weeks gestation) and involves passing a catheter transcervically into the chorion frondosum and obtaining chorionic tissue by suction. More recently CVS has been performed using a 2 mm diameter transcervical CVS forceps. The forceps are guided through the cervical canal under ultrasound guidance. Sampling is achieved by opening the forceps and closing whilst advancing the forceps further into the placenta and then withdrawing. CVS can also be performed transabdominally with a double-needle technique. However, the reports of fetal limb reduction defects following CVS before 10 weeks gestation have resulted in restriction of this procedure before 10 weeks gestation. The procedure-related loss is 2–3% in younger women but ~6% in older women. Rapid cytogenetic analysis can be made directly on the obtained tissue preparations or following 12–24-hour cell cultures. Enzyme assays for inborn errors of metabolism can be performed directly on sampled chorionic tissues. Results are available sooner than after amniocentesis, allowing for an easier first trimester termination where indicated. Occasionally, however, a discrepancy may exist between chorionic and fetal karyotype, making later amniocentesis necessary.

3. Fetal blood sampling. FBS of the umbilical vein close to its placental insertion under direct ultrasonic guidance is the commonest approach. Alternatively, blood may be sampled from the intrahepatic portion of the fetal umbilical vein. The procedure is performed after 17 weeks gestation with a procedure-related loss of approximately 1%. This procedure can be used for both diagnostic purposes (e.g. haemoglobinopathies, coagulopathies, immunodeficiency syndromes, cytogenetic and DNA studies, inborn errors of metabolism) and for monitoring fetal wellbeing or fetal therapy (e.g. monitoring acid–base status, intrauterine infection, red cell alloimmunization, immune thrombocytopenia, blood or platelet transfusion).

4. In vitro fertilization and pre-implantation diagnosis. It is now also possible to perform cytogenetic and DNA analyses from single cells obtained from human embryos as early as the eight-cell stage. The embryos can be sexed and several genetic disorders excluded before implantation.

Further reading

Handyside AH, Pattinson JK, Penketh RJA, Delhanty JD, Winston RML, Tuddenham EDG. Biopsy of human pre-implantation embryos and sexing by DNA amplification. *Lancet*, 1989; **i**: 347–9.

Jackson L. *CVS Latest News*, 1990, No 29.

Keeling JW (ed). *Fetal and Neonatal Pathology*. London: Springer-Verlag, 1987.

Nicolaides KH, Economides DL. Cordocentesis of small-for-gestational-age fetuses. In: Chamberlain GVP (ed). *Modern Antenatal Care of the Fetus*. Oxford: Blackwell Scientific Publications, 1990; 127–49.

Saling E (ed). *Perinatology (Nestlé Nutrition Workshop Series, Volume 26)*. New York: Raven Press, 1990.

Whittle MJ, Connor JM (eds). *Prenatal Diagnosis in Obstetric Practice*, 2nd edn. Oxford: Blackwell Science, 1995.

Related topics of interest

PULMONARY AIR LEAKS

Pulmonary air leaks occur when there is high transpulmonary pressure, alveolar overdistension and finally alveolar rupture. Following alveolar rupture, gas may track along the perivascular spaces into the pleura (pneumothorax), the interstitium (pulmonary interstitial emphysema (PIE)), the mediastinum (pneumomediastium), the pericardium (pneumopericardium) or through the diaphragmatic foramina into the peritoneum (pneumoperitoneum).

Pneumothorax

This is the commonest form of air leak occurring in up to 1% of all newborns though only 0.1% may be symptomatic. Pneumothoraces can occur spontaneously at birth or during resuscitation, but thereafter prevalence is increased in the presence of pulmonary disease (e.g. MAS or RDS) and assisted ventilation. Pneumothoraces are correlated with high mean and peak inspiratory pressures, long inspiratory times and breathing out of phase with the ventilator.

1. Clinical features. Large tension pneumothoraces produce sudden deterioration in the infant's condition with pallor, hypotension, bradycardia and hypoxemia. Air entry is reduced on the affected side and the mediastinum shifted away from the affected side. Pneumothoraces are bilateral in 15–20% and if unilateral, it is more commonly on the right. Pneumothoraces predispose infants to IVHs.

2. Management. Transillumination of the chest with a fibre-optic light shows increased transillumination on the affected side (but PIE may give similar appearance). Confirm by chest X-ray. In an emergency, needling both sides of the chest may produce immediate improvement. Pneumothoraces should be drained in symptomatic infants or infants receiving assisted ventilation. A chest drain (size 10–14FG) should be inserted under local anaesthesia and the adequacy of drainage and position of the drain checked by X-ray. Better drainage is often achieved if the drain is aimed anteriorly with the drain lying retrosternally. The risk of developing a pneumothorax may be reduced by using the lowest effective pressures, employing relatively fast ventilator rates with short inspiratory times and sedating active babies.

Pulmonary interstitial emphysema

PIE is primarily a disorder of preterm infants with RDS requiring high-pressure ventilation. Small airways rupture with air dissecting into the interstitium and being trapped within the perivascular sheaths of the lung. This reduces pulmonary perfusion producing a ventilation–perfusion mismatch, hypoxaemia and hypercapnia. It becomes progressively more prevalent with decreasing birthweight.

1. Clinical features. PIE commonly presents with worsening gas exchange in a ventilated infant. The X-ray is diagnostic with unilateral or bilateral cystic radiolucencies and hyperinflation. The appearances on transillumination may resemble a large pneumothorax.

2. Management. Minimize ventilation pressures and reduce PEEP to maintain satisfactory gases (allow higher $PaCO_2$ if pH is ≥ 7.25). Use heavy sedation or paralysis and employ fast ventilator rates (short inspiratory times) and remove PEEP. High-frequency oscillatory ventilation may be particularly beneficial. With unilateral PIE, place the infant on his/her side with the hyperinflated lung dependent. Selective bronchial intubation of the non-affected lung may also be useful, especially if the left lung is affected. Alternatively, for localized disease, large cysts may be artificially punctured and a chest drain left *in situ* to drain the pneumothorax.

Pneumomediastinum

With an incidence of approximately 1 in 400, this is often seen in the presence of other air leaks in preterm ventilated infants, though if isolated it is usually asymptomatic. Diagnosis is made on the chest X-ray which shows air around the cardiac silhouette and on lateral views a hyperlucent area behind the sternum. No therapy is required, drainage is usually ineffective.

Pneumopericardium

This may arise from gas tracking from the mediastinum into the pericardial sac in a sick ventilated preterm infant, producing cardiac tamponade. There is rapid clinical deterioration with bradycardia, hypotension, cyanosis and muffled heart sounds. Mortality is high. This may mimic a pneumothorax but the chest X-ray is diagnostic, with gas completely surrounding the heart. Presence of gas beneath the heart differentiates this from a pneumomediastinum, where gas cannot track beneath the heart due to the attachment of the mediastinal pleura to the diaphragm. Small asymptomatic pneumopericardia may be observed only, but if symptomatic, urgent pericardial taps should be performed (subxiphoid approach) with continuous monitoring of the cardiovascular status.

Pneumoperitoneum

This most commonly arises from perforation of the gut (mainly NEC) but may also arise from within the chest (of ventilated infants), with the gas from air leaks tracking down diaphragmatic foramina into the peritoneum. A history of gastrointestinal disease or an abnormal gas pattern on abdominal X-ray suggests a surgical pneumoperitoneum rather than a transdiaphragmatic air leak. Marked abdominal distension may be drained by a needle tap or a drain left *in situ*.

Further reading

Halahakoon CN, Halliday HL. Other acute lung disorders. In: Yu VYH (ed). *Bailliere's Clinical Paediatrics, Vol. 3/No. 1, Pulmonary Problems in the Perinatal Period and their Sequelae.* London: Baillière Tindall, 1995; 87–114.

Halliday HL. Other acute lung disorders. In: Sinclair JC, Bracken MB (eds). *Effective Care of the Newborn Infant.* Oxford: Oxford University Press, 1992; 359–84.

Rennie JM, Robertson NRC (eds). *Textbook of Neonatology,* 3rd edn. Edinburgh: Churchill Livingstone, 1998.

Spitzer AR (ed). *Intensive Care of the Fetus and Neonate.* St. Louis: C.V. Mosby, 1996.

Taeusch HW, Ballard RA (eds). *Avery's Diseases of the Newborn,* 7th edn. Philadelphia: W.B. Saunders, 1998.

Related topics of interest

Bronchopulmonary dysplasia (p. 38)
Complications of mechanical ventilation (p. 54)
Congenital diaphragmatic hernia (p. 57)
Mechanical ventilation (p. 185)
Meconium aspiration syndrome (p. 189)
Pulmonary hypoplasia (p. 261)
Respiratory distress syndrome (p. 278)

PULMONARY HAEMORRHAGE

Massive pulmonary haemorrhage represents one end of a continuum of disorders characterized by pulmonary oedema. In the initial stages, rising capillary pressure leads to a rise in interstitial fluid, resulting in fluid loss into the alveoli and finally capillary haemorrhage. A sudden onset and a high mortality are characteristic. This is now largely a disorder of preterm infants ventilated for severe RDS and often with a large PDA causing failure with reported incidences of 1–12 per 1000 live births. Between 2 and 5% of babies with RDS develop pulmonary haemorrhage. It is also seen in term infants particularly in association with severe birth asphyxia, hypothermia, severe rhesus haemolytic disease, hydrops, left heart failure, fluid overload, sepsis, coagulation disorder, maternal diabetes, hypoglycaemia and small-for-gestational-age infants. As the haemorrhagic fluid is protein rich, it inactivates surfactant, worsening gas exchange. This haemorrhagic fluid has a haematocrit of 10%. Although synthetic surfactant therapy for RDS may increase the incidence of *clinical* pulmonary haemorrhage, *pathologically* diagnosed (at autopsy) pulmonary haemorrhage is not increased. Risk factors for pulmonary haemorrhage in surfactant-treated infants include birthweight $<700\,g$, male sex, presence of a PDA, and prophylactic use of synthetic rather than natural surfactant.

Clinical features

Commonly there is a sudden deterioration accompanied by the appearance of large amounts of pink/red frothy fluid or frank blood from the infant's oropharynx, or endotracheal tube if already intubated. There may be bleeding from other sites. The infant may be pale, hypotensive, bradycardic, cyanosed, apnoeic or with gasping respirations and shocked. If in heart failure, the infant is tachycardic with an accompanying murmur (particularly with a PDA) and hepatosplenomegaly. There are widespread crepitations with reduced air entry. In surfactant-treated infants, blood-stained secretions may be the only sign.

Investigations

- FBC. Haemoglobin commonly below $10\,g/dl$.
- Clotting screen. May be normal but commonly becomes deranged following a massive pulmonary haemorrhage.
- Radiology. Chest X-ray shows a 'white-out', or may be less striking resembling RDS and there may be cardiomegaly.
- Blood gases. Hypoxia and hypercarbia with a combined respiratory and metabolic acidosis are characteristic.
- Bacteriology. Perform an infection screen (without an LP).

Management

- Urgent resuscitation is required to prevent sudden death. Endotracheal intubation for mechanical ventilation and simultaneous volume expansion with blood or plasma is a prerequisite. Also correct any underlying disorder(s). A high PEEP ($\geq 6\,cmH_2O$) and long inspiratory time ($\geq 0.5\,s$) may be beneficial.
- Transfuse FFP (10–$15\,ml/kg$) and/or cryoprecipitate as indicated, with additional vitamin K to improve coagulation.

- Restrict fluids to 60–90 ml/kg/day when in congestive heart failure, adding diuretics (frusemide 1.5 mg/kg bd) when bleeding has stopped.
- Commence broad-spectrum antibiotics following cultures.
- Correct acidosis with bicarbonate.
- Frequent suctioning (up to several times in the hour) may be required in the initial stages to prevent the endotracheal tube blocking. The suction catheter should be measured so as only to protrude ~0.5 cm past the endotracheal tube tip to avoid provoking fresh bleeding during suctioning.
- Maintain the blood pressure with infusions of colloid, blood or inotropes.
- Additional surfactant therapy when pulmonary haemorrhage has occurred after the first dose may be beneficial (though controversial!).

Prevention

- Avoid acidosis.
- Avoid asphyxia.
- Avoid hypothermia.
- Avoid hypoglycaemia.
- Avoid over-treating with surfactant.
- Correct coagulation defects.
- Suction intubated infants with care.
- Be careful to apply the above measures to growth-restricted infants as they may be particularly at risk.

Further reading

Greenough A, Morley CJ, Roberton NRC. Acute respiratory disease in the newborn. In: Roberton NRC (ed). *Textbook of Neonatology*, 2nd edn. Edinburgh: Churchill Livingstone, 1992; 385–504.

Halahakoon CN, Halliday HL. Other acute lung disorders. In: Yu VYH (ed). *Bailliere's Clinical Paediatrics, Vol. 3/No. 1, Pulmonary Problems in the Perinatal Period and their Sequelae*. London: Baillière Tindall, 1995; 87–114.

Raju TNK, Langenberg P. Pulmonary haemorrhage and exogenous surfactant therapy: a meta-analysis. *Journal of Pediatrics*, 1993; **123**: 603–10.

Related topics of interest

Acute collapse (p. 6)
Patent ductus arteriosus (p. 230)
Respiratory distress (p. 275)
Shock (p. 302)
Surfactant replacement therapy (p. 309)

PULMONARY HYPOPLASIA

This may be defined as incomplete development of the lung resulting in a reduced lung weight and distending volume. There is an associated reduction in the number of airway divisions, alveoli, arteries and veins. The true incidence of pulmonary hypoplasia is not known as it is commonly under-reported and the diagnosis frequently masked by other pulmonary disorders.

Primary pulmonary hypoplasia

This occurs in the absence of any other diseases or conditions that would impair lung development, such as oligohydramnios or absent renal function. The reported incidence is low with less than 1% of admissions to a neonatal unit being affected.

Secondary pulmonary hypoplasia

This may be 10 times more common than primary pulmonary hypoplasia and may be present in 10–15% of early neonatal deaths.

Aetiology	Several mechanisms have been postulated based on clinical observations and animal experiments. A reduction in amniotic fluid volume (e.g. chronic amniotic fluid leak before 26 weeks gestation, Potter's syndrome, or even mid-trimester amniocentesis) commonly leads to pulmonary hypoplasia. It has been postulated that prolonged thoracic compression, reduced fetal breathing movements and a reduced intrathoracic lung fluid pressure may all be mechanistically related to pulmonary hypoplasia. Reduced intrathoracic space has been shown experimentally to reduce lung development which is in accord with clinical observations (e.g. in congenital diaphragmatic hernia, pleural effusions, thoracic tumours and asphyxiating thoracic dystrophy). Drug administration to pregnant mothers, especially angiotensin converting enzyme (ACE) inhibitors, has also been associated with pulmonary hypoplasia.
Clinical features	*1. Unilateral pulmonary hypoplasia.* This is usually asymptomatic and may be a chance finding on the chest radiograph. At times, however, there may be mediastinal shift to the hypoplastic side which may be evident clinically. Associated congenital malformations (cardiac, renal, skeletal or gastrointestinal) may be the presenting complaint and greatly increase the morbidity.
	2. Bilateral pulmonary hypoplasia. Presentation is determined by severity of the disorder. The mildly affected may have persistent tachypnoea and a chest X-ray showing a bell-shaped chest with well inflated but small lungs.

With severe pulmonary hypoplasia, resuscitation may be difficult or impossible with high inflation pressures (>30cmH$_2$O), 100% O$_2$ and persisting carbon dioxide retention.

Diagnosis

- High-pressure ventilation with persisting CO$_2$ retention (as above).
- Lung function tests show a reduced functional residual capacity (FRC) – less than 60% of expected value, i.e. 16 ml/kg bodyweight.

Management

1. Prenatal. Premature rupture of membranes before 34 weeks is associated with poor outcome. Elective delivery at 34 weeks may be recommended. Intrathoracic space occupying lesions such as cysts or effusions should be drained *in utero* to prevent prolonged lung compression.

2. Postnatal. Severe pulmonary hypoplasia may be incompatible with life. Less severe pulmonary hypoplasia may best be ventilated on high rates and low mean airway pressures. Persistent pulmonary hypertension of the newborn (PPHN) may be a complicating factor, especially when there is associated lung disease (e.g. RDS, sepsis – especially group B streptococcus or meconium aspiration). High frequency oscillation and inhaled nitric oxide therapy may be beneficial. Associated congenital anomalies (e.g. congenital diaphragmatic hernia) may adversely affect the outcome. ECMO is contraindicated in severe pulmonary hypoplasia. Associated postural and limb deformities respond to physiotherapy and orthopaedic interventions.

Differential diagnosis

The following conditions may co-exist and should be considered as alternative diagnoses.

- Severe RDS.
- Group B streptococcus pneumonia.
- Primary PPHN.
- Neuromuscular disorders (e.g. myotonic dystrophy).

Prognosis

- Mortality is high especially in primary pulmonary hypoplasia (over 50%).
- Associated anomalies (e.g. renal agenesis or congenital diaphragmatic hernia) increase mortality.
- Pneumothorax and PIE followed by chronic lung disease and prolonged oxygen-dependency are likely to develop in affected preterm infants.
- Long-term lung function may recover completely during the first few years of life or remain abnormal depending on the original diagnosis.

Further reading

Chernick V, Boat TF (eds). *Kendig's Disorders of the Respiratory Tract in Children*, 6th edn. Philadelphia: W.B. Saunders, 1997.

Dinwiddie R. *The Diagnosis and Management of Paediatric Respiratory Disease,* 2nd edn. Edinburgh: Churchill Livingstone, 1997.

Halliday HL. Other acute lung disorders. In: Sinclair JC, Bracken MB (eds). *Effective Care of the Newborn Infant*. Oxford: Oxford University Press, 1992; 359–84.

Keeling JW (ed). *Fetal and Neonatal Pathology*. London: Springer-Verlag, 1987.

Milner AD, Fox G. Congenital abnormalities of the respiratory system. In: Yu VYH (ed). *Bailliere's Clinical Paediatrics, Vol. 3/No. 1, Pulmonary Problems in the Perinatal Period and their Sequelae*. London: Baillière Tindall, 1995; 171–202.

Spitzer AR (ed). *Intensive Care of the Fetus and Neonate*. St. Louis: C.V. Mosby, 1996.

Swischuk LDE. Primary pulmonary hypoplasia in the neonate. *Journal of Pediatrics*, 1979; **95:** 573–8.

Wigglesworth JS. Perinatal Pathology, 2nd edn. London: W.B. Saunders, 1996.

Related topics of interest

Complications of mechanical ventilation (p. 54)
Congenital diaphragmatic hernia (p. 57)
Persistent pulmonary hypertension of the newborn (p. 237)
Respiratory distress (p. 275)
Resuscitation (p. 282)

RENAL AND URINARY TRACT DISORDERS – NEPHROLOGY

Nephrons develop from the fifth week of intrauterine life and they are fully formed though not fully functional by 36 weeks gestation. The infant glomerulus is a third of the size of the adult glomerulus, and although the tubules are functioning by 9 weeks, they are short and immature even at term. Consequently the newborn kidney is functionally immature. The GFR and renal blood flow are low in the newborn period. After birth, GFR increases as a function of post-conceptional age rather than postnatal age. As tubular function is immature, urine-concentrating ability is limited, as is the ability to excrete a water load. Unlike term infants, preterm infants are unable to conserve sodium. The newborn kidney is therefore vulnerable to several perinatal factors which can adversely affect renal function.

Presentation of renal and urinary tract disorders

Family history
- History of an inherited renal disorder (e.g. polycystic kidney disease – autosomal recessive and dominant), Alport's syndrome (X-linked).
- History of metabolic disorder (autosomal recessive) with renal manifestation (e.g. galactosaemia, cystinosis, tyrosinosis).
- History of vesico-ureteric reflux (4% risk of reflux in first degree relatives of index patient, but 50% risk if scarring present in index case).

Antenatal history
- Abnormal kidneys on fetal anomaly scan at 17–20 weeks or later (e.g. dilated collecting system, multicystic kidney, renal agenesis).
- Oligohydramnios (renal agenesis, dysplasia, obstructed urinary tract and Potter's syndrome).
- Elevated AFP in amniotic fluid.

Perinatal history
- Placental weight >25% of birthweight congenital nephrotic syndrome, Finnish type, autosomal recessive, associated with prematurity).
- Single umbilical artery (urinary tract anomalies in ≤3%).
- Delayed micturition (99% of healthy infants urinate by 48 hours) – suggests renal under-perfusion (asphyxia, hypotension, congenital nephritis, urinary tract obstruction, renal agenesis, tubular or cortical necrosis).
- Oliguria (urinary output <20 ml/kg/day or <1 ml/kg/hour) – suggests dehydration or any of the above factors.
- Haematuria (1 in 10 newborns have transient haematuria) – distinguish from haemoglobinuria or myoglobinuria; causes include cortical and medullary necrosis, acute renal failure, asphyxia, infection.

- Proteinuria (transient proteinuria up to 45 mg/day is common) – causes include renal vein thrombosis, infection, idiopathic familial congenital nephrotic syndrome.
- Leucocyturia (>3 white blood cells (WBCs) per high power field is abnormal in a centrifuged urine sample) – suggests urinary tract infection, nephritis.
- Oedema (excessive water and salt intake, congenital nephrotic syndrome, obstructive uropathy, acute renal failure).
- Acidosis (metabolic acidosis with normal anion gap suggests renal tubular acidosis).
- Urinary tract infection (>10^5 organisms from two clean catch samples or any growth from a suprapubic aspiration sample).
- Hypertension – mainly renovascular causes, especially renal artery thrombosis.

Specific disorders

Acute renal failure

Assume an infant is in renal failure if urine output is <1 ml/kg/hour for 24 hours and/or creatinine is >88 μmol/l or urea is >7 mmol/l. This occurs in up to 1 in 10 sick newborns.

1. Prerenal failure. This is commonly due to renal under-perfusion from:
(a) Hypovolaemia
- Maternal antepartum haemorrhage.
- Fetal/neonatal haemorrhage.
- Inadequate fluid intake or increased losses (polyuria, insensible loss or gastrointestinal loss).
(b) Normovolaemia
- Asphyxia.
- Congestive cardiac failure.
- Septic shock.

2. Intrinsic renal failure. The main causes are shock and asphyxia.

- Acute tubular, medullary or cortical necrosis.
- Arterial or venous thrombosis.
- Congenital renal anomalies (e.g. agenesis, polycystic kidneys).
- Congenital infection (e.g. toxoplasmosis or syphilis) and DIC.
- Uncorrected prerenal failure.

3. Post-renal failure.
- Ureterocele.

- Pelvi-ureteric or vesico-ureteric junction obstruction.
- Urethral obstruction – (posterior urethral valves, urethral stricture, urethral diverticulum, tumours, neurogenic bladder).

Clinical features of renal failure

- Hyperkalaemia (major cause of death from cardiac toxicity).
- Hyponatraemia (dilutional).
- Hypertension (from volume overload).
- Metabolic acidosis (inability to excrete acids).
- Hyperphosphataemia and hypocalcaemia.
- Sepsis (a major cause of death).

Investigations

1. *Blood*
- U&E and creatinine.
- Glucose.
- Calcium and magnesium.
- Albumin.
- Acid–base status.
- FBC and film.
- Blood culture (full septic screen if sepsis suspected).
- Coagulation studies.

2. *Urine*
- Microscopy (casts).
- Dipstick.
- Culture.
- Urea and creatinine.
- Electrolytes.
- Osmolarity.

3. *Others*
- Renal ultrasound scan.
- Weigh infant.
- Check blood pressure.

Management

Establish the diagnosis of renal failure and differentiate between the three main causes of renal failure, as their management differs. Confirm obstructive uropathy on ultrasound examination and refer to a urologist. Distinguishing pre-renal from intrinsic renal failure may be difficult, but the following indices may be helpful. In *pre-renal failure*, urine/plasma osmolarity is >2 (<1 intrinsic failure), urine sodium <10 mmol/l (>40 mmol/l intrinsic failure), urine/plasma urea >10 (<10 intrinsic failure), fractional sodium excretion <2% (>3% intrinsic failure) and urinalysis commonly shows benign sediment (whereas red and white cells and casts are seen in intrinsic renal failure). If the state of hydration is uncertain, give a fluid challenge with colloid or normal saline (10–20 ml/kg i.v. over 30–60 min) followed by frusemide (2 mg/kg). If urine output improves (especially >10 ml/kg over 3 hours), there is renal under-perfusion and continue with careful rehydration. If fluid volume is replete but hypotensive, try an inotrope (e.g. dopamine 5–20 μg/kg/min). If fluid challenge fails, severely cut back fluids, only replacing insensible water loss plus measured fluid and electrolyte losses (weigh infant). Correct severe acidosis (pH <7.2) and hyperkalaemia (serum potassium >6 mmol/l ± ECG changes) with resonium enemas, 10% calcium gluconate (slow i.v.) or bicarbonate (i.v.). Monitor serum electrolytes regularly plus ECG. Administer calcium supplements and phosphate-binding agents as required. If plasma sodium <120 mmol/l, potassium >8 mmol/l, bicarbonate <12 mmol/l with creatinine >630 μmol/l with severe fluid overload not responding to the above measures, consider peritoneal dialysis. Treat suspected infection (after all cultures have been obtained) with non-nephrotoxic drugs. Hypertension (commonly due to fluid overload) responds to fluid restriction. As renal function improves, ease fluid and dietary restrictions and finally remove them as renal function returns to normal.

Renal artery thrombosis

This is associated with a high umbilical artery, sepsis and hypercoaguable states. Physical signs include hypertension, haematuria, proteinuria, oliguria, congestive heart failure and, if bilateral, minimal or absent renal function. Renal ultrasound scan is normal but radionucleotide ([^{131}I] Hippuran) uptake is absent. Treat hypertension aggressively as prospects for full recovery are good.

Renal venous thrombosis

This is associated with dehydration, asphyxia, hyper-osmolality, cyanotic CHD and incidence is increased in IDMs. Common signs include flank or abdominal mass, haematuria and thrombocytopenia. Ultrasonography shows an enlarged kidney with thrombus in the renal vein or extending into the inferior vena cava. Management is supportive with correction of predisposing factors and renal failure (if it develops). Prognosis is generally good.

Nephrotic syndrome

Nephrotic syndrome is rare in the newborn. Causes of neonatal nephrotic syndrome include congenital nephrotic syndrome of Finnish type, epimembranous nephropathy due to renal vein thrombosis, congenital syphilis or hepatitis B and diffuse mesangial sclerosis. In Finland prevalence is 1.2 per 10 000 births. The placenta is large (25% of birthweight, normal 18%) and clinical signs include oedema, heavy proteinuria, hypoalbuminaemia and elevated cholesterol. The proteinuria is unresponsive to immunosuppressive drugs and corticosteroids. Renal histology shows diffuse proximal tubule dilatation.

There is severe failure to thrive and frequent bacterial infections. Management is symptomatic – salt restriction, diuretics, antibiotics for sepsis and optimizing calorie intake. Penicillin therapy is curative for the nephrotic syndrome due to congenital syphilis. If diagnosis is uncertain, renal biopsy is essential for an accurate diagnosis, prognosis, guiding therapy and parental counselling.

Renal tubular acidosis (RTA)

This is a group of disorders caused by an impaired ability to acidify urine. Three types are recognized.

1. Distal RTA (type 1). This is due to impaired distal acidification (an inability to lower urine pH below 5.5 in the face of systemic acidosis). Presenting clinical features include polyuria, hypercalciuria, potassium depletion and failure to thrive.

2. Proximal RTA (type 2). This is due to impaired HCO_3^- reabsorption in the proximal tubule with a decreased renal HCO_3^- threshold.

3. Hyperkalaemic RTA (type 4). There is impaired acidification due to impaired renal ammoniagenesis. There is a normal ability to acidify urine after an acid load but net acid excretion is subnormal due to decreased NH_4^+ excretion. It is seen in infants with hypo- or pseudohypoaldosteronism.

Suspect RTA when metabolic acidosis is accompanied by hyperchloraemia and a normal plasma anion gap, i.e. $[Na^+ + K^+] - [Cl^- + HCO_3^-] = 8-16\,mmol/l$. A normal anion gap reflects HCO_3^- loss from the kidneys or gastrointestinal tract. Distinguish proximal from distal RTA from the urine anion gap: a urine sample from a patient with hyperchloraemic metabolic acidosis and a negative urine anion gap suggests proximal RTA, while a positive anion gap suggests distal RTA. Oral alkali (sodium citrate or sodium bicarbonate) is the therapy of choice for RTA with oral diuretics (thiazide or frusemide) to reduce serum potassium in type 4 RTA.

Hypertension

Hypertension is defined by systolic blood pressure >90/60 in term and >80/45 in preterm infants. Commence therapy if systolic pressure is persistently >100 mmHg and diastolic >75 mmHg. Over 75% of neonatal hypertension is secondary to renal artery thrombosis while approximately one in five may be due to renal artery stenosis. The correct cuff should be used (width $\geq \frac{2}{3}$ of upper arm length) with the infant at rest. Symptoms and signs include those of underlying disorder and hypertension itself (hypertensive encephalopathy, seizures, congestive cardiac failure). Treatment depends on the cause.

Hypertension secondary to volume overload responds to fluid restriction, diuretics (e.g. frusemide 0.5–2 mg/kg/dose 12-hourly or chlorothiazide 5–10 mg/kg/dose 12-hourly), vasodilators (e.g. hydralazine 1–5 mg/kg/day given 6-hourly, captopril 0.1–1.0 mg/kg/day given 6-hourly) or ß-blockers (e.g. propranolol 2–5 mg/kg/day given 8-hourly). Monitor electrolytes when diuretics are used. For urgent control of hypertension, i.v. nitroprusside (0.5–5 µg/kg/min) or diazoxide (3–5 mg/kg) are useful. Investigate persistent hypertension to exclude renovascular disease, coarctation of the aorta, other intrinsic renal or post-renal disease and adrenal disorders.

Further reading

Awuzu M, Hunley TE, Kon V. Pathophysiology of acute renal failure in the neonatal period. In: Polin RA, Fox WW (eds). *Fetal and Neonatal Physiology*, 2nd edn. Philadelphia: W.B. Saunders, 1998; 1691–6.

Broin LP, Satlin LM. Clinical significance of developmental renal physiology. In: Polin RA, Fox WW (eds). *Fetal and Neonatal Physiology*, 2nd edn. Philadelphia: W.B. Saunders, 1998; 1677–91.

Postlethwaite RJ (ed). *Clinical Paediatric Nephrology*, 2nd edn. Oxford: Butterworth-Heinemann, 1994.

Proesmans W (ed). *Therapeutic Strategies in Children with Renal Disease. Baillière's Clinical Paediatrics, Vol. 5, No. 4.* London: Baillière Tindall, 1997.

Related topics of interest

RENAL AND URINARY TRACT DISORDERS – UROLOGY

Polycystic kidney disease (PCKD)

This can occur as an autosomal dominant (adult polycystic disease, ADPCKD) form or an autosomal recessive form (infantile polycystic disease, ARPCKD). In ARPCKD, the main site of dilatation is the collecting tubules. The severe form is rapidly fatal at or soon after birth. An i.v. pyelogram is characteristic (mottled nephrogram and retention of contrast with delayed excretion). The kidneys are massive, and those infants surviving the first month experience increasing renal failure and hypertension. Liver biopsy shows hepatic fibrosis with biliary dysgenesis.

ADPCKD presents similarly with renal failure and reduced renal function with progressive renal insufficiency. Nephrosonography shows bilateral large and small renal cysts. Imaging studies cannot accurately distinguish ARPCKD from ADPCKD. In ADPCKD, there is usually a family history of PCKD and parents often show hepatic or renal cysts when imaged (CT or ultrasound scans). ADPCKD has a better prognosis than ARPCKD.

Renal cystic dysplasia

When unilateral, the term multicystic kidney is used. There are large cysts with little renal tissue. It is commonly detected pre-natally. Always examine the contralateral kidney carefully as anomalies (e.g. pelvi-ureteric junction (PUJ) obstruction) are common. The non-functional kidney may require surgical removal (risk of neoplasia). Renal cystic dysplasia is associated with other anomalies, such as the Zellweger cerebro-hepatorenal syndrome and Meckel–Gruber syndrome. A 99m-technetium-labelled dimercaptosuccinic acid ($[^{99m}Tc]$-DMSA) scan is required to determine whether the kidney is functional.

Renal agenesis

The complete absence of both kidneys is rare (1 in 10 000 births). There is oligohydramnios and associated pulmonary hypoplasia with Potter's facies, bowed legs, clubbed feet, no kidneys evident on prenatal scans and affected infants die perinatally or are stillborn.

Posterior urethral valves

This only occurs in males. The bladder is distended and the urine stream is poor. Diagnosis is confirmed by renal ultrasound and micturating cystourethrogram (MCUG) though most still present acutely unwell with a UTI. The immediate management consists of draining the urinary tract via an indwelling catheter, commencing broad-spectrum antibiotics and i.v. fluid and electrolyte therapy. A paediatric urologist will be required to resect the valves. Some infants, however, eventually develop renal failure and require renal transplantation.

Hydronephrosis

This is readily diagnosed antenatally (renal pelvis >8–10 mm diameter after 34 weeks) and should be confirmed postnatally (48–72 hours). If hydronephrosis is confirmed, antibiotic prophylaxis should be commenced (trimethoprim 2 mg/kg once daily) until MCUG has been performed to rule out vesico-ureteric reflux. To determine whether a dilated kidney is obstructed, [^{99m}Tc]-mercapto-acetyl-triglycerine-3 (MAG-3) with a diuretic may be helpful. If obstruction is suspected seek a paediatric urological opinion. Otherwise regular follow-up with repeat renal ultrasound scans is required with a high index of suspicion for intercurrent UTIs. In time the hydronephrosis resolves along with the need for antibiotic prophylaxis.

Hypospadias

In hypospadias, the urethral meatus may be positioned just below the glans way back at the root of the penis. In severe cases, the penis is short and curved (due to chordee) resembling a large clitoris, causing problems in assigning a sex to the infant. If both testes are present in the scrotum the infant is male, but when absent the infant could be a female with the adrenogenital syndrome, or incomplete testicular feminization may be suspected. It is vital then that the infant's karyotype, endocrine status and pelvic anatomy be ascertained (ultrasound or laparotomy) as it may be preferable to rear some 'genetic males' as 'females' if their internal genital tract is easier to convert surgically to a female configuration. Infants should not be circumcised prior to surgical repair.

Vesico-ureteric reflux

Vesico-ureteric reflux (VUR) is the consequence of an incompetent vesico-ureteric valve mechanism and may resolve spontaneously or, infrequently, lead to chronic renal insufficiency. There is an important genetic component to non-obstructive or 'idiopathic' VUR. One-third of the siblings of affected children will also have VUR, while 60% of the offspring of parents with VUR will also be affected. VUR also occurs in apparently healthy infants and children (asymptomatic VUR), the incidence falling from birth to age 4 years, and is more common in boys (4:1). VUR associated with UTI (symptomatic VUR) is, however, predominantly found in girls, with a 4:1 preponderance. VUR is more common in infants presenting with UTI (30–50%) and in infants with prenatal hydronephrosis. VUR can cause morphological (renal scars) and functional renal damage. Renal damage is more likely with gross VUR and bladder dysfunction (e.g. neurogenic bladder). Renal scars are caused by intrarenal reflux, bacterial infection (UTI) and/or obstruction acting in concert. The rapidly growing kidney (i.e. infants and toddlers) is most susceptible to morphological damage. VUR predisposes to arterial hypertension.

1. Diagnosis of VUR. MCUG, is the 'gold standard'. It visualizes the urethra, bladder and renal pelvis, permitting grading of severity of reflux. Indirect radionuclide voiding cystography (e.g. MAG-3 renogram) is less reliable and can only be used in the older continent child. MCUGs should be performed in all infants presenting with prenatal dilatation of the renal pelvis, family history of VUR, UTI and acute pyelonephritis.

2. Management of VUR. The goal of medical therapy is to avoid UTIs by using antibiotic prophylaxis and regulation of bladder and bowel emptying. The optimum duration of prophylaxis is not known but is influenced by severity of VUR, intercurrent UTIs and associated anatomical abnormalities (see below). Surgery is indicated in patients with dilating VUR (grade ≥III) whose parents prefer an operation or are non-compliant with medical treatment. However, medical and surgical treatments are almost equally effective in protecting kidneys from new damage or the progression of pre-existing damage. In 4.2% of patients, surgery is complicated by obstruction. Follow-up until VUR resolves or the risk of complications is minimal. Spontaneous resolution of VUR may be ascertained in the older continent child by indirect (i.v.) isotope cystography which avoids catheterization and minimizes exposure to radiation.

Urinary tract infection

This is confirmed by the finding of a pure growth of a single pathogen at a count of at least 10^5 colony-forming units/ml urine in at least two clean specimens of urine, or any growth from a suprapubic aspirated urine specimen. Pus cells may be present or absent. Absence of growth from an appropriately handled bag specimen can rule out UTI. The commonest predisposing factor is urinary stasis (VUR, bladder dysfunction, infrequent or incomplete voiding, outflow obstruction as in urethral valves). In the first 2–3 months of life, UTI occurs predominantly in boys, between 3–12 months of age boys and girls are equally affected, and above 1 year girls are predominantly affected.

1. Clinical features. In infants symptoms are non-specific, including:

- Fever.
- Jaundice.
- Failure to thrive.
- Feeding difficulties.

- Vomiting and diarrhoea.
- Occasionally as severe illness with cyanosis, hypotension and shock.

2. *Immediate investigations*
- Blood and urine cultures.
- FBC.
- U&E and creatinine.
- Lumbar puncture (if particularly unwell).
- Renal ultrasound scan.

Urine microscopy of a fresh uncentrifuged clean sample identifies infection (eight organisms per high power field, or 10^7 organisms/ml) and allows treatment to be started while awaiting culture results. Dipslides can also give reliable results within 24 hours.

3. *Management.* Aim to establish a prompt diagnosis, rapid treatment and detection of any underlying cause that might predispose to further infection or lead to long-term renal damage. If there is a strong suspicion of a UTI, start treatment once a clean sample has been obtained.

- Antibiotics covering common causative organisms (*Escherichia coli*, *Enterococcus* spp., *Klebsiella* spp., *Streptococcus faecalis*, *Proteus* ssp., *Pseudomonas* spp.).
- Commence initial combination (e.g. ampicillin and gentamicin) until sensitivities are available, then switch to the most appropriate antibiotic(s) for 5–7 days (uncomplicated UTI) or 10 days (systemically unwell).
- If the infant is systemically unwell, use i.v. antibiotics until the infant is improved and has been apyrexial for 24–36 hours before reverting to oral antibiotics.
- Add a third-generation cephalosporin (e.g. cefotaxime) if meningitis is suspected.
- Maintain on prophylactic antibiotics (e.g. trimethoprim 2 mg/kg once daily) until VUR is excluded.
- Monitor fluid and electrolytes in infants presenting with dehydration or systemic illness.
- Monitor BP.
- Check post-treatment urine without stopping prophylaxis. Persistence of infection, mixed infection or early recurrence with a resistant strain suggests bladder dysfunction or outflow obstruction.

4. *Follow-up investigations (several weeks later)*
- MCUG (to detect VUR).
- DMSA scan after ≥3 months (to identify renal scarring).
- Urinalysis and urine microscopy at follow-up.

- Check BP at follow-up (hypertension and proteinuria are markers of progressive renal disease).
- Continue long-term prophylaxis if reflux or scarring is present until child is 2–3 years.
- Advise parents to have infant reassessed if fever or symptoms recur despite prophylaxis.
- Reinfection with an organism sensitive to prophylactic therapy suggests non-compliance, infection with resistant organism requires full-dose treatment and adjustment of prophylaxis.
- In absence of renal anomalies, follow-up is required for at least 1 year and ideally until the child has been infection-free for 2 years.

Imaging in renal disorders

Ultrasound scan is a mandatory first-line investigation in any renal disorder. *Intravenous urography (IVU)* is the investigation of choice in elucidating suspected anatomical abnormality. *[^{99m}Tc]-DMSA* is the investigation of choice in elucidating suspected renal parenchymal damage (scars). *MCUG* is the investigation of choice in determining the presence and severity of VUR. *MAG-3 renogram* is the investigation of choice when determining the quantitative excretory function of individual kidneys and possible outflow obstruction (when a diuretic is also administered).

Further reading

Obling H. Vesico-ureteral reflux (VUR). In: Proesmans W (ed). *Therapeutic Strategies in Children with Renal Disease. Baillière's Clinical Paediatrics, Vol. 5, No. 4.* London: Baillière Tindall, 1997; 521–38.

Smellie JM. Management and investigation of children with urinary tract infection. In: Postlethwaite RJ (ed). *Clinical Paediatric Nephrology*, 2nd edn. Oxford: Butterworth-Heinemann, 1994.

Thomas DFM (ed). *Urological Disease in the Fetus and Infant: Diagnosis and Management.* Oxford: Butterworth-Heinemann, 1997.

Related topics of interest

RESPIRATORY DISTRESS

Respiratory problems, manifest as respiratory distress, are the commonest cause of admission of newborns to the neonatal unit in the perinatal period. Respiratory distress arises from inadequate *in utero* maturation of the lung and of mechanisms controlling respiration, or from disease processes present before or after birth which compromise pulmonary function. The causes and management of respiratory distress vary depending on the gestational and chronological age of the infant.

Aetiology

1. Preterm infants

(a) Respiratory
- Surfactant deficiency.
- Pneumothorax.
- Chronic lung disease.
- Pulmonary haemorrhage.
- Pulmonary insufficiency of prematurity.
- Congenital lung malformations (e.g. cystic adenomatoid malformation).

(b) Infection
- Pneumonia.
- Septicaemia.
- Meningitis.

(c) Miscellaneous
- Cold stress.
- Hypoglycaemia.

2. Term infants

(a) Respiratory
- Pneumothorax.
- Pleural effusion.
- Transient tachypnoea of the newborn.
- Meconium and other aspiration syndromes.
- Congenital malformations (e.g. cystic adenomatoid malformations, pulmonary lymphangiectasia, pulmonary hypoplasia, CDH, congenital nasolacrimal duct obstruction (congenital dacryocystocele)).
- PPHN.
- Congenital surfactant protein B deficiency.

(b) Cardiovascular
- Congenital heart defects leading to heart failure (hypoplastic left heart syndrome, obstructed total anomalous pulmonary venous drainage, severe coarctation).

(c) Infection
- Pneumonia.
- Septicaemia.
- Meningitis.

(d) Miscellaneous
- Cold stress.

- Polycythaemia.
- Maternal drugs (e.g. opiates).
- Birth trauma and birth asphyxia.
- Neuromuscular disorders (e.g. spinal muscular atrophy type 1, myotonic dystrophy).
- Inherited metabolic disease (e.g. organic acidaemias).

Clinical features

The characteristic features are tachypnoea, grunting, nasal flaring and cyanosis, which may be superseded by apnoeas or acute collapse. In addition, cardiac murmurs, abnormal peripheral pulses or signs of cardiac failure may also be present if there is an underlying congenital heart defect.

Investigations

1. Pulse oximetry. It is useful to determine the arterial oxygen saturations as a guide to the severity of hypoxaemia and the urgency of intervention.

2. Temperature. Exclude hypothermia or pyrexia.

3. Blood glucose. Exclude hypoglycaemia.

4. Arterial blood gases. This is essential to determine the degree of respiratory failure and decisions on the next most appropriate interventions to be made. Capillary or venous blood gases may be misleading in an infant with poor peripheral perfusion. Inordinate persistent metabolic acidosis may point to a metabolic disorder.

5. Chest radiograph. Rule out pneumothorax, effusions, pulmonary oedema, abnormal cardiac silhouette, congenital diaphragmatic hernia; bell-shaped chest is seen in neuromuscular disorders, and ground glass appearance with idiopathic RDS, congenital pneumonia or aspiration.

6. FBC and film. Sepsis suggested by low or high white blood cell count and thrombocytopenia.

7. Full septic screen. This should be conducted when there is a high suspicion of sepsis.

8. ECG and echocardiogram. These are conducted for suspected CHD.

Management

This is determined by the underlying diagnosis. Aim to correct acid–base disturbance and alleviate hypoxaemia and respiratory failure. Warm cold infants and correct hypoglycaemia. Preterm infants with RDS and significant hypoxaemia should be intubated for surfactant administration and mechanical ventilation. However, infants with mild RDS may be immediately extubated after surfactant administration and maintained on CPAP. More mature infants (>34 weeks gestation) with mild RDS may be managed on CPAP or headbox oxygen with recourse to mechanical ventilation when the FiO_2 exceeds 0.6, if blood gases are unsatisfactory, or there are apnoeas.

Transient tachypnoea of the newborn usually resolves with minimal support (supplemental oxygen). Unless the supplemental oxygen requirements are modest, an arterial line should be sited for blood gas monitoring in oxygen-dependent infants. Suspected sepsis should be promptly treated with an appropriate combination of broad-spectrum antibiotics until cultures are available. Pneumothoraces and symptomatic effusions should be drained appropriately and repeat radiographs performed to determine the adequacy of the procedure.

Infants with suspected CHD or malformations requiring corrective surgery are best managed in specialist centres and may require ventilation for safe transportation. PGE_1 or PGE_2 should be commenced in infants with suspected duct-dependent congenital heart lesions and a paediatric cardiology opinion sought.

Further reading

Fanaroff AA, Martin RJ. *Neonatal–Perinatal Medicine: Diseases of the Fetus and Neonate*, 6th edn. St Louis: Mosby, 1997.

Gluckman PD, Heyman MA (eds). *Pediatrics and Perinatology: The Scientific Basis*, 2nd edn. London: Arnold, 1996.

Hamvas A, Cole S, deMello DE *et al.* Surfactant protein B deficiency: antenatal diagnosis and prospective treatment with surfactant replacement. *Journal of Pediatrics*, 1994; **125**: 356–61.

Philip AGS. *Neonatology: A Practical Guide*, 4th edn. Philadelphia: W.B. Saunders, 1996.

Taeusch HW, Ballard RA (eds). *Avery's Diseases of the Newborn*, 7th edn. Philadelphia: W.B. Saunders, 1998.

Related topics of interest

RESPIRATORY DISTRESS SYNDROME

RDS, previously called hyaline membrane disease, is the single most important medical disorder in preterm infants, affecting 40–50% of all infants born before 32 weeks gestation. It is primarily a consequence of respiratory failure secondary to cardiopulmonary immaturity in preterm infants. Avery and Mead first demonstrated in 1959 that the lungs of infants with RDS were uncompliant due to surfactant deficiency. Attempts to prevent RDS have therefore concentrated on ways of enhancing the action or accelerating production of surfactant. Accelerating lung morphological maturity is also essential.

The incidence and severity of RDS is inversely proportional to gestational age (or birthweight). In infants <27 weeks gestation, RDS is almost universal and after 27 weeks but before 32 weeks, RDS may affect two in three infants. After 32 weeks RDS is less frequent and tends to be moderate regardless of other risk factors. Mortality during the acute phase is now largely confined to ELBW infants (<1000 g).

Factors influencing risk and severity

- Gender – girls have a lower risk, less severe disease and a lower mortality than boys.
- Race – black infants have a lower incidence and severity than white infants matched for age and birthweight.
- *In utero* stress – risk is lower in disorders associated with placental insufficiency (e.g. IUGR, but not pre-eclampsia).
- Multiple pregnancy increases risk of RDS (especially in second twins).
- Maternal habits – smoking, alcohol ingestion, and maternal narcotic addiction reduce the incidence of RDS in preterm infants.
- Perinatal factors – delivery by Caesarean section prior to onset of labour, asphyxia, acidosis and hypothermia all increase the risk of developing RDS.
- Diabetes mellitus – poor control increases risk of RDS.
- Genetic factors – a familial predisposition exists as well as the recently recognized surfactant protein B deficiency in congenital alveolar proteinosis.

Prevention

- Prevention of prematurity is the ideal preventive strategy.
- If premature birth is inevitable, prenatal corticosteroid therapy is the most effective currently available intervention to reduce the incidence, severity and mortality of RDS. Meta-analysis of randomized controlled trials to date shows a reduction in risk of RDS of 40–60% and a reduction in mortality of 50%. Antenatal corticosteroids reduce the risk of developing PVH and NEC and may protect against neurological abnormality. Steroids should be given to all mothers at risk of premature delivery between 23–34 weeks gestation. Treatment consists of betamethasone or dexamethasone 12 mg i.m. given 12 hours apart. Optimal benefit begins 24 hours after initiation of therapy and lasts 7 days.

- Steroid therapy for less than 24 hours still reduces the incidence of RDS, IVH and mortality.
- Despite earlier promising studies, large randomized trials of thyrotrophin-releasing hormone (TRH)–corticosteroid combination therapy have not shown additional benefit.
- Ambroxol, a bromhexine metabolite, has been reported to be effective in preventing RDS, but this needs to be confirmed in a larger randomized study.

Pathology

Lung histopathology of infants dying from RDS shows:

- Interstitial and alveolar oedema.
- Pulmonary capillary engorgement.
- Haemorrhages.
- Atelectasis in association with over-distended air spaces (gives the radiographic 'ground glass' appearance).
- Hyaline membranes (sloughed cell debris in a protein matrix formed at the junction of respiratory bronchioles and alveolar ducts).

Pathophysiology and lung mechanics

The following features characterize RDS:

- Delayed clearance of fetal lung fluid.
- Deficiency and inactivation of surfactant.
- Increased permeability of epithelial and endothelial barriers.
- Ventilation–perfusion mismatch from intra- and extra-pulmonary shunting of PBF.

Features

- Cyanosis.
- Expiratory grunt.
- Tachypnoea and nasal flaring.
- Intercostal and sternal recession.
- Reduced lung compliance with increased work of breathing.
- Abnormal gas exchange (hypoxaemia and hypercapnia) commonly requiring supplemental oxygen or assisted ventilation.
- Abnormal chest radiograph – lung reticulogranular pattern (ground glass appearance) and air bronchograms with small lung volumes.

Management

The main principles of management include:

- Provision of adequate oxygenation and blood gas exchange by administering supplemental oxygen with or without assisted ventilation, while minimizing barotrauma and volutrauma and preventing air leaks.
- Administration of surfactant, either as prophylactic therapy at birth for infants at high risk of RDS (e.g. ≤29 weeks gestation or ≤1250 g birthweight), or as early rescue therapy for established disease.

- Supporting the cardiovascular system to maintain adequate cardiac output and tissue perfusion.
- Treating sepsis with appropriate antibiotics.
- Provision of adequate fluid therapy to maintain normal electrolyte and blood glucose homeostasis.
- Preventing intracranial haemorrhage.
- Maintaining adequate temperature control.
- Avoiding unnecessary handling of the infant and providing sedation and/or analgesia.

Maintaining adequate blood gas exchange

This may be achieved by instituting CPAP or mechanical ventilation (see 'Mechanical ventilation'). Excessive CPAP may be detrimental (produces excessive FRC, reducing compliance and PBF). Mechanical ventilation may be provided as positive pressure ventilation or high-frequency ventilation. The aim of assisted ventilation should be to maintain adequate oxygenation (PaO_2 7.5–10 kPa), correct acidosis and avoid hypo- and hypercapnia.

Synopsis of surfactant therapy

Surfactant became widely available for clinical use in Europe and North America during 1989–90, and this was heralded by a marked reduction in neonatal mortality. The main benefits of surfactant therapy are as follows:

- Reduction in the incidence of pneumothoraces.
- Variable reduction in the incidence of BPD.
- Reduction in the incidence of IVH (rescue therapy with synthetic surfactants).
- Natural surfactants produce more rapid improvements in gas exchange and may be superior to synthetic surfactants in reducing mortality.
- Major reduction in neonatal mortality (overall 40% reduction).

Potential complications of surfacant therapy

- Hyperoxia – wean ventilation and oxygen accordingly.
- Maldistribution of surfactant to one lung must be avoided.
- Incidence of PDA and pulmonary haemorrhage may be increased in the extremely preterm infants. The risk of pulmonary haemorrhage may be greater with synthetic surfactants (e.g. Exosurf).
- Avoid destabilizing the infant (i.e. avoid desaturations, blood pressure perturbations and blocking the endotracheal tube) during therapy (more likely when large volumes are administered at once).
- Transmission of infectious agents (e.g. bovine spongiform encephalitis (BSE) or 'mad cow disease' in bovine-derived surfactants, which could potentially cause nvCJD in humans. Bovine surfactants are made from BSE-free herds).

- Immunological injury from the immunogenicity of surfactant proteins has not been reported. Surfactant therapy may in fact reduce this risk by reducing the alveolar-capillary leaks associated with RDS and its treatment.

Surfactant is, however, ineffective in a third of all infants treated, partly due to maldistribution and surfactant inactivation. See 'Surfactant replacement therapy'.

Further reading

Crowley P. Antenatal corticosteroid therapy: a meta-analysis of the randomized trials, 1972 to 1994. *American Journal of Obstetrics and Gynecology*, 1995; **173:** 322–5.

Jobe AH. Pathophysiology of respiratory distress syndrome and surfactant metabolism. In: Polin RA, Fox WW (eds). *Fetal and Neonatal Physiology*, 2nd edn. Philadelphia: W.B. Saunders, 1998; 1299–1313.

Kattwinkel J, Bloom BT, Delmore P *et al.* Prophylactic administration of calf lung surfactant extract is more effective than early treatment of respiratory distress syndrome in neonates of 29 through 32 weeks' gestation. *Pediatrics* 1993; **92:** 90–8.

Robertson JB, Taeusch HW (eds). *Surfactant Therapy.* New York: Dekker, 1995.

Soll RF, McQueen MC. Respiratory distress syndrome. In: Sinclair JC, Bracken MB (eds). *Effective Care of the Newborn Infant.* Oxford: Oxford University Press, 1992; 325–58.

Taeusch HW, Boncuk-Dayanikli P. Respiratory distress syndrome. In: Yu VYH (ed). *Pulmonary Problems in the Perinatal Period and their Sequelae.* Baillière's Clinical Paediatrics, Vol. 3, No. 1. London: Baillière Tindall, 1995; 71–85.

Related topics of interest

RESUSCITATION

Everyone remembers the ABCD of any resuscitation:

Airway
Breathing
Circulation
Drugs.

But the first 'A' of neonatal resuscitation is for *anticipation*. Every maternity unit must have in place equipment, guidelines and trained staff to anticipate the need to resuscitate newborn babies. At its most basic, equipment is needed to keep the baby warm, to suck out the airways and to ventilate the baby's lungs with air or oxygen. The time to prepare equipment is immediately *after* use, but check it again on arrival. The unit's guidelines must anticipate a wide variety of circumstances, relating to the complications of pregnancy and delivery and different gestations at birth. Take precautions to reduce the risk of HIV transmission at all deliveries. Staff trained in advanced resuscitation must be resident to resuscitate the unexpectedly flat baby at birth, the unbooked preterm delivery, as well as attending the deliveries of babies recognized in advance as being at some risk. These usually include:

- All Caesarean sections under general anaesthetic.
- All breech presentations.
- All multiple deliveries.
- All preterm deliveries <36 completed weeks gestation.
- All deliveries with fetal distress:
    Meconium.
    Type II dips.
    Scalp pH <7.2.
- All babies with a suspected congenital abnormality, which may cause immediate clinical problems.
- Babies born to HIV-positive mothers.

Particularly skilled resuscitators should attend deliveries of <29 weeks gestation, anticipated severe asphyxia, and known severe abnormalities or hydrops.

The aims of neonatal resuscitation can be summarised as: **WOMB**

Keep the baby **W**arm.
Ensure **O**xygenation.
Return the baby to the **M**other.
Encourage early **B**reast-feeding.

At birth assess the heart rate, respiratory effort, tone and colour. This will help you decide what help, if any, is needed. Do not expose the baby unnecessarily. Remember the order of resuscitation:

Airway
Breathing
Circulation
Drugs.

| Airway | The head should be in a neutral position – neither flexed nor over-extended – and the jaw gently pulled forward to stop the tongue obstructing the back of the pharynx. |

Airway

The head should be in a neutral position – neither flexed nor over-extended – and the jaw gently pulled forward to stop the tongue obstructing the back of the pharynx.

Breathing

- If the breathing is shallow or irregular, but the heart rate >100, recheck the airway, stimulate gently and give facial oxygen.
- If respiratory effort is absent, or the heart rate <100, or the baby is persistently cyanosed, start ventilation with a face mask and T-piece. After checking the airway, an initial breath of 3 s at 20–30 cmH$_2$O followed by regular breaths of 1s should create an FRC and allow the baby to take over the breathing. If the baby does not respond, be ready to intubate. Check whether the mother has recently had opioid analgesia, and if so, be ready to give i.m. naloxone.
- Once intubated, give an initial breath of 3 s, and then regular 1s breaths. Babies with very stiff lungs may need higher initial pressures to inflate them, but with increased risk of pneumothoraces and other air leaks.
- Most babies respond rapidly to ventilation after intubation, but some do not. Likely reasons are that the tube is in the oesophagus or the right main bronchus, or blocked, or too small a tube has been used in a large baby. Some features of the baby may make resuscitation difficult or impossible. In general, these babies will be either very preterm (unventilatable and unresuscitatable), abnormal with pulmonary hypoplasia or severely asphyxiated.
- If the endotracheal tube is definitely in the right place, and some chest movements are seen, but the baby remains profoundly bradycardic, the circulation must also be supported.

Circulation

- ECM is performed in a ratio of five compressions to one breath, at a rate of 100–120 compressions per minute.
- While one resuscitator looks after the airway and breathing, the second circles the neonate's chest with his/her hands so that the two thumbs lie over the lower third of the sternum, just below the nipple line. Alternatively, the baby can be laid flat on a firm surface and massaged with two fingers over the lower sternum.
- Compressions should indent the chest by 2–3 cm, or about half the antero-posterior diameter of the chest.
- If, with combined ventilation and ECM, the baby still does not pick up, adrenaline should be given.

Drugs

- Only use drugs after adequate ventilation and ECM fail to improve the baby's condition.
- Only four drugs are essential: adrenaline, bicarbonate, glucose and naloxone. *Table 1* gives dose information for these.

Table 1. Drug doses for resuscitation

Drug	Dose	Route	Comments
Adrenaline (1 in 10 000)	0.1 ml/kg then 1 ml/kg (10 µg/kg then 100 µg/kg)	i.v.	Repeat dose or give via UVC if inserted
	1 ml/kg	Endotracheal	
Sodium bicarbonate	2 mmol/kg (2 ml/kg of 8.4%)	i.v.	Slowly over 5 to 10 min, diluted to 4.2% in 5% glucose
Glucose	0.2 g/kg (1 ml/kg of 20%)	i.v.	
Naloxone	100 µg/kg	i.m.	Not for babies of opiate-dependent mothers

- There is no place for calcium and atropine, which have not been shown to be effective in neonatal resuscitation.
- The *only* indication for naloxone is depression from maternal analgesics.
- Adrenaline can be put down the endotrachael tube for persistent bradycardia or asystole.
- Bicarbonate should not be used routinely, but only for severely asphyxiated babies, to whom it should be given as a slow infusion, not as a bolus.
- A small dose of glucose will give a bolus to the heart.

Special groups of babies

1. Preterm and low birthweight.

- Keep the baby warm!
- Ask for theatre/delivery room temperature to be increased. Work under overhead heater in draught-free area.
- Dry rapidly while assessing baby's state. Change wet sheets for warm dry ones.
- Keep exposure to a minimum. Use a pre-warmed transport incubator to transfer the baby to the NICU.

2. Caesarean section babies

- Fetal lungs secrete fluid. This is reversed in term babies by catecholamine surges during labour – then the lungs are compressed in the birth canal, and only small amounts of fluid are left in the lungs prior to the first breath.
- Caesarean section babies have excess lung fluid at birth and may 'drown' if it is not aspirated. If intubation is needed, suck out the trachea before ventilating.

3. Meconium-stained liquor. Approximately 8–10% of babies are born through meconium-stained liquor. Aspiration of this can lead to MAS with potentially fatal consequences. Light meconium staining seldom causes problems and intubation and suction are unnecessary, but for babies delivered through heavily stained liquor with or without particulate matter, a combined midwifery–paediatric approach is used.

1. The oropharynx is sucked out when the head is delivered either on the perineum or through a Caesarean incision.
2. The resuscitator visualizes the cords and sucks out the trachea, either by inserting an FG10 suction catheter through the cords or by passing a catheter down through the endotracheal tube. Suction pressures of up to 100 mmHg are used through as large a catheter as possible.
3. If necessary, standard resuscitation can now start with a reduced chance of forcing meconium into the lungs with the first few positive pressure breaths.

There is no evidence that either compression of the chest after birth or saline lavage during resuscitation are beneficial.

4. *Hydrops fetalis.* See 'Hydrops fetalis'.

5. *Infants of HIV-positive mothers*
- The safest way to deliver infants of HIV-positive mothers is by Caesarean section.
- Resuscitation should be as atraumatic as possible with minimal damage to the baby's mucosa, thus reducing the risk of infection by infected maternal blood.
- Resuscitators should wear gloves, plastic aprons, gowns, and appropriate footwear and eye protection.
- No mouth-operated suction should be used.
- Once the baby is stable, wash off maternal blood and *only then* give i.m. vitamin K. This is to reduce the risk of infecting the infant.

6. *Extremely preterm babies at the threshold of viability.* Resuscitation of the very preterm infant is both technically and ethically difficult. The legal age of viability in the UK is 24 weeks gestation, but some infants of less than 24 weeks survive, and for some gestation is uncertain. Units should have specific guidelines for the care of women in established labour at (say) 20–23 weeks when delivery is inevitable. A possible set of guidelines is offered below.

- On admission, the obstetric registrar is informed. When established labour is diagnosed and gestation confirmed as 'X' or above, the paediatric registrar is informed and management of the case agreed by both teams. (In the author's unit, 'X' is 23 weeks, a figure chosen after audit of outcomes and the EPICure study.)

- If unbooked and/or gestation is uncertain, the paediatric registrar will be present at birth. Active resuscitation will occur unless the baby is *very* small and immature.
- The plan of management is discussed with the parents by the obstetrician and recorded in the mother's notes.
- The management will fall into one of the following categories:

(a) No active resuscitation

No monitoring.

Choice of appropriate analgesia.

Appropriate and sensitive support is given to the parents.

The paediatrician will not be present at delivery.

The baby is given to the parents to hold. He/she will stay with the parents until there are no signs of life – unless otherwise requested.

(b) Active resuscitation

No continuous electronic monitoring – because no emergency section will be performed.

Intermittent auscultatory monitoring – some babies die during labour, and they will not be resuscitated if this is confirmed and there is no heartbeat at birth.

Nursed in delivery room with resuscitation equipment.

Senior paediatricians must attend to assist resuscitation.

Starting intensive care does not mean it has to be continued.

(c) Termination of pregnancy for fetal abnormalities

Stopping resuscitation in asphyxiated babies
- On available evidence, it is reasonable to stop if a baby has no spontaneous respiratory effort after 30 min of appropriate resuscitation.
- In the absence of a heartbeat, it is reasonable to stop after 10 min of appropriate resuscitation.

Further reading

American Academy of Pediatrics/American Heart Association. *Textbook of Neonatal Resuscitation*. Dallas: American Heart Association, 1994.

Ginsberg HG, Goldsmith JP. Controversies in neonatal resuscitation. *Clinics in Perinatology*, 1998; **25:** 1–15.

Royal College of Paediatrics and Child Health/Royal College of Obstetricians and Gynaecologists. *Resuscitation of Babies at Birth*. London: BMJ Publishing, 1997.

Related topics of interest

RETINOPATHY OF PREMATURITY

Retinopathy of prematurity (ROP) is a disorder of the developing retinal vasculature in which the normal progression of the newly forming vessels (vasculogenesis) is interrupted, resulting in the development of new abnormal blood vessels (neovascularization), which may heal by completely involuting with normal vascularization of the retina (regression) or progress to a chronic phase (cicatricial ROP) with scarring, retinal detachment and visual loss. In 95% of cases, ROP regresses spontaneously, but progressive disease is the leading cause of blindness in preterm infants.

Epidemiology and natural history

Over the past two decades the incidence of ROP has increased due to the increasing survival of ELBW infants (birthweights <1000 g). The NIH-sponsored multicentre trial of cryotherapy for ROP (CRYO-ROP Study), carried out on an estimated 15% of all births in the USA in which the infants weighed less than 1251 g, has provided insight into the epidemiology and natural history of ROP.

- Some degree of ROP developed in <10% of those weighing >1500 g at birth, 47% weighing 1000–1250 g at birth, 78% weighing 750–999 g at birth and 90% of those <750 g birthweight.
- In >90%, the condition regressed and healed before the onset of blinding disease, with only 6% of all infants developing severe disease ('threshold ROP') requiring treatment.
- When left untreated ~50% developed visual loss but cryotherapy reduced the incidence of unfavourable outcome by ~50% among infants at threshold.
- The most preterm infants were more susceptible to ROP.
- The timing of the development of threshold ROP was related to post-conceptional age (median 37 weeks) rather than chronological (postnatal) age.
- Cryotherapy reduced the incidence of blinding disease.

Aetiology and risk factors

- The aetiology of ROP is multifactorial.
- The degree of immaturity of the eye is the most important risk factor.
- The second strongest factor is oxygen therapy. A correlation exists between ROP and the concentration and duration of oxygen therapy, but wide variations in arterial oxygen tension may be a greater risk factor than the absolute level of hyperoxia. ROP has occurred in infants who never received supplemental oxygen, term infants with cyanotic CHD, and rarely even in stillborn infants.
- Severe ROP develops in the sickest infants (i.e. correlates with asphyxia, acidosis, shock, sepsis, blood transfusions, IVH, PVL, BPD).

Classification

- Once the retina is fully vascularized, ROP can no longer develop.

In 1984, the International Classification of ROP (ICROP) was introduced, allowing the location, severity and extent of disease to be described accurately. It was updated in 1987 to include the sequelae of ROP.

- *Disease location* is described by the use of three distinct zones of the retina centred on the optic disc. Zone 1 is the area closest to the optic disc; zone 3 is the most peripheral region and denotes complete vascularization to the edge of the retina; zone 2 is intermediate.
- *Extent of disease* is recorded in clock hours of retina involved.
- *Disease severity* is divided into five stages. In stage 1, a visible demarcation line is seen separating vascular from avascular retina. In stage 2, a ridge develops from the line in stage 1 (the mesenchymal arterio-venous shunt). In stage 3 disease, there is extraretinal fibrovascular proliferation with new vessels projecting from the ridge or retina (neovascularization) into the vitreous. Stage 4 is partial retinal detachment, and stage 5 is total retinal detachment.
- 'Plus' (+) disease denotes disease progression with increasing dilation and tortuosity of the arterioles and a vitreous haze, and can occur at any stage of disease.

Screening

- Screening aims to identify infants at risk for severe disease and those who would benefit from the available therapies.
- ROP rarely develops before 4–6 weeks after birth. Prethreshold (moderate) disease occurs at approximately the same post-conceptional age (37 weeks); the more mature infants are younger chronologically when they develop threshold disease.
- Current UK guidelines for ROP screening include the following criteria: any baby ≤1500 g birthweight or ≤31 weeks gestational age, although it has been suggested that these be altered to <1250 g birthweight or ≤29 weeks gestation.
- Two-weekly (or more frequent) follow-up examinations are performed till complete retinal vascularization occurs.
- Once retinal vessels reach zone 3 (the most peripheral zone), severe ROP and visual sequelae are unlikely, whereas when severe disease (stage 3+) occurs in zone 1, prospects for vision are poor even with treatment.
- Stage 1 and 2 disease spontaneously regresses in 95% of cases. At stage 3+, 50% of disease regresses spontaneously, the other half progressing to retinal detachment without treatment.
- Stage 3+ is the threshold for treatment.

Treatment	• The treatment of choice is retinal ablative therapy of the peripheral avascular retina with cryotherapy or laser therapy. • Cryotherapy reduces the incidence of adverse sequelae in severe disease by 50%. • Retinal ablation eliminates the angiogenic stimulus for the abnormal neovascularization produced in the avascular region. The peripheral retina is sacrificed in order to preserve the already vascularized retina and the macula in particular. • Cryotherapy involves freezing the avascular portion of the retina (plus the sclera and choroid) under local or general anaesthetic. • Adverse effects include conjunctival and eyelid oedema, subconjunctival haemorrhage, retinal and preretinal bleeding, apnoeas, bradycardias (oculocardic reflex with eyelid pressure), desaturations and respiratory and cardiorespiratory arrest. • Diode indirect laser photocoagulation is equally effective, safer and easier to apply, especially for zone 1 disease which is difficult to reach with a cryoprobe. Laser therapy is better tolerated with fewer systemic complications, less ocular destruction, more discrete retinal scars and less discomfort for the infants. • Partial (stage 4) or total retinal detachment (stage 5) has a poor prognosis for vision as therapy (scleral buckling and vitrectomy) is ineffective.
Prevention	• Supplemental antioxidants (e.g. vitamin E) are ineffective. • There is no safe range for arterial oxygen tensions though it is recommended that arterial PO_2 be maintained <10 kPa. • Surfactant therapy has indirectly increased the incidence of ROP through increased survival of ELBW infants. • Inositol and vitamin A supplementation are reported to reduce the incidence of ROP.
Long-term outcome	*1. Sequelae of progressive ROP* • Progressive ROP leads to severe visual impairment or total visual loss. • Late retinal detachments may still occur after initial successful treatment. *2. Sequelae of regressed ROP* • Generally, the higher the stage at the time of regression the worse the sequelae, which include myopia (nearsightedness), visual field defects, strabismus, amblyopia, glaucoma and late retinal detachments.

- ROP severity is also strongly associated with the development of strabismus (squint) with crossed eyes (esotropia) being the most common.
- Should the eyes be unequally affected, the infant may suppress the use of the worse eye and develop a lazy eye (amblyopia), which should be aggressively treated to preserve binocular vision.

Further reading

Hunter BG, Mukai S. Retinopathy of prematurity: pathogenesis, diagnosis and treatment. *International Ophthalmology Clinics*, 1992; **32:** 163–84.

Report of a Joint Working Party of the Royal College of Ophthalmologists and the British Association of Perinatal Medicine. Retinopathy of prematurity: guidelines for screening and treatment. *Early Human Development,* 1996; **46:** 239–58.

Watts JL. Retinopathy of prematurity. In: Sinclair JC, Bracken MB (eds). *Effective Care of the Newborn Infant.* Oxford: Oxford University Press, 1992; 617–39.

Ziavras E, Javitt JJ. Retinopathy of prematurity. In: David TJ (ed). *Recent advances in paediatrics, No. 13.* Edinburgh: Churchill Livingstone, 1995; 177–91.

Related topics of interest

SEDATION AND ANALGESIA ON THE NEONATAL INTENSIVE CARE UNIT

Although neonatal intensive care relies heavily on the use of sophisticated and expensive instrumentation for the constant remote monitoring of sick infants, several other necessary procedures require the infants to be directly handled. Many of these procedures (e.g. tracheal intubation, insertion of chest drains, arterial and venous cannulation and phlebotomy) are stressful, unpleasant and painful. It is now accepted that even the most immature of infants mount physiological responses to procedures, manifest as tachycardia or bradycardia, and hypoxaemic or hypertensive episodes. In addition, there are constant environmental stresses, such as excessive noise and light.

The provision of adequate analgesia and sedation to sick infants is not only kind but positively beneficial. The agitated and struggling infant on assisted ventilation is more likely to be suboptimally ventilated, develop a pneumothorax or intracranial haemorrhage, self-extubate or accidentally disrupt i.v. access lines. By carefully tailoring the doses of analgesics or sedatives each infant receives, the maximum benefits may be obtained while minimizing the side-effects.

Assessment of pain

Pain is difficult to assess, especially in the ventilated infant where the classic behaviour responses to pain, such as crying and distinct facial expressions, are obscured by strapping and the endotracheal tube obscures the baby's face. Blood pressure and heart rate have a poor correlation with the degree of agitation or pain. However, a more objective clinical score has been validated in non-ventilated preterm infants, which incorporates body movements as well as facial expression and cry (Neonatal Infant Pain Score or NIPS), and a new score has recently been designed for use in ventilated babies.

Management of pain and agitation

Analgesia or a sedative should be administered *prior* to undertaking procedures (not after several failures!) depending on the procedure and anticipated pain or discomfort.

1. Morphine. This is widely used as both an analgesic and a sedative. Morphine inhibits nociceptive reflexes by mimicking endogenous endorphins. Following a loading dose of 100–200 μg/kg (over 1.5–2 hours), a continuous infusion of 10–40 μg/kg/hour provides steady levels of analgesia and sedation for the ventilated infant. Morphine infusions reduce the stress response to ventilation in preterm infants. Side-effects include respiratory depression, bradycardia, hypotension (histamine release), urinary retention, decreased gastric motility, drug tolerance and physical dependence. Morphine is metabolized in the liver and excretion is renal (slower in preterm infants). To avoid withdrawal symptoms, after >1 week therapy wean gradually. Long-term follow-up studies up to the age of 5–6 years do not show adverse neurodevelopmental effects in preterm infants who received morphine for sedation during mechanical ventilation.

2. Diamorphine. Diamorphine is more lipid soluble than morphine, and has a more rapid onset of sedation and less hypotensive effects. Its side-effects profile is similar to morphine. The loading dose is 120 µg/kg (over 2 hours) followed by a continuous infusion of 15 µg/kg/hour.

3. Fentanyl. This is a synthetic opioid 80–100 times more potent that morphine. It has a more rapid onset of action (peak effect in 1–2 min when given i.v.), and a short half-life with very few haemodynamic effects (decreased histamine effects). Following a loading dose of 1–4 µg/kg, a continuous infusion of 1–2 µg/kg/hour provides effective analgesia. Side-effects include a higher rate of withdrawal symptoms, a more rapid development of tolerance and chest wall rigidity with rapid large-dose infusions.

4. Paracetamol. This is well suited for minor discomfort or pain (e.g. after immunizations) and may be repeated 4–6-hourly at a dose of 10 mg/kg/dose.

5. Ketamine. Ketamine is a fast-acting phencyclidine derivative which is both a sedative and potent analgesic. Its effects are apparent within 1–2 min and last 5–10 min. The standard dose is 0.5–1 mg/kg followed by a continuous infusion at 5–20 µg/kg/min. Ketamine increases heartrate, cardiac output, BP and CBF.

6. Midazolam. This short-acting, water-soluble benzodiazepine is a commonly used sedative especially in ventilated infants. It is metabolized in the liver and excreted in the urine. It has a rapid onset (1–5 min) but the half-life in neonates is 6–12 hours. Clearance is reduced and half-life increased in neonates compared to older infants. The loading dose is 100–200 µg/kg and the continuous infusion rate is 1–2.5 µg/kg/min. Concurrent administration of fentanyl with midazolam may produce dystonic movements and hypotension.

7. Chloral hydrate. Chloral hydrate is a hypnotic and sedative agent well tolerated by neonates at 30–50 mg/kg. The parent drug and its active metabolite trichloroethanol have long half-lives and therefore a potential for accumulation with repeated dosage. It has no respiratory depressant or analgesic effects. Side-effects include cardiac arrhythmias, gastrointestinal irritability and paradoxical agitation. Trichloroethanol may compete with bilirubin for hepatic glucuronidation.

Toxic effects from prolonged use include hypotension, renal failure, CNS depression and carcinogenicity.

8. Massage. The stress response may also be reduced by non-pharmacological means, e.g. stroking or massage.

Muscle relaxation

Routine muscle relaxation is not advocated. However, some critically ill ventilated infants may benefit from paralysis, e.g. mature infants with ventilator asynchrony or CDH. Complications of paralysis include deterioration of gas exchange, obscuring seizures, pain or agitation, tissue oedema, muscle contractures and myopathy. Muscle relaxants should be given concurrently with analgesics, as infants would still feel pain.

1. Suxamethonium. This has the most rapid onset of action (1 min) and shortest duration of action (4–6 min), making it ideal for emergencies. It may be used to facilitate intubations. The dose is 2 mg/kg i.v. or 4 mg/kg i.m. The onset of action is slower (2–3 min) and duration of action longer (10–30 min) when given i.m.

2. Pancuronium. Pancuronium is metabolized in the liver and excreted in urine (delayed excretion in renal failure). It raises BP, cardiac output and heartrate. The dose is 100 μg/kg i.v. (effective in 3 min and lasting 60 min).

3. Vecuronium. Vecuronium has few cardiovascular side-effects and is metabolized and excreted by the liver (in bile), although in neonates renal excretion is important. The dose is 100 μg/kg i.v. (effective in 2 min and lasting 30 min) followed by infusion of 1–3 μg/kg/min.

Further reading

Alexander SM, Todres ID. The use of sedation and muscle relaxation in the ventilated infant. *Clinics in Perinatology*, 1998; **25**: 63–78.

Bucher H-U, Bucher-Schmid A. Treating pain in the neonate. In: Hansen TN, McIntosh N (eds). *Current Topics in Neonatology, No. 1.* London: W.B. Saunders, 1996; 85–110.

Lawrence J, Alcock D, McGrath P, Kay J, MacMurray SB, Dulborg C. The development of a tool to assess neonatal pain. *Neonatal Network*, 1993; **12**: 59–65.

Sparshott M. *Pain, Distress and the Newborn.* Oxford: Blackwell Science, 1996.

Related topics of interest

SEIZURES

A seizure is a sudden paroxysmal depolarization of a group of neurones resulting in a transient alteration in neurological state. This may involve abnormal sensory, motor or autonomic activity, with or without a change in conscious level. Seizures generally are indicative of another underlying disease process and very few are idiopathic (2–5%). Seizures are a fairly common occurrence in the neonatal period with an incidence of 1–3 per 1000 live births at term. The incidence may be up to 50 times greater in preterm infants. The incidence of electrographic but clinically silent seizures is unknown, but up to 80% of electrographic seizures may be clinically silent especially in preterm infants. The primary objective of any intervention is to control the seizures, determine causation and rapidly correct any treatable causes as this may improve prognosis.

Seizure types

There are four types of clinical seizures: subtle, tonic, clonic and myoclonic. Each can be focal, multifocal or generalized.

1. Subtle seizures. The most common variety (~50% of all seizures), manifested by apnoea, eye fluttering and deviation, staring, sucking and chewing, cycling, boxing, unstable blood pressure and tachycardia.

2. Clonic seizures. Making up ~20–30% of all seizures, these are more common in preterm infants and are typified by rhythmic jerky movements (1–4/s) with consciousness usually preserved. They may be focal, suggesting a focal underlying lesion, such as cerebral artery infarction (but may also result from metabolic derangements), or multifocal.

3. Myoclonic seizures. Contributing ~15% of all seizures, these are rapid isolated jerks especially of the upper limbs, signifying metabolic or major structural derangement. They may be focal, multifocal or generalized.

4. Tonic seizures. Making up ~5% of all seizures, these are typified by sustained focal or generalized posturing of the body, such as tonic extension of all limbs, pronation of arms and clenching of fists. Generalized tonic seizures often signify more serious pathology, for example severe IVH.

It is important to distinguish jitteriness and apnoeas from seizures. Jitteriness is characterized by a symmetrical tremor of the extremities (spares the face) occurring at a higher frequency (5–6/s) than clonic movements. Jitteriness can be induced by an external stimulus and ceases with gentle restraint. Apnoeas may be a manifestation of subtle seizures, especially in term infants and when the apnoea is not accompanied by bradycardia and is associated with staring, eye opening or deviation of eyes.

Aetiology

1. Hypoxic–ischaemic encephalopathy (HIE). This is the commonest cause, accounting for half of the cases of neonatal seizures. Moderate HIE tends to present with subtle and clonic seizures, while severe HIE may present with myoclonic and tonic seizures. The seizures present in the first 24 hours.

2. CNS infection. Prenatal or perinatal infection may account for up to one in five cases of neonatal seizures. The commonest bacterial pathogens are group B streptococcus, *E. coli* and *Listeria* sp. Herpes simplex encephalitis and other pre-natal infections should also be excluded.

3. Intracranial haemorrhage/infarction. Following birth trauma in terms infants, subarachnoid and subdural haemorrhages may cause seizures independently from any co-existing asphyxia. IVHs with or without periventricular haemorrhagic infarction can cause generalized tonic seizures. The above causes may account for 10–15% of neonatal seizures.

4. Metabolic derangements. These may account for 1 in 10 neonatal seizures, the commonest being hypoglycaemia, hypocalcaemia, hypomagnesaemia and hyper- or hypo-natraemia. IMD (e.g. urea cycle defects, aminoacidurias and organic acidopathies) though rare should be considered when there is a positive family history, persistent acidosis, unusual odours or seizures unresponsive to conventional therapy. Rarely, IMD may present with severe recurrent seizures (myoclonic and clonic) and a burst-suppression EEG pattern, and early myoclonic encephalopathy. Pyridoxine dependency is a rare autosomal recessive defect in gamma-aminobutyric acid (GABA) synthesis which presents with early onset refractory seizures which are abolished by administering pyridoxine (50–100 mg).

5. Maternal drug addiction. Neonatal drug withdrawal is an important cause of neurological dysfunction though only 1 in 20 will develop seizures. Methadone withdrawal seizures may occur as late as 3 weeks though most other drugs produce symptoms earlier (<3 days). Cocaine abuse may predispose to prenatal cerebral artery infarction.

6. CNS malformation. Brain malformations are associated with an increased incidence of seizures. A rare syndrome, early infantile epileptic encephalopathy, may present with severe early tonic seizures, and a burst-suppression EEG pattern. It is associated with a very poor outcome.

7. Familial. Benign familial neonatal convulsions is an autosomal dominant condition presenting with clonic seizures on day 2–3 and resolving within the first 6 months of life. The infant is normal between seizures, investigations show no abnormalities and subsequent development is normal.

8. *Miscellaneous.* During quiet sleep some infants may have bilateral synchronous myoclonic jerks beginning in the first week and resolving within 2 months, i.e. benign neonatal sleep myoclonus. The EEG is normal during and between the events. Normal outcome is expected. Another benign form of neonatal seizures with multifocal clonic seizures has a peak age of onset at 5 days and resolves by day 15 (the 'fifth day fits'). The cause is unknown.

Investigations

1. *Primary investigations*
- Blood glucose.
- U&E, calcium, magnesium.
- Blood gases.
- Blood culture and CSF culture.
- Cranial ultrasound scan.
- EEG.

2. *Secondary investigations*
- Maternal and neonatal drug screen.
- Congenital infection screen (maternal and fetal TORCH serology).
- Metabolic screen (serum lactate, ammonia, amino acids, urine organic and amino acids).
- MRI or CT scanning.
- Cerebral function monitoring.
- Therapeutic trial of pyridoxine.

Management

The aim is to detect the underlying cause and give appropriate specific therapy and control the seizures. Although seizures *per se* could cause further neuronal compromise, it is unclear how important this is in the clinical situation as this has to be balanced against the potential deleterious effects of anticonvulsant therapy. One pragmatic approach is to control frequent (>3 seizures/hour) or prolonged seizures (>3 min duration) especially if they adversely affect systemic blood pressure or respiration. As many anticonvulsants cause respiratory depression and impair myocardial function, blood pressure and respiratory activity should be monitored.

Drug therapy

1. *Phenobarbitone.* This is a very effective first-time monotherapy controlling up to 70% of all seizures. Loading dose is 20 mg/kg i.v. (may be repeated, giving a total of 40 mg/kg) and maintenance is 6 mg/kg/day (given 12-hourly). Half-life is 3–8 days and the serum therapeutic level is 90–180 mmol/l. Phenobarbitone is a free-radical scavenger and reduces calcium entry after ischaemia.

2. Clonazepam. This second-line drug is most useful when seizure control is poor. The loading dose is 100–200 μg/kg (i.v. over 30 s) followed by an infusion of 10–30 μg/kg/hour. Convert to oral once-daily dose when seizure control is achieved. Other benzodiazepines such as lorazepam may also be useful. Diazepam has a very short duration of action and marked respiratory depressive effect making it unsuitable for long-term therapy.

3. Phenytoin. This is useful for securing short-term seizure control and not for long-term use as it causes myocardial depression and has very variable metabolism. Loading dose is 20 mg/kg (i.v. at <1 mg/kg/min).

4. Paraldehyde. The loading dose is 200–400 mg/kg i.v. or rectally followed by an infusion of 15–150 mg/kg/hour (0.3–3 ml/kg/hour of a 5% solution). Protect from light and if plastic syringes are used change 12-hourly. Paraldehyde is metabolized by the liver and lungs (not affected by impaired renal function) and has a short half-life (12–24 hours).

Prognosis
The underlying cause determines the prognosis. The prognosis is poor with brain malformations, intractable seizures, generalized myoclonic or tonic seizures, burst-suppression or persistent low-voltage EEG states and persisting neurological abnormalities on examination.

Further reading

Bernes SM, Kaplan AM. Evolution of neonatal seizures. *Pediatric Clinics of North America*, 1994; **41:** 1069–104.
Evans D, Levene M. Neonatal seizures. *Archives of Disease in Childhood*, 1998; **78:** F70–5.
Scher MS. Seizures in the newborn infant: diagnosis, treatment, and outcome. *Clinics in Perinatology*, 1997; **24:** 735–72.
Volpe JJ. *Neurology of the Newborn*, 3rd edn. Philadelphia: W.B. Saunders, 1995.
Wasterlain CG, Vert P (eds). *Neonatal Seizures*. New York: Raven Press, 1990.

Related topics of interest

SEXUAL AMBIGUITY

Genetic sex is determined at fertilization. The fetus develops a female *gonadic sex* unless a testis-determining factor (TDF) is present. The sex-determining region Y gene (SRY) on the short arm of the Y chromosome fulfils this role. When a testis develops, it secretes testosterone and Müllerian inhibitor substance (MIS). Testosterone acts on the Wolffian ducts to produce male internal genitalia, the vas deferens, epididymis and seminal vesicles. Externally, the androgen target cells convert testosterone into dihydrotestosterone (DHT) with the enzyme 5α-reductase. DHT stimulates the development of the male external genitalia, the penis and scrotum. MIS leads to the regression of the Müllerian ducts that would have developed into internal female genitalia in the absence of a testis. Thus a *phenotypic sex* is normally established by the end of embryogenesis, but when this has an uncertain appearance at birth, the baby is considered to have ambiguous genitalia. *Sex of rearing* is determined more by what can be realistically achieved with the anatomy and hormones (and the likely effect of puberty) than by karyotype.

At birth

1. The parents. The birth of a seemingly well infant but with indeterminate sex can cause unimagined anxiety and distress to the parents, and if badly managed, can irreparably damage the doctor–parent relationship. The usual cry of 'It's a boy!' or 'It's a girl!' is painfully absent for the parents of most babies with ambiguous genitalia, though some will have a sex assigned by the birth attendant, and this may later prove to be wrong. Therefore the first issue is to help the parents. Honesty is vital: uninformed guesses about the sex of the baby are devastating if wrong. The discussions with the parents should include the following statements:

(a) The sex that the baby is destined to be is not yet clear. They should be shown their baby's anatomy and simple drawings of sex organ development.

(b) The problem can be solved, and a definite sex assigned.

(c) In the meantime, the baby should not be named and the registration of the birth should be delayed until a sex has been assigned.

(d) Any attempt to assign 'the most likely sex' must be resisted. The baby should always be called 'baby', not 'he', not 'she' and certainly not 'it'!

Parents will want to know how long it will be before a sex can be assigned. It is better to suggest a week or so and to have an answer in 4 or 5 days, rather than the opposite, which parents find unbearable. To avoid confusion, the supervision of all such infants should be under one senior physician, who should be responsible for organizing the investigations and communicating the results of the same to parents.

2. The baby. Assessment includes:

- Checking the family history for similar babies, presence of hypospadias or cryptorchidism, and infertile aunts.
- Neonatal or infant male deaths (congenital adrenal hyperplasia (CAH) with salt loss).
- Assessment of phallic size, the presence/absence of midline fusion of the labia/scrotum, position and size of gonads if any are palpable, and the position of the urethral orifice.
- Physical examination for other congenital abnormalities.

3. Investigations. These should be performed urgently and the initial investigations should include:

- *Chromosomes* that can be sent immediately after birth or from cord blood.
- Plasma *17-hydroxyprogesterone (17-OHP)* to exclude CAH. As this is raised in all newborns, sampling has to be delayed for 48 hours (normal value <18 nmol/l). It remains elevated in ill and preterm babies, and this may cause diagnostic confusion.

These two investigations may be all that is necessary because 90% of ambiguous genitalia recognized at birth in the UK are secondary to virilization of a female (46XX) from CAH, with an autosomal recessive inheritance. The incidence of CAH in the UK is 1 in 10 000, with >95% of cases due to 21α-hydroxylase deficiency (of which there are several allelic forms), wherein very high levels of 17-OHP are found. It is also the only life-threatening form, as salt loss and consequent collapse can occur within a few weeks of birth in those with a severe deficiency. The experienced clinician may suspect other problems if characteristic or unusual changes are apparent, and request additional tests.

Classifying the problem

1. Female pseudohermaphroditism. These infants have a normal female karyotype, ovaries and Müllerian structures but a masculine external genitalia appearance. The most common cause of this virilization of a genetically female fetus is CAH, and in the UK this is nearly always due to a deficiency of 21α-hydroxylase, although 11β-hydroxylase ($\sim 5\%$) and 3β-hydroxysteroid dehydrogenase (3β-HSD) deficiency (<5%) can also cause it. About 50% of 21α–hydroxylase deficiency cases have salt loss. *Figure 1* shows the steroid biosynthetic pathways involved, and *Table 1* presents some enzyme defects with their clinical outcomes. Other causes of female virilization are very rare; they include drug ingestion and masculinizing tumours in the mother or fetus.

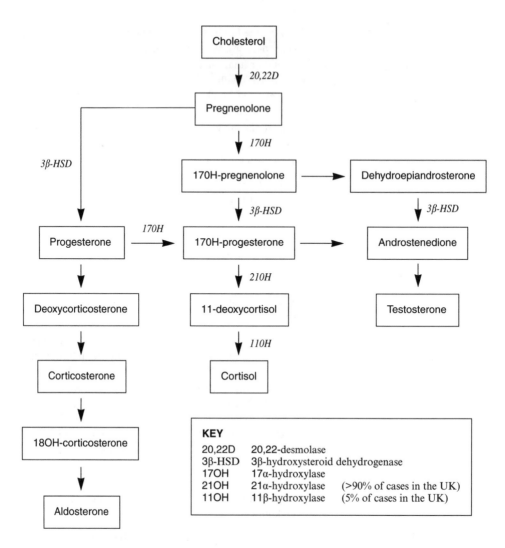

Figure 1. Simplified steroid biosynthetic pathways

Table 1. Summary of the effects of specific enzyme defects

Defect	Virilization in girls	Incomplete masculinization of boys	Salt loss	Hypertension
20,22D	No	Yes	Yes	No
3β-HSD	Yes	Yes	Yes	No
17OH	No	Yes	No	Yes
21OH	Yes	No	50% Yes	No
11OH	Yes	No	No	Yes

2. *Male pseudohermaphroditism.* There is incomplete virilization of a genetic male with testes. This may be due to:

(a) Impaired metabolism of androgens by peripheral tissues
- 5α-reductase deficiency is an autosomal recessive defect, in which the internal male organs (testosterone-dependent) develop normally, but the external genitalia (DHT-dependent) are ambiguous, and the phallus is small.
- Testicular feminization: androgen receptor/post-receptor defects in which the end organs do not respond to the androgens present as a spectrum of abnormalities, from an apparently normal female (but sometimes with bilateral inguinal hernias with a testis in them) to an infertile male.

(b) Impaired testosterone production (rare)

3. *Abnormal gonadal differentiation*
- True hermaphroditism occurs when an individual has both testicular tissue with seminiferous tubules and ovarian tissue with follicles. They may combine as an ovotestis or be separate gonads. Some present at birth with abnormal genitalia, others only at puberty when secondary sexual characteristics do not develop normally. Eighty per cent are XX, 10% XY, 10% mosaic.
- Asymmetrical gonadal dysgenesis – a testis on one side and streak gonad on the other.
- XX males frequently have the SRY gene translocated to the paternal X chromosome.

Further reading

Hughes IA. Management of congenital adrenal hyperplasia. *Archives of Disease in Childhood*, 1988; **63**: 1399–1404.

Levine LS, Pang S. Prenatal diagnosis and treatment of congenital adrenal hyperplasia. *Journal of Pediatric Endocrinology*, 1994; **7**: 193.

McGillivray BC. Genetic aspects of ambiguous genitalia. *Pediatric Clinics of North America*, 1992; **39**: 307–17.

Warner GL, Hughes IA. The clinical management of ambiguous genetalia. In: Brook CGD (ed). *Clinical Paeditric Endocrinology*, 3rd edn. Oxford: Blackwell Science, 1995.

Related topics of interest

Acute collapse (p. 6)
Congenital malformations and birth defects (p. 70)
Postnatal examination (p. 244)
Prenatal diagnosis (p. 253)

SHOCK

Shock constitutes a medical emergency where prompt and appropriate action can lead to a full recovery, whereas delayed though appropriate action may be inadequate to save the patient's life. A state of shock implies a generalized inadequacy of blood flow and tissue perfusion throughout the body, resulting in tissue damage. It can develop insiduously or rapidly progress to an irreversible stage.

Shock may be categorized according to its aetiology into septic, hypovolaemic, cardiogenic, anaphylactic and neurogenic. Despite the varied aetiology, the clinical features are remarkably similar.

Clinical features

- Generalized pallor.
- Ill looking.
- Cold peripheries.
- Poor capillary refill.
- Weak or impalpable pulses.
- Tachycardia and hypotension.
- Cyanosis and mottled skin.
- Tachypnoea and/or laboured breathing.
- Metabolic or mixed acidosis.
- CNS depression and hypotonia.

Management

Resuscitative measures must be instituted before any detailed examination.

1. Improve oxygen delivery to tissues
- Administer oxygen by face mask or bagging.
- Intubate and ventilate if there is severe respiratory distress, respiratory failure or marked acidosis.

2. Improve cardiac performance
- Restore circulating blood volume if hypovolaemic (administer 15–20 ml/kg of 4.5% albumin, FFP, blood or normal saline, then reassess).
- If not hypovolaemic, give a 10 ml/kg volume challenge (colloid or normal saline) to increase venous return.
- Improve myocardial contractility by:
- (a) Correcting acidosis
  Commence artificial ventilation and/or administer $NaHCO_3$ (or THAM) if pH <7.25, and reassess.
- (b) Administering inotropes
  Dopamine infusion (5–20 μg/kg/min) preferably via central line as there is risk of tissue necrosis.
  Adrenaline infusion (0.1–1 μg/kg/min) if in severe shock.

3. Determine the likely cause by reviewing risk factors
- Suspect *infection* in the presence of preceeding temperature instability, fever or hypothermia, long lines, feed

intolerance and respiratory instability (e.g. apnoeas). Promptly institute antibiotics (empirically) following appropriate cultures (blood, urine and CSF).

- Suspect *cardiac cause* in the presence of gallop rhythm, pulse differential (brachial/femoral), cardiomegaly, murmur(s), hepatosplenomegaly, lung crackles or cyanosis. Beware of cardiac tamponade especially with indwelling central lines and muffled heart sounds. Perform echocardiography and remove central line immediately if tamponade is confirmed. Aspirate pericardial effusion.
- Suspect a *pulmonary cause* in the presence of reduced breath sounds (tension pneumothorax), vomitus or blood in oropharynx (aspiration of vomitus or pulmonary haemorrhage), tachypnoea and grunting.
- Suspect *anaphylactic reaction* if drugs and/or blood products have recently been administered or are currently being administered. Discontinue any ongoing parenteral medications or blood products and give adrenaline (1:10 000 at 0.1 ml/kg i.v. – minimum 1 ml). May repeat this after 5 min. Hydrocortisone (5–10 mg/kg i.v.) may be given in a severe reaction. Observe patient over the next 24 hours.
- Suspect *intra-abdominal cause* in the presence of abdominal distension and/or bilious vomiting (NEC ± perforation) – place a nasogastric tube and empty the stomach to decrease risk of aspiration.
- Suspect *adrenal insufficiency* if hyponatraemic, hyperkalaemic, ± hypoglycaemic and dehydrated.

Investigations
- Arterial blood for acid–base balance and blood gases, FBC, coagulation studies, U&E, creatinine and glucose.
- Chest X-ray and abdominal X-ray (with abdominal signs).
- Infection screen (urine, blood, ± CSF culture). LP may be delayed. Remove suspect vascular lines and send tips for culture. Swab any surgical wounds or infected sites.
- Echocardiography (with cardiac signs).
- Cranial ultrasound scan (intracranial haemorrhage).

Further reading

Donn SM, Faix RG (eds). *Neonatal Emergencies*. Mount Kisco, NY: Futura Publishing Co, 1991.

Related topics of interest

SKIN DISORDERS

The skin structure of a full-term neonate is the same as that of an adult, apart from the dermis which is thinner. All four layers of the epidermis are present by 24 weeks gestation but the epidermis is much thinner in preterm infants <34 weeks, in particular the stratum corneum (outer layer). Barrier function is poor with the potential for high water losses and increased absorption of topical applications.

Physiological skin lesions:

- Milia.
- Vernix caseosa.
- Harlequin colour change.
- Cutis marmorata.
- Physiological scaling.
- Sucking blisters.
- Sebaceous gland hyperplasia.
- Lanugo hairs in preterm.

Vesiculopustular lesions The majority of neonatal skin lesions are vesiculopustular and lesions fall into four categories – transient rashes, infections and infestations, genodermatoses and naevoid disorders. The history of appearance and distribution of lesions is helpful in differentiating between these causes.

1. Transient rashes
- *Miliaria.* Due to blockage of the eccrine sweat ducts. If blockage is superficial then clear, thin-walled vesicles (miliaria crystallina) are seen, whereas itchy red papules (miliaria rubra) are present if the blockage is lower down in the epidermis. They are typically seen in the first 2 weeks of life.
- *Erythema toxicum neonatorum.* Present in up to 50% of neonates and typically presents in the first 48 hours of life. Skin lesions range from erythema to urticarial papules and pustules which contain eosinophils. It may recur beyond the first month of life.
- *Transient neonatal pustulosis.* Commoner in neonates with black skins. Superficial fragile pustules containing neutrophils are present at birth and rupture easily (sometimes *in utero*) to leave a pigmented macule with a collarette of scale. Macules may last for 3 months.
- *Infantile acropustulosis.* Presents in the first 3 months of life. Recurrent crops of itchy 1–4 mm vesiculopustules containing neutrophils and sometimes eosinophils are typically seen on the hands and feet. Lesions cease by the second or third year.
- *Eosinophilic pustular folliculitis.* A rare condition with male predominance. Lesions may be present at birth and

come in recurrent crops of white/yellow pruritic papules which tend to affect the scalp, hands and feet.

- *Neonatal acne.* Relatively common, particularly closed comedones on the nose, forehead and cheeks. Open comedones, inflammatory papules and pustules may occur. It tends to resolve within 1–3 months without scarring.

2. *Infections and infestations*
- Bacterial – impetigo, staphylococcal scalded skin syndrome.
- Herpes virus infections – HSV, VZV, CMV.
- Fungal – candida, pityrosporum.
- Parasitic – scabies.

3. *Genodermatoses*
- *Epidermolysis bullosa (autosomal dominant and recessive).* A group of inherited disorders with an abnormal tendency to blister formation. The severity depends on the level of cleavage in the skin.
- *Incontinentia pigmenti (X-linked dominant).* Usually presents in the first few days of life with vesiculobullous lesions. These last for a few weeks and are followed by warty papules. It is usually lethal *in utero* in males.

4. *Naevoid disorders*
(a) Urticaria pigmentosa (mastocytosis)
- Reddish-brown macules which urticate when rubbed may be present shortly after birth. Lesions usually resolve by puberty.
(b) Naevi
- Salmon patches are flat pink lesions present at birth usually on the upper eyelids, glabella or nape of the neck. They gradually fade although 10–20% of those on the neck may persist.
- Port wine stain (naevus flammeus). This deep red/purple lesion is present at birth and does not change with time.
- Strawberry marks are usually not present at birth but develop in the first few weeks, initially as a flat lesion and subsequently becoming raised and red.
- Sebaceous naevus. This is an oval or linear yellow–orange warty lesion typically affecting the scalp. There is a risk of neoplastic change after puberty.
- Giant pigmented naevus (bathing trunk naevus). This extensive brown pigmented naevus is present at birth and carries a risk of malignant melanoma. Treat by dermabrasion in the first week of life.
(c) Congenital ichthyoses
- Collodian baby. The baby is red and covered in a shiny translucent membrane.

- Harlequin fetus. Thick plaques with fissures cover the body surface.

It is important to start treatment without delay. Nurse in a high-humidity incubator and apply a greasy emollient such as white soft paraffin and liquid paraffin in a 50:50 mixture to the skin every 2 hours. Fluid requirements may be as high as 200–250 ml/kg and need close monitoring.

(d) Neonatal lupus erythematosus
- This presents within the first few weeks of life as an erythematous scaly rash, typically around the eyes, and may be associated with heart block. There may be no history of SLE in the mother but there is placental passage of antibodies most commonly anti-Ro (anti-SSA).

(e) Developmental abnormalities
- Aplasia cutis. There is localized absence of skin most commonly affecting the posterior scalp. An ulcer is present at birth and heals slowly with scarring.
- Amniotic band deformities.

Further reading

Harper J. *Handbook of Paediatric Dermatology*, 2nd edn. London: Butterworth-Heinemann, 1990.

Rook A, Wilkinson DS, Ebling FJG, Champion RH, Burton JL (eds). *Textbook of Dermatology*, 5th edn. Oxford: Blackwell Scientific, 1992.

Van Praag MC, Van Rooij RW, Folkers E, Spritzer R, Menke HE, Oranje AP. Diagnosis and treatment of pustular disorders in the neonate. *Paediatric Dermatology*, 1997; **14:** 131–43.

Related topics of interest

STRIDOR

Stridor is the noise produced on inspiration or expiration due to abnormal narrowing of the upper airway (trachea or larynx). Inspiratory stridor is more common. The aetiology is varied, including both congenital and acquired causes. Persistent stridor in the neonatal period requires investigation.

Aetiology

1. Subglottic stenosis. This may result from the trauma of endotracheal intubation especially if prolonged, or may be congenital. Inspiratory and expiratory stridor is present.

2. Laryngomalacia. This is due to floppy aryepiglottic folds and inspiratory stridor predominates and is worsened by lying in a supine position but relieved by lying prone. The cry is normal. This is the least serious of causes and generally improves with growth.

3. Vocal cord palsy. This is associated with respiratory distress, inspiratory stridor and difficulties in feeding.

4. Tracheal compressions. This may be external (e.g. vascular strictures from double aorta or anomalous vessels) or internal (e.g. subglottic haemangiomas and papillomas) producing inspiratory and expiratory stridor. Subglottic haemangiomas commonly co-exist with cutaneous haemangiomas.

5. Miscellaneous. Laryngeal clefts, webs and other rarer congenital malformations may also produce stridor, respiratory distress and feeding difficulties. Some rare disorders, for example Pelizaeus–Merzbacher disease may also be associated with stridor.

Clinical features

- Very mild stridor may not be associated with obvious physical signs.
- Moderate to severe stridor is accompanied by tracheal, sternal and intercostal recession.
- Severe stridor is not influenced by posture.
- Tachycardia may be a sign of impending collapse.
- The obligatory excess respiratory work in moderate to severe stridor may cause failure to thrive.
- Cutaneous capillary haemangiomas may be associated with subglottic haemangiomas.

Investigation

- Pulse oximetry.
- Anterior–posterior chest X-ray and lateral view of neck.
- Barium swallow (vascular rings).
- Fibreoptic laryngoscopy.
- Microlaryngoscopy.
- CT scan (vascular rings).

Management   Laryngomalacia generally improves over time, but where there is serious hypoxaemia, surgery may be required (e.g. supraglottic trimming) but it may be difficult to avoid tracheostomy. Systemic steroids may be used with benefit to treat significant subglottic haemangiomas and post-extubation stridor. Congenital laryngeal and tracheal anomalies may require specialist surgical correction. Vascular rings may require resection or re-arrangement. Rarely, tracheostomy may be required.

Further reading

Chernick V, Boat T. *Kendig's Disorders of the Respiratory Tract in Children*, 6th edn. Philadelphia: W.B. Saunders, 1997.

Dinwiddie R. *The Diagnosis and Management of Paediatric Respiratory Disease*, 2nd edn. Edinburgh: Churchill Livingstone, 1997.

Freeland AP. The laryngologist in the neonatal unit. In: Gray RF, Rutha J (eds). *Recent Advances in Otolaryngology*. Edinburgh: Churchill Livingstone, 1988; 109–24.

Quiney RE, Gould SJ. Subglottic stenosis: a clinicopathological study. *Clinical Otolaryngology*, 1985; **10**: 315–27.

Richardson ME. *Otolaryngology (Pediatric Volume)*, 3rd edn. St. Louis: C.V. Mosby, 1998.

Related topics of interest

Complications of mechanical ventilation (p. 54)
Congenital malformations and birth defects (p. 70)
Intubation (p. 170)
Respiratory distress (p. 275)

SURFACTANT REPLACEMENT THERAPY

In 1980, Fujiwara and co-workers were the first to show a benefit from intra-tracheal surfactant instillation in preterm babies with RDS. They used a modified bovine surfactant; other natural surfactants have been derived from bovine or porcine lungs and human amniotic fluid. Synthetic surfactants are composed mainly of dipalmitoyl phosphatidylcholine (DPPC, or 'lecithin') that lowers surface tension, and a spreading agent such as tyloxapol and hexadecanol or unsaturated phosphatidyl glycerol. Presently they do not contain surfactant proteins.

Early trials of both natural and synthetic surfactants showed a reduction of about 40% in mortality from RDS and a similar reduction in pneumothoraces compared to control babies who did not receive surfactant. The incidence of IVHs is not greatly affected, but PDA, pulmonary haemorrhages and apnoeas are slightly more frequent in surfactant-treated babies. PDA and pulmonary haemorrhages both result from an early lowering of pulmonary vascular resistance, which increases pulmonary flow and left-to-right shunting through the duct and so fills up the pulmonary vasculature. Pulmonary haemorrhage – best thought of as pulmonary haemorrhagic oedema – is seen in about 4% of surfactant-treated babies. Delayed ventilator pressure weaning may help reduce the incidence. Apnoeas occur more frequently as babies come off the ventilator sooner.

After these early studies, further questions were asked about the use of surfactants in babies with respiratory distress. It is now clear that:

- Early treatment with surfactant is better than late.
- Natural surfactants are more effective than synthetic ones.
- Surfactant therapy benefits babies with meconium aspiration. It may also be beneficial in congenital pneumonia, CDH, PPHN, pulmonary haemorrhage, as a transient therapy in infants with congenital deficiency of the surfactant-associated protein SP-B, and in the 'adult' (or 'acute') respiratory distress syndrome (ARDS) where natural surfactants (which contain SP-B and SP-C) may be superior to synthetic surfactants (which do not contain proteins).

The timing of surfactant treatment has been divided into:

1. Prophylactic surfactant given at birth or before respiratory distress develops.
2. Early treatment given as soon as moderate respiratory distress develops in a baby and preset thresholds are passed – e.g. a mean airway pressure of 7 mbar or FiO_2 >40%.
3. Late treatment (rescue therapy) given only when severe RDS is present.

Late treatment is the least effective of these approaches, and is no longer used. The debate now is whether babies at risk should receive surfactant at birth or just as early as possible during respiratory distress, perhaps even being intubated solely for surfactant administration, then extubated and put on nasal prong CPAP if their disease is mild. There is little doubt that preterm babies who receive surfactant within minutes of birth benefit more than those who receive it early in the disease, even if this is only 1–2 hours later. The cost of giving it at birth to all babies of (say) <32 weeks is prohibitive because only 20–40% of the more mature babies in this group would go on to need ventilation and surfactant. They are the most numerous, and also those least likely to die and/or develop chronic lung disease. The clinical benefits and the benefit/cost ratio increase inversely with gestational age, so many units give surfactant at birth only to babies between 23–24 weeks and 27–28 weeks gestation. Others give it to all babies

<32 weeks gestation as soon as they are intubated, whether that is at birth, or some time later if they develop respiratory distress.

Head-to-head trials have compared natural with synthetic surfactants. Compared to those treated with the synthetic surfactant, babies treated with a natural one had odds ratios (OR) of 0.8 for neonatal mortality, 0.86 for the combined end-point of chronic lung disease and death, and 0.53 for pulmonary air leaks (not every commercially available surfactant has been evaluated in such trials). Natural surfactants also act more quickly. This is because of the presence of the surfactant-associated proteins SP-B and SP-C that help in the adsorption and spread of the surfactant. SP-A and SP-D are removed during the extraction process. Both play a role in host defence mechanisms, and SP-A is involved in the local recycling of surfactant. To date, head-to-head clinical trials comparing two natural surfactants with each other (e.g. Survanta™ versus Infasurf™, or Survanta™ versus Curosurf™) have not shown major differences in long-term outcome (e.g. mortality and chronic lung disease) between these preparations.

The phospholipid content of a normal surfactant pool has been estimated to be approximately 100 mg/kg bodyweight. Preterm infants with RDS may have only 5 mg phospholipid per kg. Most surfactant manufacturers recommend doses of 100 mg phospholipid per kg bodyweight suspended in 3–5 ml of saline per kg. Manufacturers' dosing and redosing recommendations have ranged from a relatively restrictive use to a more liberal use (e.g. multiple doses given every 6 hours if the baby remains intubated and requiring >30% oxygen). On average, two to three doses are given, but in conditions characterized by surfactant inactivation, multiple doses may be more effective. Respiratory disease in term infants causes abnormalities in surfactant metabolism. Meconium displaces and inhibits surfactant, and the increased capillary permeability in pneumonia leads to surfactant inactivation by fibrin. Treatment is aimed at reversing or overwhelming this pathology. Optimal dosing schedules for this have yet to be established, but 6-hourly aliquots of 150–200% of the normal dose, starting soon after birth, have been used in some trials.

Further reading

Barrington KJ, Finer NN. Care of near-term infants with respiratory failure. *British Medical Journal*, 1997; **315**: 1215–58.

Findlay RD, Taeusch HW, Walther FJ. Surfactant replacement therapy for meconium aspiration syndrome. *Pediatrics*, 1996; **97**: 48–52.

Fujiwara T, Maeta H, Chida S *et al.* Artificial surfactant therapy in hyaline membrane disease. *Lancet*, 1980; **i**: 55–9.

Halliday HL. Natural versus synthetic surfactants in respiratory distress syndrome. *Drugs*, 1996; **51**: 226–37.

Kattwinkel J. Surfactant: evolving issues. *Clinics in Perinatology*, 1998; **25**: 17–32.

Kattwinkel J, Bloom BT, Delmore P *et al.* Prophylactic administration of calf surfactant extract is more effective than early treatment of respiratory distress syndrome in neonates of 29 through 32 weeks' gestation. *Pediatrics*, 1993; **92**: 90–8.

Long W (ed). Surfactant replacement therapy. *Clinics in Perinatology*, 1993; **20(4)**.

Morley CJ. Systematic review of prophylactic versus rescue surfactant. *Archives of Disease in Childhood, Fetal and Neonatal Edition*, 1997; **77**: F70–4.

Robertson B. New targets for surfactant therapy: experimental and clinical aspects. *Archives of Disease in Childhood, Fetal and Neonatal Edition*, 1996; **75**: F1–3.

Related topics of interest

Mechanical ventilation (p. 185)
Meconium aspiration syndrome (p. 189)
Persistent pulmonary hypertension of the newborn (p. 237)
Pulmonary haemorrhage (p. 259)
Respiratory distress syndrome (p. 278)

SURGICAL EMERGENCIES

In a minority of deliveries, the newborn infant may require acute life-saving intervention for cardio-respiratory support or immediate and rapid assessment for a variety of congenital anatomical defects that require urgent attention. The greatest assets in dealing with any infant with a problem in the immediate newborn period are anticipation and a team approach. Anticipation of a problem is commonly based on antenatal diagnosis by ultrasonography. When there is ample warning before the delivery, the assembled team can best decide on the timing, route and site of delivery. Infants with complex congenital defects will require transfer to a tertiary paediatric surgical centre. Maternal transfer to an appropriate maternity unit facilitates the infant's postnatal care. Despite all the advances in antenatal diagnosis, some newborn infants may still be found to have unexpected anomalies requiring urgent surgical attention. In addition, previously well neonates may also develop acute medical disorders requiring urgent surgical attention.

Conditions presenting at birth

Abdominal wall defects

- Gastroschisis.
- Ectopia vesicae.

Management
- Cover the defect(s) with dry sterile dressing and/or plastic covering (e.g. cling film).
- Obtain venous access and administer colloid to support the circulation – if necessary.
- Administer an infusion of 10% dextrose to maintain normal blood glucose.
- Obtain blood from infant and mother for blood grouping and cross-matching.
- Refer to a paediatric surgical service.

Anomalies of the gastrointestinal tract

- Oesophageal atresia.
- TOF.
- Small bowel obstruction (e.g. duodenal or ileal atresia) with or without perforation.

Management
- Withhold oral feeds.
- Obtain venous access and maintain normal blood glucose by administering an infusion of 10% dextrose.
- Nasogastric suctioning to decompress the stomach and constant oropharyngeal suctioning to clear pharyngeal secretions (oesophageal atresia).
- Obtain maternal and infant's blood for grouping and cross-matching.
- Refer to a paediatric surgical service.

Urological anomalies

- Posterior urethral valves.
- Severe bilateral hydronephrosis.
- Ureteric rupture and urinary ascites.
- Bilateral pelvi-ureteric junction/vesico-ureteric junction obstruction.

Management
- Confirm prenatal findings with postnatal ultrasound scan.
- Catheterize infants suspected of having posterior urethral valves.
- Obtain urgent MCUG and refer to paediatric urologist.
- For suspected bilateral pelvi-ureteric/vesico-ureteric junction obstruction and ureteric rupture, refer immediately to a paediatric urologist. Commence prophylactic i.v. antibiotics.

Cardiac anomalies

As most of these anomalies are not diagnosed until referral to a specialist paediatric cardiology centre, early referral to such a centre is therefore desirable. A handful of lesions require early surgical intervention if chances of survival are to be enhanced. The main conditions are:

- HLHS.
- Coarctation of the aorta/interrupted aortic arch.
- Obstructed total anomalous pulmonary venous drainage.
- TGA with intact ventricular septum.
- Pulmonary atresia with intact ventricular septum.
- Complex congenital heart lesions.
- Tricuspid atresia.

It is essential to commence a PGE_1 infusion (0.05–0.1 μg/kg/min) in infants suspected of having duct-dependent lesions at the earliest opportunity. Correct metabolic acidosis and commence treatment for heart failure (if present) with diuretics (e.g. frusemide 1–2 mg/kg/dose). Intubation and mechanical ventilation may be necessary. Once the infant is stabilized, transfer to a paediatric cardiac centre.

Specific disorders

1. Congenital diaphragmatic hernia. If previously diagnosed antenatally, avoid bagging to prevent aeration and expansion of intrathoracic bowel. Intubate immediately at birth. Proceed to surgery when the infant has stabilized (see 'Congenital diaphragmatic hernia').

2. Torsion of the testes. This is a real emergency as the affected testis must be operated on within a few hours or it becomes non-viable. The affected testis is higher, often larger and, if recently twisted, very tender. This may occur prenatally, in which case the enlarged bluish testis is non-tender. Urgent exploration is required to untwist the testis, if still viable, or orchidectomy, if non-viable, with orchidopexy being performed on the contralateral side.

Conditions presenting later

These are mainly gastrointestinal in nature and are summarized below:

- Intra-abdominal perforation with peritonitis.
- Strangulated hernias (inguinal, femoral).
- NEC.
- Volvulus.

Occasionally a variety of other acute medical conditions may arise and require an urgent surgical input. These include acute thromboembolic phenomena, accidents with vascular lines (e.g. snapped central intravascular lines with a retained distal portion), major subdural haemorrhages, serious post-operative wound dehiscence, and serious accidental injuries.

Management
- Commence nasogastric drainage to decompress the abdomen.
- Withhold oral feeds and commence infusion of a dextrose electrolyte to maintain normal blood glucose.
- Administer analgesia as a continuous i.v. infusion whenever infants are, or are likely to be, in pain.
- If surgery is likely to result in significant blood losses, obtain infant's blood for grouping and cross-matching.
- Administer colloid to support the circulation (where necessary).
- Unless an expert opinion is already available on site, transfer to an appropriate paediatric surgical service.

Further reading

Black JA, Whitfield MF. *Neonatal Emergencies: Early Detection and Management*, 2nd edn. Oxford: Butterworth-Heinemann, 1991.
King LR. *Urologic Surgery in Infants and Children*. Philadelphia: W.B. Saunders, 1998.
O'Neill Jr JA, Rowe MI, Grosfeld JL, Fonkelsrud EW, Coran A. *Pediatric Surgery*, 5th edn. St Louis: Mosby, 1998.

Related topics of interest

Congenital diaphragmatic hernia (p. 57)
Herniae (p. 108)

Necrotizing enterocolitis (p. 195)
Neonatal surgery (p. 200)

THERMOREGULATION

Thermoregulation is the ability to maintain a normal body temperature in varying environmental conditions and temperatures. When these protective homeostatic mechanisms are overcome, body temperature rises or falls outside the normal range. The thermal stresses a baby may have to deal with include:

- Excessive cooling from evaporation, radiation, convection and conduction.
- Excessive heating from high environmental temperatures and humidity, radiant heaters and over-wrapping.

Cooling

There is a clearly established relationship between hypothermia and increased mortality and morbidity, and prompt attention to temperature control is mandatory. Hypoxia reduces the ability of the baby to respond to a cold stress, so the asphyxiated baby and/or the baby with respiratory distress are at particular risk. Evaporation of amniotic fluid from the skin of a newborn baby is a common cause of cooling immediately after birth, even in tropical environments or warm rooms. Such evaporation can drop a term baby's temperature as much as 2°C in 15 min. Rapid drying and wrapping reduce this fall, but many commercially available radiant heaters will not. Heat is radiated from a naked baby who is a 'hot spot' radiating heat to its cooler surroundings. Significant radiant heat loss occurs from the head, so dressing a baby includes putting a hat on. Convective and conductive heat losses in a dressed baby are minimal, providing bedding and clothes are at body temperature when put on, and the baby is not in a draught, which would also increase evaporative cooling.

Preterm and small-for-dates babies are particularly prone to hypothermia because of their:

- High surface area to body size ratio.
- Lack of subcutaneous adipose tissue that helps insulate the body.
- Poor energy stores and limited brown fat deposits.

Babies respond to cooling with:

- Reduction of heat loss by peripheral vasoconstriction and the assumption of the fetal position to reduce the exposed surface area.
- Extra heat production. This involves the release of noradrenaline that acts locally in the brown fat deposits to stimulate lipolysis and hence heat production. For this to be successful there must be adequate oxygenation of the tissues and a good circulation. Glucose will also be metabolized for heat production and hypoglycaemia must

therefore be avoided. Newborn infants cannot warm themselves through shivering.

Thermoneutrality

A baby with a normal temperature who is trying neither to increase heat production, nor to increase heat loss, is said to be in a *thermoneutral* environment. Incubators should therefore be capable of providing a thermoneutral environment for a range of babies at different ages. The environment must be defined not just in terms of temperature but also humidity, convection (draughts) and surrounding radiant heat sources. A well, week-old, 3.5 kg baby needs lower environmental temperatures than a small, extremely preterm one on the first day, when temperatures in excess of 37°C and high humidity in a draught-free environment may be necessary if the baby is naked.

Over-heating

Larger babies can become overheated under phototherapy lamps, radiant heaters, inside closed incubators or if over-wrapped in a warm room. As best their circumstances allow, they will respond to this by:

- Increased heat loss through peripheral vasodilatation and increasing the exposed surface area by adopting a 'sun-bathing' posture.
- Sweating. However, term babies are able to achieve only a modest increase in cooling through sweating – much less than children or adults – and preterm babies have even more limited sweating. If the child is over-swaddled, then the response to heat stress can be very limited and the baby becomes hyperthermic.
- Panting. This limited response to heat stress which persists for some weeks after birth, together with the inability to wriggle free of bedclothes and clothing, contributes to the risk of cot-death in over-swaddled babies.

Further reading

Brück K. Neonatal thermal regulation. In: Polin R, Fox WW (eds). *Fetal and Neonatal Physiology,* 2nd edn. Philadelphia: W.B. Saunders, 1998; 676–702.

Okken A, Koch J (eds). *Thermoregulation of Sick and Low-birthweight Neonates.* Berlin: Springer, 1995.

Sinclair JC. Management of the thermal environment. In: Sinclair JC, Bracken MB (eds). *Effective Care of the Newborn Infant.* Oxford: Oxford University Press, 1992; 40–58.

Related topics of interest

TRACE MINERALS AND VITAMINS

Eight trace minerals are nutritionally essential for humans: chromium, copper, iodine, iron, manganese, molybdenum, selenium and zinc. They play vital roles in several metabolic pathways. Clinical deficiencies have been described for six of the minerals. As accretion of trace minerals occurs during the last trimester of pregnancy, prematurity is associated with low stores at birth and the premature infant is at increased risk of developing trace mineral deficiencies.

Chromium

Chromium is involved in glucose homeostasis and this is the only biological role postulated for this micromineral. Chromium deficiency has not been described in infants. Human milk has 0.3–0.5 µg chromium/l and the chromium content of preterm human milk is unknown. The recommended enteral chromium intake is 0.1–0.5 µg/kg/day, and 0.05–0.2 µg/kg/day (0.2 µg/kg/day in the preterm infant) parenterally. There are no data to justify intakes higher than that received by the breast-fed infant.

Copper

Copper is contained in several enzymes including cytochrome oxidase and is required for connective tissue formation, myelinization and iron utilization. The most abundant copper-containing enzymes are the superoxide dismutase enzymes, which protect cell membranes against oxidative injury. Caeruloplasmin, representing 60% of the copper in plasma and the interstitial fluids, is a weak oxidase and primarily transports copper from its storage sites in the liver and muscles. Deficiency state (copper <40 µg/dl and caeruloplasmin <15 mg/dl) is associated with hypotonia, osteoporosis and fractures, pallor, sideroblastic anaemia resistant to iron therapy, neutropenia, decreased pigmentation of skin and hair, failure to thrive, diarrhoea, hepatosplenomegaly, skin rashes akin to seborrhoeic dermatitis, psychomotor retardation and lack of visual responses.

Therapy is with 1% copper sulphate solution giving 0.6–0.8 mg copper/kg/day. The copper content of early preterm mother's milk is 0.8 mg/l, falling to 0.6 mg/l by 4 weeks. Formula feeds contain 0.01–1.4 mg copper/l. The recommended enteral copper intake for term and preterm infants is 120–150 µg/kg/day, and 20 µg/kg/day parenterally. Withhold copper in the presence of cholestasis.

Iodine

Iodine is essential for normal thyroid function. Iodine deficiency depresses the production of thyroid hormones especially thyroxine. In geographic regions where dietary iodine is <15 µg/kg/day, endemic goitre may occur. Endemic cretinism may result from maternal iodine deficiency, with 5–15% of cases of endemic neonatal goitres developing overt cretinism. Preterm infants are more susceptible to both iodine deficiency and excess due to impaired compensatory mechanisms. Such infants may also absorb excess iodine through their skin from povidone-iodine- and alcohol-iodine-containing skin-cleansing agents. Bovine milk-based formulas contain 50 µg iodine/l, preterm formulas 50–146 µg/l and breast milk 70–90 µg/l. The recommended enteral iodine intake is 30–60 µg/kg/day with a parenteral intake of 1.0 µg/kg/day (both term and preterm infants). Based on these recommendations, an exclusively breast-fed preterm infant should receive iodine supplementation as their intakes would fall below the 30 µg/kg/day lower limit.

Iron

The total body iron is ~75 mg/kg which is the same for term and preterm infants. Iron is present in the fetus as haemoglobin iron, tissue iron (myoglobin and iron-containing enzymes) and storage iron (as ferritin and haemosiderin in the liver and spleen). The iron content of human milk falls from 1 mg/l to <0.5 mg/l during the first 6 months of lactation, but iron levels in preterm breast milk are similar to those in term breast milk. Iron absorption and utilization is better with human milk than with bovine milk or formula milk. Consequently, exclusively breast-fed term infants do not require iron supplementation for the first 6 months of life, whereas formula-fed infants are commonly started on iron-enriched formula from birth. VLBW infants remain iron replete until their birthweight has doubled, commonly at age 2 months. The recommended iron supplementation dose is 2 mg/kg/day up to a maximum of 15 mg/day, which should be started at 4–8 weeks in preterm infants and continued for the rest of the first year. If total parenteral nutrition is provided exclusively for the first 2 months of life, parenteral iron will be required at 0.1–0.2 mg/kg/day.

Manganese

Manganese deficiency has not been described in humans. It acts as an activator of the gluconeogenic enzymes pyruvate carboxylase and isocitrate dehydrogenase, protects mitochondrial membranes through superoxide dismutase (a manganese-containing enzyme), and activates glycosyl transferase which takes part in mucopolysaccharide synthesis. Preterm infants may be at increased risk of toxicity. The manganese content of human milk is ~5 µg/l with formula milks containing 0–340 µg/l. The recommended enteral manganese intake for term and preterm infants is 0.75–7.5 µg/kg/day, and 1.0 µg/kg/day parenterally.

Molybdenum

In mammals, molybdenum is essential for the function of three enzymes: aldehyde, xanthine and sulphite oxidases. Sulphite oxidase is required for the disposal and excretion of sulphur, while xanthine oxidase is required for the terminal oxidation of purines and their excretion as uric acid. Molybdenum deficiency has not been described in preterm infants. The molybdenum content of human milk is $\sim 2\,\mu g/l$ but the molybdenum content of preterm milk is not known. The recommended enteral molybdenum intake for term and preterm infants is $0.3\,\mu g/kg/day$, and $0.25\,\mu g/kg/day$ parenterally (but only when on long-term total parenteral nutrition).

Selenium

The only established physiological role of selenium is as an integral part of the selenium-dependent enzyme glutathione peroxidase. Selenium protects cell membranes from peroxidase damage through detoxification of peroxides and free radicals. Selenium and vitamin E have overlapping functions. Deficiency produces myopathy, cardiac failure and haemolytic anaemia. Clinical selenium deficiency has not been described in the preterm infant although a biochemical deficiency occurs. Low hepatic selenium stores at birth predispose the preterm infant to deficiency. The selenium content of mature human milk is $20\,\mu g/l$ (falling to $15\,\mu g/l$ by 3–6 months), while colostrum contains twice as much selenium. Preterm human milk contains $24\,\mu g$ selenium/l, while formula milks contain $7–14\,\mu g/l$. The recommended enteral selenium intake for preterm infants is $1.3–3\,\mu g/kg/day$ (breast-fed infants receive $\sim 3\,\mu g/kg/day$). The recommended parenteral selenium intake is $1.5–2.0\,\mu g/kg/day$ ($2\,\mu g/kg/day$ for the preterm infant). Parenteral intake should be reduced in infants with renal impairment.

Zinc

Zinc is essential for humans, playing especially important roles in cell growth and development. It is found in 200 metalloenzymes including RNA and DNA polymerase, alkaline phosphatase, erythrocyte carbonic anhydrase and several other enzymes associated with haem synthesis, protein metabolism and carbohydrate and energy metabolism. It is essential for cell division and for insulin activity. The normal plasma zinc level is $>70\,\mu g/dl$. Zinc is better absorbed from human milk than from bovine or formula milk. Colostrum has a high zinc content. The zinc content of formula milk is higher than that of human milk. Excretion is via faeces except in the parenterally fed infant where the primary excretory route is renal.

Clinical zinc deficiency is manifest by decreased appetite, failure to thrive, hair loss, poor wound healing, skin lesions and depressed immunity. Plasma zinc levels and alkaline phosphatase activity are subnormal. A deficiency state acrodermatitis enteropathica (autosomal recessive) due to defective zinc absorption leads to a scaling pustular/erythematous rash around the mouth, ears, fingers, toes and anogenital region, diarrhoea and failure to thrive with low plasma zinc. Therapy is with zinc sulphate, 1–3.5 mg zinc/day. The recommended enteral zinc intake is 1 mg/kg/day (720–1400 µg/kg/day for preterm infants), and 400 µg/kg/day parenterally.

Vitamins

1. Vitamin A. This is required for synthesis of rhodopsin and other retinal pigments and also for maintenance of epithelial membranes. It is degraded by light and is stored in the liver with tightly regulated excretion, bound to retinol-binding protein. Deficiency may predispose to chronic lung disease, susceptibility to infection, xeropthalmia and blindness. An excess produces irritability, brittle bones, dry skin, loss of hair and raised intracranial pressure. The recommended intake of vitamin A in term infants is 333 IU/kg/day and 1500–2800 IU/kg/day (450–840 µg/kg/day) in preterm infants.

2. Pyridoxine (B6). Pyridoxine serves as a cofactor for several reactions involved in the synthesis, interconversion (e.g. transamination and decarboxylation) and catabolism of amino acids. Deficiency causes convulsions, weakness, anaemia and dermatitis. The recommended oral intake is 150 µg/100 kcal with the parenteral intake being 1.0 mg/day (term infants) and 0.18 mg/kg/day (preterm infants).

3. Vitamin C. Has a role in collagen synthesis and amino acid metabolism, catecholamine synthesis, carnitine synthesis, iron absorption and it protects against hyperphenylalaninaemia and hypertyrosinaemia in the newborn period. A supplement of 200 µg/day is recommended.

4. Vitamin D. Natural vitamin D (D_2 from plants or D_3 synthesized in the skin) is converted to 25-hydroxyvitamin D (25-OHD) in the liver and then in the kidney into the active metabolite 1,25-dihydroxyvitamin D (1,25-$(OH)_2D$) which increases calcium and phosphorus absorption from the gut. Preterm infants have lower stores of vitamin D at birth and a greater need for skeletal mineralization. With adequate phosphorus and calcium, 400–600 IU vitamin D/day should suffice.

5. Vitamin E. The generic term for a number of tocopherol compounds. It is an antioxidant which inhibits the naturally occurring peroxidation of cell membrane polyunsaturated fatty acids by scavenging free radicals. The physiological effects of vitamin E include facilitation of normal phagocytosis, haem synthesis and prevention of anaemia. The proposed pharmacological effects have included the prevention of retinopathy of prematurity, IVH and BPD, but these remain unproven. High doses produce toxicity and may be associated with sepsis and NEC. Preterm infants should receive 5–25 IU/day oral vitamin E.

6. *Vitamin K.* This is required in the synthesis of clotting factors II, VII, IX and X by the liver. A single dose of 1 mg i.m. (0.5 mg for preterm infants) is protective against haemorrhagic disease (vitamin K deficiency bleeding, VKDB). If given by mouth for VKDB, two oral doses of 2 mg in the first week is enough for formula-fed babies, but for those exclusively breast-fed a third dose of 2 mg is given at 1 month of age.

7. *Folic acid (pteroylglutamic acid).* A water-soluble vitamin that functions as a coenzyme donor and acceptor of one-carbon units in nucleotide and amino acid metabolism. It is required by enzyme systems which synthesize RNA, DNA and some amino acids (e.g. serine). Deficiency produces neutrophil hypersegmentation, megaloblastic changes, poor growth (disturbed DNA synthesis may alter cell division in several tissues), and in severe cases macrocytic anaemia and hypotonia. The human milk content of folate increases with advancing lactation, averaging 50 µg/l (range 26–141 µg/l). The recommended dietary allowance for folic acid is 25 µg/day for infants from birth to 6 months. For VLBW infants, an enteral intake of 25–50 µg/kg/day is recommended until 40 weeks post-conceptional age, whereupon 4 µg/100 kcal (the minimal recommended intake for term infants) should suffice. Preterm infants fed on preterm formulas and term formula-fed infants on at least 150 ml/kg/day should meet their daily requirements. However, preterm infants fed human milk may benefit from folate supplementation of at least 50 µg/day. The recommended parenteral folic acid intake is 56 µg/kg/day for preterm infants and 140 µg/kg/day for term infants.

Further reading

Greene HL, Hambidge KM, Schandler R, Tsang RC. Guidelines for the use of vitamins, trace elements, calcium, magnesium, and phosphorus in infants and children receiving total parenteral nutrition. Report of the Subcommittee on Pediatric Parenteral Nutrient Requirements from the Committee on Clinical Practice Issues of the American Society of Clinical Nutrition. *American Journal of Clinical Nutrition*, 1988; **48**: 1324–42.

Litov RE, Combs GF. Selenium in pediatric nutrition. *Pediatrics*, 1991; **87**: 339–52.

Specker BL, DeMarini S, Tsang RC. Vitamin and mineral supplementation. In: Sinclair JC, Bracken MB (eds). *Effective Care of the Newborn Infant*. Oxford: Oxford University Press, 1992; 162–77.

Tsang RC, Lucas A, Uauy R, Zlotkin S (eds). *Nutritional Needs of the Preterm Infant: Scientific Basis and Practical Guidelines*. Baltimore: Williams & Wilkins, 1993.

Related topics of interest

Bronchopulmonary dysplasia (p. 38)
Fluid and electrolyte therapy (p. 87)
Neonatal surgery (p. 200)
Nutrition (p. 221)

TRANSFUSION OF BLOOD AND BLOOD PRODUCTS

Sick preterm infants frequently require blood transfusions in the first weeks of life due to significant cumulative losses from repeated blood sampling. In preterm infants, the amount of blood loss may easily equal or exceed the infant's circulating blood volume. Older preterm infants often require transfusion at a later time for anaemia of prematurity. Large acute blood losses or cumulative chronic losses in the mature infant may also require transfusion to replace the blood volume. In the immediate newborn period, transfusions aim to bring the haemoglobin back to the original normal level, while in the later period the haemoglobin is maintained at 12–14 g/dl (PCV ≥40%). While blood transfusion has been made considerably simpler and safer, it still carries some risks for the infant.

Indications for early transfusion
- Significant anaemia at birth.
- Significant acute haemorrhage.
- Iatrogenic blood losses (cumulative sampling losses for diagnostic purposes).
- Exchange transfusion.
- Prenatal haematological disorders (e.g. rhesus isoimmunization).

Indications for late transfusion
- Symptomatic anaemia of any cause (producing tachycardia, apnoeas, feeding difficulties and poor weight gain).
- Surgery with significant blood loss.
- Severe sepsis.
- Severe NEC.

Requirements for neonatal blood transfusion
- Blood used should have been screened for infection with CMV, HIV, HBV and hepatitis C virus (HCV).
- Blood and blood products should also be free from bacterial infection (approximately 16% of transfusion fatalities reported by the United States FDA between 1986 and 1991 were due to bacterial contamination).
- Use of small subunits derived from one pack (octopus or satellite units) is encouraged to reduce donor exposure.
- In immediate newborn period, maternal blood is required to ensure compatibility.
- For massive transfusions (e.g. ECMO or exchange transfusion) fresh whole blood less than 48 hours old or reconstituted whole blood (washed packed red cells and FFP) is required.

Potential complications
- Hematomas from extravasation of blood during transfusion.
- Metabolic acidosis from large transfusions with stored blood (blood pH falls with storage).
- Hypocalcaemia and hypomagnesaemia (citrate binding in citrate phosphate dextrose (CPD) or CPDA-1 units).

- Hypernatraemia (high sodium of blood stored in CPD).
- Hyperkalaemia (serum potassium rises in stored blood).
- Heart failure from rapid or large-volume transfusions.
- Hypothermia from transfusing blood directly out of the refrigerator (4–6 °C), and also apnoea, hypotension and hypoglycaemia.
- Mechanical haemolysis due to passage of erythrocytes through fine cannulae (or peristaltic infusion pump!).
- Transmission of infection (HIV, CMV, HBV, HCV, malaria, syphilis and other bacterial infections).
- Sensitization to red cell antigens (older infants).
- Transfusion reaction due to incompatible blood.
- Transfusion-associated graft-versus-host disease (TA-GVHD) – rare but rapidly fatal with a mortality >90% (may be prevented in infants receiving large transfusions by irradiating the blood prior to transfusion which inactivates the T lymphocytes responsible for TA-GVHD).

Transfusion reactions

There are two important serological differences between infants and older children or adults. First, infants have IgG antibodies derived from the maternal circulation which gradually decline during the first few months of life. Second, infants have a poor response to antigenic challenges such as allogenic red cell antigens. Thus when transfused with red cells that differ from their own, infants do not respond by making alloantibodies until after the third month of life. Any antibodies detected in a newborn's blood sample are maternal in origin. Therefore, if an infant's initial antibody screen is negative, blood of an appropriate blood group can be issued to the infant without the need for further typing or cross-matching for the first 3 months of life.

Transfusion reactions are therefore relatively rare in the newborn period, but when they occur they may be life-threatening. A transfusion reaction may be immediate or occur after several days or weeks. Immediate reactions include fever (often due to antileucocyte antibodies), allergic reactions (anaphylaxis or urticaria), acute haemolysis and a haemorrhagic state. Delayed reactions include the development of haemolysis and sensitization to red cell antigens, making later cross-matching more difficult and predisposing the infant to more transfusion reactions. An acute haemolytic reaction due to incompatible blood is serious as it can result in acute renal failure and DIC. Symptoms include fever, bleeding and shock. The transfusion must be discontinued, blood bank notified and the blood pack returned to the blood bank along with 3–5 ml of the infant's blood (clotted sample), and BP and urine output should be monitored. Treat shock, if present, appropriately (see

'Shock'). The vast majority of transfusion reactions are due to clerical errors and can therefore be avoided by careful double-checks. Note that acute haemolytic transfusion reactions *do not* occur in the very young infants. They also do not manifest delayed haemolytic transfusion reactions as they do not produce antibodies to allogenic erythrocytes. Isohaemagglutinins (the naturally occurring antibodies against other blood groups), which are responsible for acute haemolytic transfusion reactions, are detectable in <50% of infants at age 6 months.

Donor–recipient blood group compatibility

Infant's blood group	Compatible donor red cells	Compatible donor plasma
O	O	AB, O, A, B
A	O, A	AB, A
B	O, B	AB, B
AB	O, A, B, AB	AB

Special considerations

Occasionally, strongly held parental beliefs against the transfusion of blood or blood products make for potentially difficult management, particularly in the very preterm infant. Where possible it is desirable to be mindful of the parents' wishes, as the parents will assume the care of the infant following discharge from the unit. Blood sampling for diagnostic purposes should be reduced to the minimum. Erythropoietin administration reduces the need for late transfusions. Where the need for a blood transfusion is overwhelming and parents still object to a blood transfusion, it may be necessary to initiate legal proceedings, making the infant a ward of court. See 'Special note', p. 326.

Other blood products

1. *Human albumin.* This may be used to support the circulating blood volume at 10–20 ml/kg (4.5% albumin), or for dilutional exchange (20–30 ml/kg). In oedematous states, 25% salt-poor albumin may be used to increase the plasma oncotic pressure. Some 4 ml of 25% salt-poor albumin provides 1 g of albumin.

2. *Fresh frozen plasma.* FFP may be used for supporting the circulating blood volume (10–20 ml/kg), treating haemorrhagic states (e.g. DIC, vitamin K deficiency) and for dilutional exchange (20–30 ml/kg).

3. *Cryoprecipitate.* This is used to replace clotting factors and correct bleeding states including fibrinogen deficiency (or fibrinogen <1 g/l). It may therefore be used in haemophilia A,

von Willebrand's disease and dysfibrinogenaemia. A unit or bag is sufficient for an infant. An average of 80 units of factor VIII activity is present in each 5–10 ml bag.

4. Platelet concentrate. One unit of platelets (30–50 ml/unit) raises the platelet count by 50 000. Give platelets to correct life-threatening bleeding or severe thrombocytopenia (platelet count <20 000/mm³), as one unit of platelets, or give up to 20 ml/kg.

Special note: All blood-products carry the theoretical risk of transmitting infection (and currently in the UK, new variant Creutzfeldt–Jakob disease, nvCJD). To August 1998, there had been 27 recorded deaths from nvCJD. The issue of plasma product safety arose when three of the first 23 nvCJD victims were identified as blood donors. This theoretical risk may be reduced by using plasma products from populations not affected by nvCJD (e.g. USA). A recent estimate of the risk of infection from transfusion of a unit of blood derived from a repeat whole blood donor gave a risk of 1 in 64 000 for HBV, 1 in 103 000 for HCV, and 1 in 493 000 for HIV (US data).

A recent report has suggested an increased risk of mortality in critically ill patients who received human albumin for hypovolaemia or hypoalbuminaema.

Further reading

Cohen AC, Manno C. Transfusion practices in infants receiving assisted ventilation. *Clinics in Perinatology*, 1998; **25:** 97–111.
Dolan G. Blood and blood product transfusion. In: Lilleyman JS, Hann IM (eds). *Paediatric Haematology*. Edinburgh: Churchill Livingstone, 1992; 431–56.
Hann IM, Gibson BES, Letsky EA (eds). *Fetal and Neonatal Haematology*. London: Baillière Tindall, 1991.
McClelland DBL (ed). *Handbook of Transfusion Medicine*, 2nd edn. London: HMSO Publications, 1996.
Nathan G, Orkin SH. *Nathan and Oski's Hematology of Infancy and Childhood*, 5th edn. Philadelphia: W.B. Saunders, 1997.
Vengelen-Tyler V (ed). *Technical Manual of the American Association of Blood Banks*, 12th edn. Arlington: American Association of Blood Banks, 1995.

Related topics of interest

Anaemia (p. 9)
Bleeding disorders (p. 25)
Blood pressure (p. 34)

Neonatal surgery (p. 200)
Shock (p. 302)

TRANSPORT OF SICK NEONATES

Of the approximately 150 million infants currently born each year worldwide, the vast majority have no access to the level of neonatal care that they may require. Some infants may therefore require transfer to centralized or regional centres for specialized care. These include preterm infants, newborns with cardiac or surgical problems, and those with complex congenital malformations. In the UK, approximately 1% of all births (i.e. 10 000 infants) may require transfer in the neonatal period. Furthermore, 1 in 10 attempts to transfer may be unsuccessful due to lack of space (the majority being for infants of birthweight <1500 g). Infants declined admission to centres offering a more appropriate level of care have a higher morbidity and mortality. However, inter-hospital transportation of high-risk infants is also fraught with potential dangers and complications which may further increase morbidity or mortality. It is now accepted that infants transferred under controlled conditions with skilled assistance have a reduced morbidity and mortality and have reduced requirements for intensive care. When time permits, the transfer of the pregnant mother to a more appropriate perinatal centre is associated with a more favourable neonatal outcome. However, transfer *in utero* with a mother in early labour is associated with increased risk of obstetric and maternal complications, including the unplanned delivery of an infant during transit. Neonatal transportation is therefore a serious undertaking, the success of which requires skilled personnel, appropriate equipment, good communication and organization. The goal of neonatal transport is to provide outborn infants with the same quality of care during transit as they would receive in a level III neonatal unit.

Equipment for neonatal transport

The equipment used for neonatal transport should meet the needs of VLBW infants through to the large term infants with surgical or medical problems. It should be easy to operate, light, robust and securely mounted to the transport system. There should be a reliable battery providing ample back-up power for all vital equipment.

1. Transport incubator. This should be double-walled and able to provide a stable thermal environment despite variations in external temperature.

2. Ventilator. This should be simple to use yet reliable and preferably designed for transport use. It should allow visualization of the ventilator settings being used, and the oxygen concentration being delivered.

3. Drug and fluid administration equipment. The 50 ml syringe pump devices are probably the most appropriate and three to six may be needed.

4. Pulse oximeter.

5. Oxygen analyser.

6. Suction devices. These should preferably be battery operated and with adjustable pressure.

7. Emergency equipment. For intubation, needle aspiration of the chest and chest drain insertion along with Heimlich valves, hand ventilation, cannulation for i.v. access, a portable cold-light source and standard resuscitation drugs.

8. Medications. Some neonatal units may not have the following medications available at all times and it is preferable for the transport team to carry their own supplies: these include plasma, surfactant, dobutamine, dopamine, morphine, pancuronium, midazolam, and PGE_1 or PGE_2.

9. Mobile telephone. This may be very helpful in case of difficulties in transit.

Stabilization before transportation

The cornerstones of ideal neonatal transportation are the maintenance of an optimal temperature and normal or near-normal physiological parameters and the minimization of unexpected adverse events. For a smooth transfer requiring minimal intervention *en route*, the infant *must be* stabilized before departure. Stabilization is the correction or treatment of processes that, left unaltered, may lead to a deterioration in the infant's status. Infants transferred after adequate stabilization have a lower morbidity and mortality. Stabilization should assess the adequacy of gas exchange and oxygenation, circulation (perfusion and BP), thermoregulation, acid–base balance and metabolic control.

Checks before departure

- Secure airway and check position of endotracheal tube by radiographs.
- Assess adequacy of ventilation by the transport equipment by performing arterial blood gases prior to departure. If surfactant has been administered, wait for at least 30 min before performing arterial blood gases to determine the need to reduce ventilatory support before the transfer.
- Assess adequacy of intravascular access sites and set up 'reserve' access sites if necessary.
- Check that BP and blood glucose are satisfactory.
- Ensure infant is well covered, insulated and warm, leaving only part of the face exposed for monitoring.
- Ensure analgesia and sedation will be adequate during transport.
- Collect all the relevant maternal and infant historical data and results of recent laboratory and radiological investigations.
- Inform your intended destination of your departure so that the receiving team are prepared for the infant, specifying any preparations which may be required in advance.

During transportation

- Use full remote monitoring of temperature, heart rate, oxygen saturation and BP.
- Avoid opening the incubator and exposing the infant to cold air.

- Ensure ambulance cabin heating and lighting are adequate.
- Depending on the duration of the trip (e.g. ≥ 2 hours) or the occurrence of adverse events, additional monitoring (e.g. blood glucose measurements) may be required.

Checks on arrival

- Take infant's temperature and re-warm if hypothermic.
- Perform arterial blood gases and adjust ventilation and/or correct significant metabolic acidosis accordingly.
- Check BP and augment it if necessary.
- Check blood glucose and correct hypoglycaemia if present.

Transport of infants <1000 g birthweight

As these infants have a greater morbidity and mortality, their safe transport requires greater vigilance and proficiency of the transporting team. Most of these infants will require assisted ventilation during transfer and they are more likely to deteriorate during transportation. They are more vulnerable to cold stress, hypoglycaemia and endotracheal tube blockage (due to narrow tube size 2–2.5 mm). When contemplating the transfer of extremely preterm infants (22–24 weeks gestation) and the outcome appears unfavourable, it may be preferable for the baby to stay with his/her parents and not undergo transfer and ultimately die in transit or in a distant hospital away from the parents.

Transport of surgical newborns

Four out of five infants requiring surgery in the newborn period are stable term infants, and most commonly have an abnormality of the gastrointestinal tract. The essentials of successful transfer remain the same but with the following additional requirements.

- Stabilization before transport is vital. This will include placement of a nasogastric tube for decompression of the stomach (especially in the presence of intestinal obstruction), prevention or correction of hypothermia, provision of i.v. fluids to prevent hypoglycaemia and replace abnormal fluid losses, securing the airway (ventilation may be required in ~15% of cases) and adequate dressing for exposed viscera (e.g. gastroschisis).
- All the relevant records including results of laboratory investigations and X-rays should accompany the infant.
- A maternal blood sample (10 ml clotted blood) should be forwarded to facilitate cross-matching.
- Obtain consent for the operation from the mother (if parents are not married, father's consent may not be valid).
- Administer vitamin K (i.m. or i.v.).

Transport of newborns with cardiac disorders

In addition to the details already given above, infants suspected of having duct-dependent lesions should be commenced on PGE_2 (10–20 ng/kg/min for stable unventilated infants and

50–100 ng/kg/min for sick, ventilated infants). The lowest possible supplemental oxygen concentration should be used in infants with suspected duct-dependent lesions. Metabolic acidosis should be corrected and inotropes commenced in hypotensive infants and diuretics in infants with congestive cardiac failure. Unstable infants should be intubated for transfer.

Air transport

Though less common in the UK due to the distances involved, air transport may be essential when long distances are involved, a rapid response time is required, adverse traffic and road conditions exist, and where international transfers are required. Commonly, helicopters are used for distances of 30–400 miles and fixed-wing aircraft for distances of >400 miles. It is even more important to stabilize the infant before transportation by air as the incidence of complications may be greater (20–40%). Special problems peculiar to air transport may be encountered, in particular vibration and decompression. Air collections (e.g. pulmonary air leaks) enlarge and may cause clinical deterioration. The risk of hypothermia is increased (temperature falls by 2 °C for every 1000 feet rise).

Avoiding adverse events

- Check transporting equipment daily to minimize unexpected equipment failure during transportation.
- Inexperienced staff should not be assigned to transport sick infants unless accompanied by more experienced staff.
- Regular audits of transport and review of the conduct and outcomes of transport facilitate remedial steps to avoid future recurrence of adverse events.
- The continuing education and training of all members of the transport team is essential.

Dealing with parents

Parents should be given accurate information they can easily understand on the condition of their infant and the need for transfer. They should be reassured that transfer is in the best interests of their baby and the mother should 'rejoin' her infant at the earliest opportunity.

Further reading

Jaimovich DG, Vidyasagar D (eds). Transport medicine. *Pediatric Clinics of North America*, 1993; **40** (2).
Mir NA (ed). *Manual of Neonatal Transport*. Manchester: E. Petch Printers, 1997.

Related topics of interest

VOMITING

Vomiting occurs at certain periods in almost all infants in the neonatal period. Minor vomiting during or after feeds is physiological and universal. However, when it becomes persistent, projectile and large in volume, a pathological cause is more likely. Bilious vomiting should always be regarded as abnormal.

Aetiology

- Excessive feeding.
- GOR.
- NEC.
- Sepsis (including UTI).
- Oesophageal anomalies (e.g. pharyngeal cleft).
- Intestinal obstruction (especially if vomiting is bilious).
- Gastric outlet obstruction (especially pyloric stenosis, incidence 3 in 1000, male:female ratio 4:1).
- Drug induced – some enteral medication may increase the risk of vomiting (e.g. chlorothiazide), as may the administration of several medications at the same time along with feeds.
- Metabolic disorder (IMD, e.g. galactosaemia (urine-reducing substances-positive)).
- Feed intolerance (e.g. cows' milk protein intolerance).
- Gut malrotation.
- Hiatus hernia.
- Hydrocephalus.

Investigations

- U&E.
- Abdominal radiograph.
- Oesophageal pH monitoring.
- Barium swallow and follow-through examination (oesophageal anomalies and gut malrotation).
- Abdominal ultrasound scan (gastric outlet obstruction).
- Arterial blood gases (alkalosis with pyloric stenosis, persistent acidosis with IMD).
- Infection screen (blood, urine ± CSF culture).
- Metabolic screen (urine amino and organic acids, plasma amino acids, NH_3, lactate).

Management

A pragmatic approach should be adopted in managing vomiting. The above list of investigations is certainly not necessary for every vomiting infant. Vomiting is often transient and attention to the frequency and volume of feeds is sufficient to improve the symptom. If reflux is suspected, 24-hour oesophageal monitoring should be performed. Alternatively a barium swallow may be performed. Although this is less sensitive, it has the advantage of simultaneously excluding gut malrotation and gastric outlet obstruction. Where such a facility is not available, a trial of antireflux therapy and feed thickeners may be curative and diagnostic. Avoid administering emetic drugs before feeds and spread out oral medication administration over the day, discontinuing any unnecessary medications. Feed intolerance is not as common as imagined, especially in the newborn period. It should be considered, however, when simple remedies have failed to improve the vomiting in the presence of a relevant family history. A soya-based formula (e.g. Wysoy, Farley Health Products), or one of the elemental formulae (e.g. Pregestimil, Mead Johnson) may then be tried.

Where the vomiting is persistent with mild-to-moderate abdominal distension, stop oral feeds and obtain an abdominal X-ray. If this is satisfactory but vomiting recurs on introducing feeds, commence an i.v. dextrose–electrolyte infusion and rest the gut for 1–3 days before trying enteral feeding again. This is more likely to occur in the growth-retarded infant. The serum electrolytes may occasionally give an indication as to the cause of vomiting (uraemia of renal failure; hyponatraemia in adrenal insufficiency; hypokalaemia in paralytic ileus; hypochloraemic alkalosis in pyloric stenosis). When vomiting is projectile, perform a test feed (peristalsis may also be visible in pyloric stenosis). Presentation may occur as early as the first week. If a test feed is inconclusive but the clinical picture is highly suggestive of pyloric stenosis, proceed to an abdominal ultrasound examination or barium swallow ('string sign' seen in pyloric stenosis). A low-grade pyrexia may suggest infection and the need for an appropriate infection screen including urine microscopy.

Bilious vomiting, even with an unremarkable abdominal X-ray, should be regarded as abnormal and a surgical opinion sought. Similarly, an infant with a tense, tender and silent abdomen probably has a 'surgical abdomen' (NEC, intestinal obstruction and/or perforation) and requires a surgical review.

Further reading

Black JA, Whitfield MF. *Neonatal Emergencies: Early Detection and Management*, 2nd edn. Oxford: Butterworth-Heinemann, 1991.
Lister J, Irving IM (eds). *Neonatal Surgery*, 3rd edn. London: Butterworths, 1990.
Philip AGS. *Neonatology: A Practical Guide*, 4th edn. Philadelphia: W.B. Saunders, 1996.

Related topics of interest

Abdominal distension (p. 1)
Gastro-oesophageal reflux (p. 90)

Hirschsprung's disease (p. 110)
Necrotizing enterocolitis (p. 195)

INDEX

Congenital diaphragmatic hernia, 57–60, 313
  ECMO in, 59
  gastro-oesophageal reflux in, 60
  high frequency ventilation in, 59
  nitric oxide in, 59
  pulmonary hypoplasia in, 57, 59
Congenital heart disease – congestive heart failure,
      61–64
  atrioventricular septal defect, 62
  cardiomyopathies, 62
  coarctation of the aorta, 36, 62
  critical aortic stenosis, 62
  hypoplastic left heart syndrome, 6, 62, 68
  interrupted aortic arch, 6, 62
  patent ductus arteriosus, 62, 230–233
  total anomalous pulmonary venous drainage, 63, 68
  transient myocardial ischaemia, 62, 68–69
  truncus arteriosus, 62
  ventricular septal defect, 62
Congenital heart disease – cyanotic defects, 65–69
  double inlet left ventricle, 68
  double outlet right ventricle, 68
  Ebstein's anomaly, 68
  pulmonary atresia, 68
  pulmonary stenosis, 68
  tetralogy of Fallot, 68
  transposition of the great arteries, 68
  tricuspid atresia, 68
  truncus arteriosus, 68
  univentricular heart, 68
Congenital malformations and birth defects, 70–71
Congenital surfactant protein B deficiency, 275
Creatine phosphokinase, 214, 216
Cystic fibrosis, 1, 198
  meconium ileus and, 1, 198
  screening for, 198

Death of a baby, 72–74
  post-mortem, 7, 73
Discharge planning and follow-up, 75–77
Disseminated intravascular coagulation, 26
Duodenal atresia, 49

Endotracheal tube, 3
  blockage, 3, 6
  dislodged, 3, 6
Erythema infectiosum, 155
Erythropoietin, 9, 11, 99
Extracorporeal membrane oxygenation, 78–79, 262
  nitric oxide and, 78
  oxygenation index and, 78
Extreme prematurity, 80–83,
  handicap and, 81
  survival and, 80

Faecal chymotrypsin, 198
Feeding difficulties, 84–86, 242
Fluid and electrolyte therapy, 87–89
Folic acid, 321
  neural tube defects and, 203

Galactosaemia, 163, 180, 331
Gastro-oesophageal reflux, 90–92, 331
  bronchopulmonary dysplasia and, 91
  endoscopy in, 91

medical treatment, 91
Nissen fundoplication and, 92
oesophagitis in, 90
pH monitoring in, 90, 331
Gastroschisis, 253, 329
Germinal matrix-intraventricular haemorrhage,
    93–96
  classification, 94
  periventricular haemorrhagic infarction and, 95
  post-haemorrhagic hydrocephalus, 95
  prevention, 94
Gestational age
  appropriate for, 165
  assessment of, 19–20
    antenatal ultrasound, 19–20
    Ballard assessment, 20
    Dubowitz assessment, 19
    lens examination, 20
    nerve conduction studies, 20
  large for, 165
  small for, 165
Glanzmann's disease, 27
Glucose-6-phosphate dehydrogenase deficiency,
    173–174
Growth hormone, 30, 165, 168

Haemolysis,
  immune, 9
  non-immune, 9
Haemolytic disease, 97–100
  exchange transfusion in, 99
Haemorrhage, 9
  fetal, 9
  intra-abdominal, 6, 11
  intracranial, 4, 11, 16, 21
  intraventricular, 7, 21
  periventricular, 21
  pulmonary, 6, 259–260
  subaponeurotic, 21
  subarachnoid, 21
  subdural, 21, 22
Haemorrhagic disease of the newborn, 27
Head size, 101–102
  large head, 101
  small head, 102
Heart murmurs in neonates, 103–104
  innocent, 103
  pathological, 103
Hepatitis
  hepatitis A, 179
  hepatitis B, 105–107, 133, 179, 245
    immunization, 106
    prophylaxis, 106
  hepatitis C, 179
  hepatitis D, 179
Herniae, 108–109
  epigastric, 109
  inguinal, 108
  umbilical 108
Hirschsprung's disease, 1, 49, 110–113
  enterocolitis in, 111, 112
  intestinal obstruction in, 110
  neuronal intestinal dysplasia and, 112
  nitric oxide in, 110
  rectal biopsy in, 112